Epidemic Malaria and Hunger in Colonial Punjab

This book documents the primary role of acute hunger (semi- and frank starvation) in the 'fulminant' malaria epidemics that repeatedly afflicted the northwest plains of British India through the first half of colonial rule. Using Punjab vital registration data and regression analysis, it also tracks the marked decline in annual malaria mortality after 1908 with the control of famine, despite continuing post-monsoonal malaria transmission across the province.

The study establishes a time-series of annual malaria mortality estimates for each of the 23 plains districts of colonial Punjab province between 1868 and 1947 and for the early post-Independence years (1948–1960) in (East) Punjab State. It goes on to investigate the political imperatives motivating malaria policy shifts on the part of the British Raj. This work reclaims the role of hunger in Punjab malaria mortality history and, in turn, raises larger epistemic questions regarding the adequacy of modern concepts of nutrition and epidemic causation in historical and demographic analysis.

Part of The Social History of Health and Medicine in South Asia series, this book will be useful to scholars and researchers of colonial history, modern history, social medicine, social anthropology, and public health.

Sheila Zurbrigg is a physician and independent scholar based in Toronto, Canada. Her health history research investigates rising life expectancy in South Asian history in relation to food security. She has served as Short-Term Epidemiologist for the World Health Organization, Smallpox Eradication Program, Uttar Pradesh and as Coordinator, Village Health Worker Program, Madurai, Tamil Nadu, India. She has also held appointments as Adjunct Professor, International Development Studies, Dalhousie University, Halifax, Nova Scotia, Canada; Visiting Scholar, York University, Toronto, Canada; and Visiting Scholar, Jawaharlal Nehru University, New Delhi, India. Her work with traditional village midwives in rural Tamil Nadu (1975–1979) led to analysis of child survival in contemporary India in relation to food security and conditions of women's work. In 1985, she turned to South Asian health history research, funded by the Social Sciences and Humanities Research Council (Ottawa), and is currently investigating the epistemic shifts leading to loss of understanding of the role of acute hunger in the region's malaria mortality history. Among her forthcoming work is her second monograph *Uncoupling Disease and Destitution: The Case of South Asian Malaria History*.

The Social History of Health and Medicine in South Asia
Series editors: Biswamoy Pati
Formerly at Department of History, University of Delhi, India

Mark Harrison
Director of the Wellcome Unit for the History of Medicine and Professor of the History of Medicine, University of Oxford, UK

Since the late 1990s, health and medicine have emerged as major concerns in South Asian history. The Social History of Health and Medicine in South Asia series aims to foster a new wave of inter-disciplinary research and scholarship that transcends conventional boundaries. It welcomes proposals for monographs, edited collections and anthologies which offer fresh perspectives, innovative analytical frameworks and comparative assessments. The series embraces diverse aspects of health and healing in colonial and postcolonial contexts.

Colonial Modernities
Midwifery in Bengal, c. 1860–1947
Ambalika Guha

Society, Medicine and Politics in Colonial India
Edited by Biswamoy Pati and Mark Harrison

Epidemic Malaria and Hunger in Colonial Punjab
Weakened by Want
Sheila Zurbrigg

For more information about this series, please visit: www.routledge.com/The-Social-History-of-Health-and-Medicine-in-South-Asia/bookseries/SHHM

Epidemic Malaria and Hunger in Colonial Punjab
Weakened by Want

Sheila Zurbrigg

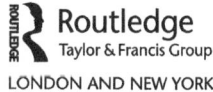

Routledge
Taylor & Francis Group

LONDON AND NEW YORK

First published 2019
by Routledge
2 Park Square, Milton Park, Abingdon, Oxon OX14 4RN

and by Routledge
605 Third Avenue, New York, NY 10017

First issued in paperback 2020

Routledge is an imprint of the Taylor & Francis Group, an informa business

British Library Cataloguing-in-Publication Data
A catalogue record for this book is available from the British Library

Library of Congress Cataloging-in-Publication Data
A catalog record has been requested for this book

ISBN 13: 978-0-367-73248-6 (pbk)
ISBN 13: 978-0-8153-8511-0 (hbk)

Typeset in Sabon
by Apex CoVantage, LLC

For Philip and for Daniel and Gabe

Contents

Figures

Tables

Preface and acknowledgments

To set out to write a history of malaria mortality in colonial South Asia required much innocence on my part with regard to the work entailed. My gratitude is immense for the many people who kept me inspired through the very long process.

I thank first the Social Sciences and Humanities Research Council of Canada for three rounds of support as a private scholar, research and stipend funding that made possible initial forays into the very large, and largely uncharted, body of malaria research records from the colonial period of British India and allowed time to access the vital registration and administrative data that form the base of the study. I hope the trust that was extended to an untested scholar may at last be seen as justified in some portion in these pages.

I am grateful for interest expressed from the start by anonymous referees for this work. I have deep regret that Ian Catanach, who generously agreed to identify himself, has not lived to see the project completed. As well, for other colleagues and friends who gave crucial encouragement and support in the earlier days: the late Nigel Crook at the School of Oriental and Asian Studies; Bill Owen, medical librarian at Dalhousie University, Halifax, Nova Scotia; and the late John Farley, Professor Emeritus of Biology, Dalhousie University. I have often wondered whether I could have persisted had it not been for John's interest and uncomplaining feedback on first drafts of many chapters.

As an independent researcher, one has advantages of greater time and flexibility to pursue questions in detail, and to incorporate further key questions as they present themselves. A drawback has been that as the scope of the study expanded, so too did competing commitments – to family, teaching, and world events. A further drawback has been lack of regular links with South Asian scholars. This has meant reliance to a large extent on published work. Much of this study was necessarily a solitary task because so little of the malaria primary sources had yet to be researched or malaria mortality history itself explored. But certainly, I would have benefitted from more direct feedback in broader areas, and I look forward to critical commentary on the work. The roots of this project go deep. Its origin lies in five years of privileged acquaintance with many of the traditional midwives of Ramanathapuram (Ramnad) district in rural southern Tamil Nadu, women who allowed me a glimpse of their health care and midwifery skills and their daily wage lives as agricultural labourers. Returning to Canada in 1980, I found a development literature that attributed mortality decline in the 'global south' to the transfer of modern medical techniques. It did not ring true: my initial work in rural Uttar Pradesh in the mid-1970s with the WHO smallpox eradication program, and subsequently in Ramnad district, had revealed a dire lack of accessible general health care services, despite a skeletal building in each rural district. In time I found myself setting down to paper one particularly compelling account conveyed to me earlier by the midwife of Veer-anendal village, one common enough but also encapsulating powerfully the constraints faced by the rural poor in accessing basic health care and the larger barriers to child care and nourishment posed by intense poverty. Meena's response to my retelling (in *Rakku's Story*) of her account ultimately pushed me some years later to consider what the historical record might also reveal – how the historical 'Rakku's story' might read.

The 'handle' came when I was alerted to the existence of a remarkable 1911 study of epidemic malaria mortality in British India: S.R. Christophers's *Malaria in the Punjab*, cited by Ira Klein in his 1973 article, 'Death in India, 1871–1921.' I am extremely grateful to Professor Klein for this. The 1911 study *did* ring true. But beyond its conclusions regarding epidemic malaria and foodgrain prices, the study brilliantly demonstrated the value of the colonial vital registration data for South Asian health history research – an insight Tim Dyson encouragingly would confirm to me soon after. Along with the relative invisibility of quantitative analysis of malaria mortality within epidemic historiography, I was puzzled by this time also by the near absence of analysis of the key post-1920 period of beginning South Asian mortality decline. These 'gaps' drew me in further, prodded by a growing sense of how much understanding seemed to have been lost. But it left me pondering as well the larger epistemic questions as to *how*.

Many, many people have contributed to this study. Feedback from Neeladri Bhattacharya on my initial writing was invaluable, as was his own extensive writing on the colonial agricultural economy of Punjab.

Generous encouragement from Jose Antonio Ortega Osona mid-way through was equally important, as was Jean Drèze's, who continues to take the unfreedom of food and livelihood precarity seriously in his intelligent and unswerving analysis and activism on contemporary hunger in India. I thank them greatly. Interest from Prabhu Mohapatra and Sumit Guha was an important boost as well. Throughout, the critical contemporary health analysis of Imrana Qadeer, Mohan Rao, and Debabar Banerji at the Centre for Social Medicine and Community Health, Jawaharlal Nehru University has been, and remains, an important touchstone, though they may often have wished a much quicker completion of this historical 'chapter.'

For many Madurai friends who made possible my introduction to the subsistence realities of the Ramnad rural landless poor, my gratitude is abiding – first perhaps for the late Prof. K.A. Krishnamurthy for his humanity and unflagging support – paediatrician-in-spirit to all of Tamil Nadu's rural children. The practical experience of those years was made possible for me by the dedication, translating guidance, and priceless friendship of Anusuya Andichamy and Shahnawaz Ghouse. With deep gratitude I remember Janaki Ramaswamy and her family for their extraordinary care and shelter through the initial Madurai years, and the encouragement of her elder brother, Dr. G. Venkataswamy, much honoured ophthalmologist in the State.

Personal funding support during these years came from the Canadian International Development Agency and the remarkable Head of its Health Division, Bill Jeanes. His personal interest in the Ramnad rural health project was critical, and I remember his support fondly. I would like to acknowledge, as well, the practical insights of David Morley at the Institute of Child Health, UK. His 'Road to Health' card, a simple growth chart, made hunger 'visible' to me in the young children of Ramnad district, and also its consequences – a card Meena and Puliyoor village midwife, Rakku, astutely described as a child's horoscope.

For encouragement and onerous editing support for my early efforts in putting pen to paper, I am profoundly indebted to John Desrochers and the late John Maliekal of the Bangalore Social Action Trust. It was their inspiring activism that convinced me to pursue the Ramnad midwives' insights into an understanding of the broader determinants of health.

The published work of many historians provided essential stepping stones as I struggled to place the expanding questions and historical sub-disciplines into a larger whole. Though I remain a novice with respect to most South Asian historiography, here I mention several works pivotal for this study. They include Arup Maharatna's empirical confirmation of the shift in famine relief effectiveness evident in the 1907–1908 United Provinces. As well, David Arnold's exploration of the key political moment in 1918 when response to foodgrain exports and starvation desperation turned from sporadic grain riots to systematic confrontation.

Crucial also for comprehending the demise in understanding of the 'human factor' in malaria historiography has been Christopher Hamlin's scrupulous analysis of the wider epistemic content of Edwin Chadwick's 1842 Sanitary Report and its contribution to the 'uncoupling of disease and destitution' within modern public health and epidemic thought. It is a story with parallels a century later with respect to malaria in South Asia. His scholarship has largely kept me afloat navigating the at times 'recondite' historiography of Western epidemic theory and historiography.

My gratitude to Douglas Hay and Jim Phillips is immeasurable for their painstaking feedback on the study overview, and for their insistent assurance of its coherence. I am deeply indebted to Paul Antze for his interest, constant encouragement, and patience over the long years, and to Rosemary Jeanes Antze for her friendship, and for sharing an appreciation of south Indian food equal to my own.

For taking on the task of statistical work for the study, and leading me to understand it, my heartfelt thanks go to Linda Pereira, John Fahey, Brian Eastwood, Barbara Lacey, Margaret Harnish, and Wade Blanchard, variously of the Biostatistics and Mathematics departments at Dalhousie University, Halifax. And more recently, Matt Kowiger, Heather Krause (Centre for Social Innovation, Toronto), and Erika Mulder and Carys Craig of York University.

And then there are the miraculous archivists and librarians of Dalhousie University's Killam library. My respect and gratitude are immense for Gwyn Pace, Joe Wickens, Kellie Hawley, Marlyn McCann, Catherine Pickett, Christine Hatton, Shirley Vail, Clare Cheong, and Johnelle Sciocchetti. Their expertise in pursuing obscure reports has helped fill crucial gaps over the very long way – work that truly keeps human experience from the dustbin fate of history. I thank also the staff at the India Office Library, now housed within the British Library, for many summers of assistance, and as well the staff of the National Archives of India.

Through the often-lonely work, the enduring friendship and medical integrity of Carol Buck, Barbara Lent, Sandi Witherspoon, and Paul and Sandra Odegaard have been a strength and bridge between continents. I thank Christine Davidson for her friendship, also Jeanette

Neeson for her great encouragement and appreciation of the importance of subsistence history. By their enormous and unwavering engagement in the global present, Betty 'Pete' (Peterson) and Dale Hildebrand have kept me connected to the world through the long years of historical preoccupation. Betty, with her own archivist ways, has understood it all, and has been in many ways my 'oxygen.' Fatima and Ismail Cajee, Carolyn van Gurp, Alexa McDonough, Brooks Kind, and Lisl Fuson have sustained me through the toughest writing times through their deep friendship, peace passion and camaraderie, and complete involvement in our larger society. To Heidi Williams, bedrock inspirer to whom I owe my own critical engagement with the world, countless hours of early editing help, and very much else, my gratitude is endless.

For their forbearance with an often-preoccupied mom, for their constant moral support and indispensable computer skills ever ready at hand, and for the joy they give, I thank with greatest pride Daniel and Gabe.

Above all, my gratitude, impossible to convey, is for Philip, life partner whose support in all ways has allowed this (his)story to see the light of day. His encouragement, stellar historical sense, editing skills, and patience beyond all reason, lie at the core of my initiating the study, navigating its daunting academic terrain, and prevailing.

Abbreviations and acronyms

AJTMH	*American Journal of Tropical Medicine and Hygiene*
AJPH	*American Journal of Public Health*
BEI	Board of Economic Inquiry (Punjab)
BWF	'Black-water fever,' *Sci. Mem. Med. Sanit. Dep.*, 1908.
BMA	British Medical Association
BMJ	*British Medical Journal*
CDR	crude death rate (per 1000)
CEHI	*Cambridge Economic History of India*
DNB	*Oxford Dictionary of National Biography*
EPW	*Economic and Political Weekly*
FCR	*Famine Commission Report*
FDR	fever death rate
GOI	Government of India
GOI-PHC	*Annual Report of the Public Health Commissioner with the Government of India* [1922–1947]
GOI-SCR	*Annual Report of the Sanitary Commissioner with the Government of India* [1868–1921]
GoP	Government of Punjab
ICMR	Indian Council of Medical Research
IESHR	*Indian Economic and Social History Review*
IJM	*Indian Journal of Malariology*
IJMR	*Indian Journal of Medical Research*
IMG	*Indian Medical Gazette*
IMR	infant mortality rate (per 1000 live births)
IMS	Indian Medical Service
IRFA	Indian Research Fund Association
JIH	*Journal of Interdisciplinary History*
JMII	*Journal of the Malaria Institute of India*
JTM	*Journal of Tropical Medicine*
JTMH	*Journal of Tropical Medicine and Hygiene*

LN	League of Nations
LNHO	League of Nations Health Organization
LNMC	League of Nations Malaria Commission
LNMC-India report	*Report of the Malaria Commission on its Study Tour of India*, Geneva, 1930.
MAS	*Modern Asian Studies*
MD	*Malaria in the Duars* (1909)
MP	'Malaria in the Punjab,' *Sci. Mem. Off. Med. San. Dep.*, 1911
NMCP	National Malaria Control Programme
PLGP	Proc. of the Lieutenant-Governor of the Punjab, in the Home Dept (Sanitary)
PLRA	*Report of the Land Revenue Administration of the Punjab* (Lahore: Govt Printing)
PLRA Ext.	Extracts of the Deputy Commissioner reports
PP	*Parliamentary Papers*
PPHA	*Report on the Public Health Administration of the Punjab* [1922–1947]
PPWIB	*Annual Report, Public Works Dept., Irrigation Branch* (Punjab).
PSCR	*Report on the Sanitary Administration of the Punjab* [1867–1921]
RCAI	*Report of the Royal Commission on Agriculture in India*
RMCRS	*Reports to the Malaria Committee of the Royal Society*
RMSI	*Records of the Malaria Survey of India*

Sci. Mem. Off.
   Med. San. Dep. Scientific Memoirs by Officers of the Medical and Sanitary Departments of the Government of India (New Series)
Season and Crops Report
   Report on the Season and Crops of the Punjab [1901–1944]

Stat. Abst.	*Statistical abstract relating to British India* (London: HMSO, 1840–1920)
Trans. Bombay Congress	*Transactions of the Bombay Medical Congress, 1909*
TRSTMH	*Transactions of the Royal Society of Tropical Medicine and Hygiene*

Glossary

anthropophilic propensity of the female mosquito to seek blood meals from humans rather than animals

bonification agricultural improvement programs advanced by early 20th-century Italian malaria workers in malarious regions

case fatality rate the proportion of deaths within a designated population of 'cases' (people with a medical condition), over the course of the disease

chowkidar village watchman

crescents term for the falciparum malaria gametocyte observed in infected red blood cells

crude death rate annual number of deaths from all causes per 1,000 population

dacoity banditry, armed robbery

dalit term for the lowest ('out-caste') level in Hindu social hierarchy

doab tract lying between two major tributaries of the Indus or Ganges river [*do* – two, *ab* – water]

epizootic an epidemic disease in a non-human animal population

gametocyte the sexual reproductive stage of the malaria parasite, transmitted from the human host to the female vector mosquito during its blood meal

holoendemic a state of nearly year-round malaria transmission resulting in high levels of acquired immunity in the local population such that clinical symptoms of malaria infection are minimal amongst all but young children

hyperendemic highly intense but seasonal malaria transmission, associated with high parasite and spleen (splenomegaly) rates (>50 per cent), with acquired immunity levels sufficient to keep regular re-infection largely asymptomatic in adults and older children

kharif agricultural season from April 15 to October 15

lakh   one hundred thousand
parasite rate   that proportion of persons found with microscopically
   confirmed parasites in the bloodstream (parasitemia)
protozoa   a single-celled microscopic animal with a defined nucleus
rabi   agricultural season from October 15 to April 15
rupee   16 *annas*; one *anna* (approx. one British pence) = four *paise*;
   one *paise* = three *pies*
sardar   labour recruiter
seer   0.93 kg, or 2.06 lb
spleen rate   generally defined as the per cent of children under the age
   of 10 years in a population with an enlarged spleen (splenomegaly)
splenomegaly   enlargement of the spleen sufficient to be palpable
   below the left rib cage
sporozoite   the infective stage of the malaria parasite that is passed to
   the human host from the salivary glands of the female mosquito
   during a blood meal
tahsil   a revenue administration division, made up of several *thanas*
takavi   government agricultural loans
thana   a subdivision of a rural district, under a sub-inspector of police
zaildar   local Indian revenue agent for the Punjab colonial government
zamindar   landowner who leases land for cultivation by tenant
   farmers
zoophilic   propensity of the female mosquito to seek blood meals
   from animals rather than humans
zymotic   a 19th-century term for acute febrile infectious diseases
   believed to be caused by atmospheric vapours (miasma) resulting
   from fermentation of organic matter

1   Introduction

A large portion of the population was greatly weakened by want; [and the 1877 drought] was followed in 1878 and 1879 by a dreadful epidemic of fever.
— *Gurgaon District Gazetteer*, 1884, p. 132

The multifaceted history of malaria illuminates fundamental aspects of human history.
— C.E. Rosenberg, 'Foreword,' in R. Packard, *The Making of a Tropical Disease*, 2007, ix

Little could the village *chowkidars* (watchmen) of the Indian subcontinent have known when they began reporting weekly deaths and births in the late 1860s to the local *thana*[1] offices of the British colonial administration that they were contributing to a body of data which would provide far-reaching insights into human health history.[2] In recent decades the analytic importance of the South Asian vital registration records, based upon the reports of these low-status rural functionaries, has been increasingly recognised by historical demographers.[3] This study of epidemic malaria history employs these data from one region of British India, gathered from the 36,000 villages and towns of the northwestern province of Punjab, to explore the impact of changes in food security on malaria mortality decline and beginning rise in life expectancy across the later colonial and early post-colonial period.

From the mid-19th century through to the early 1920s, mortality levels across much of India were extremely high, with life expectancy in the low to mid-twenties. Recurring famine and epidemic crises were reflected in low, or sometimes negative, demographic growth. Among these 'epidemics of death,' malaria figured pre-eminently, typically as a surge in autumnal fever deaths following the monsoon rains. This mortality profile began to change quite fundamentally from the early decades of the 20th century. Decline in mortality crises after 1920 brought a sustained, if modest, rise in life expectancy, a transition captured with some clarity in the provincial sanitary records, annual reports in which the vital registration data were published. Though the precise timing and extent of mortality decline differed among the major provinces of British India, by the third decade of the 20th century, a trend of increasing survival rates is evident for the Indian subcontinent as a whole (Figure 1.1).[4]

For more than a century following the late 19th century identification of specific disease microbes, demographic and epidemic historians have debated the relative roles of economic factors (rising living standards) versus environmental (sanitation/public health) and modern medical measures in explaining the secular rise in human life expectancy in the modern world. The question has been phrased roughly thus: to what extent has mortality decline resulted from changes in exposure to infectious disease (i.e., transmission of infection) and improved medical treatment, relative to the effect of rising human host resistance to disease through increasing food security?

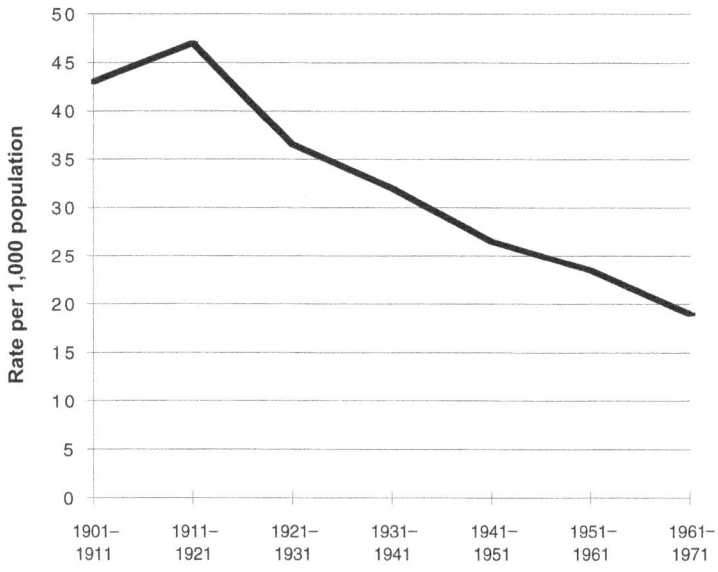

Figure 1.1 Decadal crude death rate, India, 1901–1971

Source: *Census of India*.

In a rather different form, this same question poses itself in the pages of the sanitary records of British India, here expressed as a quiet dichotomy running through the 80 years of vital registration records. One 'voice' prefaces each annual report with data on local (provincial) harvest conditions, price levels of staple foodgrains, and prevailing employment and wage rates, information sanitary officials deemed key to interpreting general conditions of public health (mortality) and epidemic patterns for the year. A second voice, within the body of these same reports, interprets epidemic patterns according to prevailing medical theories of disease transmission. Through much of the 19th century, for example, post-monsoon 'fever' mortality was explained in classic terms of 'miasma' – poisonous vapours emanating from rotting organic matter following the monsoon rains[5] – an explanation which shifted seamlessly in the early 20th century to post-monsoon entomological conditions conducive to breeding of the malaria mosquito vector. Though separate, the two views, economic and miasmic-entomological, often came together at times of food crises, when sanitary officials described such fever epidemics in terms of 'malaria merely reap[ing] a harvest prepared for it by the famine.'[6]

Both voices remained in the provincial sanitary ledgers and the burgeoning Indian malaria research literature through the final years of British rule to 1947. By the mid-20th century, however, the economic view had receded from the medical sub-discipline of malariology in India, and more completely so from the international literature. But by this point, so too had the virulent form of malaria: the severe epidemics and classic 'saw-tooth' pattern of mortality that had once featured so prominently on the South Asian vital landscape had markedly declined after 1920, including in Punjab, the region most 'notorious' in the Indian subcontinent for its epidemic malaria burden.[7] Here, the abrupt cessation of malaria transmission with residual insecticide (DDT) spraying in the early 1950s would have only marginal impact on prevailing death rates in the post-Independence state, the historical epidemic mortality impact of the disease having been largely tamed four decades earlier with the political imperative of famine control (Figure 1.2).

Such a picture of South Asian malaria history – the highly lethal form of the disease receding well before modern methods of malaria transmission control – is one at odds with current understanding of mortality decline in the post-colonial 'developing' world. Preoccupation with powerful new medical technologies of vector control that emerged in the immediate post-World War II era, combined with shifts in core epidemiological concepts and language relating to both disease

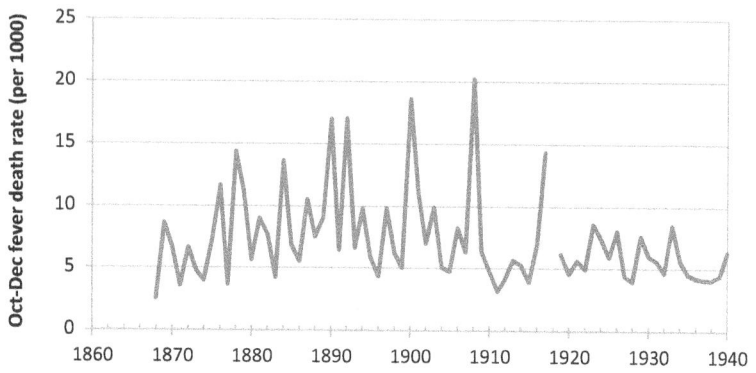

Figure 1.2 Mean annual Oct.–Dec. fever death rate, 23 plains districts, Punjab, 1868–1940

*Note: See ch. 3 for an explanation of Oct.–Dec. fever death rate as an estimate of annual malaria mortality. 1918 is omitted since malaria deaths are indistinguishable from influenza mortality.

Source: *Report on the Sanitary Administration of the Punjab*, 1868–1921; *Report on the Public Health Administration*, Punjab, 1922–1940.

and hunger over the preceding century, together have constrained analysis, and left the history of malaria mortality decline in the Indian subcontinent largely unrecognised and unwritten. This study is an attempt to reclaim some of this lost history. It seeks to understand more clearly the role of acute hunger in contributing to the so-called fulminant form of malaria in one corner of colonial India, Punjab province (Figure 1.3). It asks how this understanding came to be lost, and what a more complete South Asian malaria, and hunger, historiography can contribute to our understanding of human health history. It is perhaps fitting, if ironic, that the illiterate village *chowkidars*, who often came from the least food secure, low- or out-caste sections of their communities, should have provided the data essential to recovering this history.

Significance of 'Malaria in the Punjab' (1911)

In September 1911, the Indian government formally released the results of an official inquiry conducted two years earlier into the causes of the 1908 malaria epidemic in Punjab province, an epidemic which in the space of three brief months had left 300,000 people dead

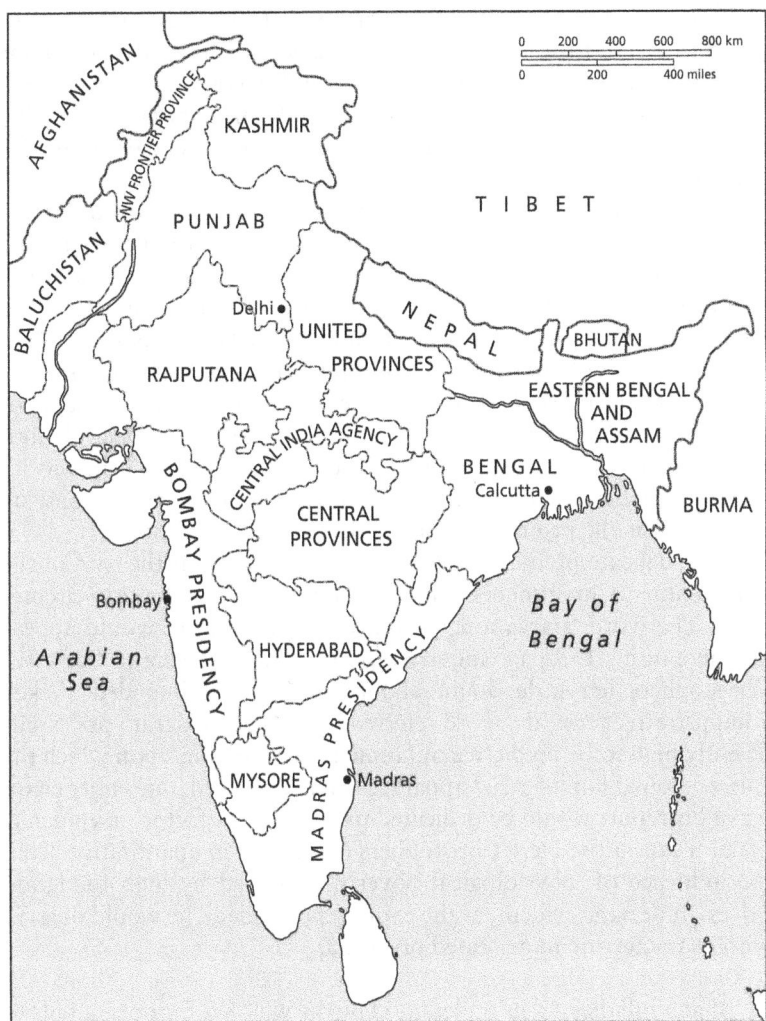

Figure 1.3 India in 1909

Source: E. Kolsky, *Colonial Justice in British India* (New York: Cambridge University Press, 2010), p. 188, Map 5.1.

Note: All maps included in this book are historical in nature and have been used for representative purposes. The international boundaries, coastlines, denominations, and other information shown do not necessarily imply any judgement concerning the legal status of any territory or the endorsement or acceptance of such information. For current boundaries, readers may refer to the Survey of India maps.

and brought the economy of this northwestern region of the subcontinent to a standstill. The determining causes of the epidemic, Major S.R. Christophers concluded in his cautious but comprehensive report, *Malaria in the Punjab*, were 'excess rainfall and scarcity. . . . [T]he former is an essential, whilst the latter is an almost equally powerful influencing factor.'[8]

That malarial fever was associated with the annual monsoon rains was hardly a new revelation within the echelons of the British Indian sanitary administration. Long before Ronald Ross's 1897 confirmation of the role of mosquitoes as vector in malaria transmission, the relationship between malarial fever and the yearly monsoon rains had been evident to colonial officials, interpreted as triggered by 'miasmatic' vapours from rain-soaked soils. In the semi-arid northwest plains of Punjab, a region where annual malaria transmission was sharply limited to the immediate post-monsoon period, this relationship was all the more evident. More remarkable in the inquiry's conclusions, by contrast, was the prominence given to economic conditions.

In the delicate political climate of the British Raj at the turn of the 20th century, Christophers's choice of terms was assiduously circumspect. The word 'starvation,' or indeed even 'hunger,' would appear nowhere in his 135-page inquiry report. Yet in referring to 'scarcity,' Christophers left little doubt about the meaning intended. A key administrative term, the word referred to market foodgrain prices sufficiently high to be predictive of famine, a designation upon which the entire colonial famine relief apparatus hinged. Indeed, one entire chapter of his report would be dedicated to the 'human factor' in epidemic malaria causation. Here Christophers chronicled in quantitative detail the influence of 'physiological poverty' triggered by high foodgrain prices. 'It became evident, as the enquiry proceeded,' he would observe with characteristic understated precision,

> that a full dietary, as understood by the well-fed European, falls to the lot of but few of the poorer classes, and that in times of scarcity these are accustomed to adapt themselves to circumstances *by proportionately restricting the amount of the food they take.*[9]

Tucked quietly into the text of the 1911 report, this observation bore profound implications for British Indian rule. It was, in effect, explicit acknowledgement of the lethal impact of episodic soaring prices ('scarcity') which increasingly had been triggered by the entry of Indian foodgrains onto the international grain market over the preceding half-century.

Malaria in the Punjab is a remarkable document for many reasons. Some relate to the study itself; others, to the larger importance of malaria in the region's health, demographic, and political history. Epidemiologically, the report is the most rigorous analysis of epidemic malaria ever conducted in India, a quantitative investigation of not a small localised malaria 'outbreak,' but rather of a vast regional epidemic extending over a territory of some 100,000 square kilometres.[10] The study is remarkable also in that it was conducted scarcely a decade after Ronald Ross's elucidation,[11] in southern India, of the mosquito as vector in malaria transmission. Exploration of the complex microbiological factors underlying malaria transmission, though still in its early stages, already dominated malaria research, and in this work Christophers was a leading figure. *Malaria in the Punjab*, and his previous work at the Punjab military cantonment at Mian Mir, would in fact lay much of the foundation of modern entomological and epidemiological understanding of the disease.

Key to the study's analytic rigour was Christophers's use of the province's vital registration data. Systematic recording of monthly deaths in the towns and villages of Punjab dates from 1867. Deaths, and from the early 1880s also births, were reported weekly by the village *chowkidar* to the nearest *thana* police station,[12] and there compiled in monthly statistics recorded under a limited range of disease categories that included smallpox, cholera, 'fever,' 'bowel complaints,' and later plague. If not entirely complete, reporting in Punjab province by the final decades of the 19th century had attained remarkably high levels. In some districts such as Ludhiana, coverage was estimated at 93 to 97 per cent by the turn of the century.[13] The annual sanitary reports thus represent a unique data series, one spanning many decades of extremely high, pre-demographic-transition mortality levels, and continuing across the post-1920 period of South Asian mortality (crude death rate) decline.

Cause-of-death data contained in the annual sanitary reports, on the other hand, were much more problematic. Often half or more of all deaths were recorded under a general 'fever' heading, a catch-all category Christophers referred to as 'merely a great residuum of undiagnosed causes of death.'[14] Christophers recognised, however, that the distinctive seasonal pattern to the major epidemic diseases of the Indian subcontinent made it possible to distinguish specific diseases from one another within the monthly mortality returns. Malarial deaths could be identified as a characteristic post-monsoon rise in fever deaths that peaked in October of each of the 41 years between 1868 and 1908. Both in the shape of its mortality curve and in its timing, this autumnal rise was a pattern distinctive to malaria.[15] The value of the vital registration data, in other words, lay not in accuracy of medical diagnosis but rather in the regular monthly recording of deaths. Christophers's inquiry would become the first major epidemiological study where the analytic potential of these data was fully exploited, making possible detailed geographical mapping of 1908 epidemic mortality rates across the province in relation to local topography, rainfall, and harvest patterns.

Malaria in the Punjab was remarkable also for its analytic scope. Christophers was seeking as broad a canvas as possible upon which to examine the relationship between malaria transmission and malaria mortality: the goal, to tease apart the factors underlying the transformation of an endemic disease into the 'malaria cyclone' visited upon the province in 1908, a form he would come to term 'fulminant' malaria.[16] 'Endemic malaria certainly exists, but it is the mortality from the epidemic disease,' he stressed, 'which gives to malaria in the Punjab such prominence.'[17] Christophers's use of the term 'epidemic disease' here refers to a marked increase in lethality (case fatality rate) from 'ordinary' (endemic) transmission rather than to a qualitatively different type of malaria (strain of parasite) transmitted.

> We know that as a result of some epidemics certain areas have lost in a single year as much as one-seventh of their population and have received a set back to their natural increase of population which it has taken decades to rectify. . . . [W]ithin its own realms no disease has a more profound effect upon population than malaria. . . . But of how exactly malaria acts we have very little accurate statistical knowledge.[18]

To this end, Christophers made extensive use of a range of other administrative reports dealing with irrigation, land surveys, and crop returns as well as district gazetteers. Those scientific questions for which little information was available in the literature he took upon himself to investigate directly. His laboratory and field research encompassed not just entomological conditions, but also soil, hydrological, social, and agricultural conditions, attempting to bring all together in a single analytic frame. This breadth to the study was all the more remarkable given the dominant focus of medical scientists at the time. Ronald Ross's confirmation of the role of mosquitoes in malaria transmission a decade earlier had very quickly directed professional medical attention towards the entomological dimensions of vector-borne 'tropical disease' transmission. Christophers himself was at the forefront of this research in India, but he did not limit himself to the vector side of the epidemic equation, going on to explore associated social and economic conditions with as much rigour as ecological and entomological factors. 'The researches of Celli in Italy and of Dr. Bentley and myself in India,' he argued in the final pages of his Punjab report, 'show the necessity of considering the conditions affecting the human host as well as those affecting the numbers and life generally of the mosquito. In dealing with epidemic conditions . . . this is especially necessary.'[19]

If pursuit of economic dimensions to epidemic malaria behaviour was unusual within the medical world of 1911, these broader questions were hardly unprecedented within the annals of the colonial administration. Soaring malaria mortality had repeatedly been documented in relation to the South Asian famines of the late 19th century, in Punjab and across the subcontinent. Indeed, if the 1908 epidemic stood out, it did so not for the novelty of the economic context, but rather because the year had *not* been one of officially designated famine. Foodgrain prices across the province had been high in the months leading up to the 1908 autumn epidemic, but overt destitution as assessed by resort to famine 'test works' had failed to reach levels sufficient to trigger enactment of the provincial Famine Code,[20] unlike in the neighbouring United Provinces.

Looking back over the previous four decades of Punjab sanitary records for the province, Christophers could see that severe fever epidemics had occurred in virtually all years of high foodgrain prices whether or not famine had been formally declared. Indeed, with the exception of recent plague mortality, most years of very high crude death rates were years of soaring grain prices as well as fever (malaria) mortality. '[W]e cannot help being struck by the fact that if we take the summit of the curve in each case it will be found to coincide with an epidemic. . . . This sequence carried out with such regularity can scarcely be accidental.[21]

It was this pattern that would prompt Christophers to extend his investigation into the general phenomenon of epidemic malaria and grain prices ('scarcity') in the region. Employing available techniques of statistical analysis, and creating some of his own, he attempted to quantify the relationship he saw between annual foodgrain prices, monsoon rainfall, and fever mortality as far back as the provincial vital registration records would permit.

It was in this work, it appears, that he came to recognise the special opportunity that Punjab malaria epidemicity offered for quantitative epidemiological analysis of the factors underlying malaria lethality more generally. Throughout South Asia, a general association existed between the annual monsoon rains and malarial fevers. However, in most regions of the subcontinent, malaria transmission extended well beyond the immediate post-monsoon period, a function of the continuously warm and humid tropical and subtropical climate. Thus, malaria deaths in a given year tended to overlap seasonal mortality patterns of other common infectious diseases. By contrast, malaria transmission in the Punjab plains generally was sharply limited to the final weeks of the southwest monsoon (July–September) rains and the several weeks immediately following.[22] Landlocked, and with low annual rainfall, the region was subject to climatic extremes, with freezing temperatures in winter and dry heat reaching up to 50 degrees Celsius the pre-monsoon months of May and early June, conditions that sharply limited mosquito longevity. Except for the period during and immediately following the summer monsoon, atmospheric humidity was too low and temperatures too extreme to allow sufficient time for malaria parasite development inside the mosquito vector and thus effective transmission.

It is this distinctly identifiable character to malaria mortality in the plains of Punjab that continues to make the study of malaria in this region methodologically so important for historical epidemic research. In the process, *Malaria in the Punjab* would become the first epidemiological investigation into the *general* relationship between economic conditions and malaria mortality in South Asia, and quite possibly the only comparable study in the world. 'Broadly speaking,' Christophers concluded, 'malaria [has] been the main agent which brought to a head in actual mortality the effects produced by the great economic stresses.'[23]

Malaria, famine, and imperialism

In undertaking such an investigation, Christophers, and ultimately the colonial government, was walking an extraordinarily fine line. The questions raised by the Punjab inquiry challenged fundamental economic doctrines of classical political economy that to date had buttressed half a century of colonial economic policy. Publication of *Malaria in the Punjab* in 1911 marked a critical juncture for the British Raj where the human cost of *laissez-faire* economic doctrine, through its effect on foodgrain prices, was momentarily being laid bare through public documentation of its impact on the lethality of endemic disease. Penned by a most loyal and trusted servant to the imperial crown, the 1911 Punjab study offered scientific 'proof' of a relationship long evident to famine and provincial sanitary commissioners. In doing so, as will be argued in chapter 7, it strengthened those voices urging the colonial government to step back from its rigid adherence to non-interference in food supply and price behaviour, and from its contradictory subsidisation of grain exports. Preventing starvation, many had come to conclude, was the only way to contain the 'disastrous' malaria epidemics plaguing the region, and the increasing public and international opprobrium associated with them.

Recent scholarship on Western imperial history has begun to revisit the series of later 19th-century famines that swept across diverse continents under European colonial rule. Among such work, Mike Davis's panoramic study of the famines of 1876–1878 and 1896–1900 in South Asia, China, and Brazil traces these events in relation to global rainfall patterns under El Niño and La Niña influence. In each continent, however, famine severity was primed, he concludes, by the undermining of traditional food security and grain storage systems triggered by the commercialisation of agriculture and channelling of local agricultural production onto newly globalised foodgrain markets.[24]

The impact of these two major famine periods can readily be seen in Punjab as well, in soaring epidemic malaria mortality patterns in both 1878 and 1900. But the 'fulminant' epidemics of Punjab were not limited to these two periods of exceptional 'global' drought. The malaria epidemics of 1878 and 1900 appear simply as two examples among a series of price-related severe epidemics marking the first six decades of direct British rule. Punjab malaria history suggests, in other words, that the mortality crises of this period were a more general phenomenon and indicate in turn a greater role for colonial political economy in the 'Victorian holocausts' of the period than for climatic events.

Ultimately, *Malaria in the Punjab* is remarkable, therefore, as well for its political context. No small irony attaches to the fact that the scarcity-primed malaria epidemics of Punjab were occurring in a province renowned as the 'breadbasket' of the British Indian empire, the showcase for the technological development that empire was bringing to the subcontinent through vast engineering feats of canal irrigation. Punjab was the arena and symbol of enlightened colonial rule. Of equal importance to the British Raj, Punjab's grain-export earnings constituted a major contribution to the fiscal base upon which the solvency of the imperial project rested.[25] All the more disquieting, then, that the 1907–1908 agricultural year of severe drought and 'scarcity' and ensuing epidemic malaria was also one in which almost 2 million tons of foodgrains had been exported from the province.[26] Thus for hunger to be openly addressed in an official inquiry as a major factor in the malaria toll in Punjab, of all provinces, was hardly a message the British Raj could have relished. The notoriety of these 'terrible visitations' in Punjab[27] was all the more embarrassing in the prevailing climate of political unrest in the province, further fuelled by the growing nationalist movement.[28]

Why particular diseases come to merit official and epidemiological attention at certain times is, of course, a question central to public health historiography, as demonstrated in Christopher Hamlin's in-depth account of the emergence of Edwin Chadwick's 1842 Sanitary Report in Britain.[29] In the case of epidemic malaria in Punjab, the simplest explanation for administrative attention was growing concern over the cost of economic disruption. Train service across the province during the autumn malarial months of 1908 frequently had had to be suspended, 'to the great financial loss not only of the department but also of commercial and agricultural interests generally,' while at Amritsar '[f]or many weeks labour for any purpose was unprocurable . . . [with] almost the entire population . . . prostrated.'[30]

But the identification of anopheline mosquitoes as the vector of malaria a decade earlier had brought imperatives from another direction as well. Virtually overnight, the colonial sanitary administration faced soaring medical expectations to be 'doing something' about the mosquitoes which transmitted the deadly malaria parasite. Pressures were mounting, even more embarrassingly, at home from within the British medical profession. Scathing criticism of colonial government inaction on the mosquito front soon was coming from Ross himself,[31] retired from the Indian Medical Service in 1899 and by 1901 a globally renowned medical Nobel laureate for his 1897 work, and his teaching at the Liverpool School of Tropical Medicine. Ross's indictment of colonial sanitary competency, however, was not restricted to unsuccessful mosquito control efforts at the Punjab military cantonment at Mian Mir, the site of the first systematic attempt between 1902 and 1908 to interrupt malaria transmission in rural India through mosquito destruction. Early on in those efforts, irrigation canals had been identified as bountiful sources of the incriminating malaria vector, *An. culicifacies*. Ross's insistent call for abolition of all irrigation channels at the cantonment thus cut a broader swath, casting an unsettling shadow on the vast and still expanding network of Punjab canals.

Moreover, international scrutiny of sanitary conditions in India through this period was already intense following the outbreak of plague in Bombay in 1896, an epidemic that had followed the rail routes exporting grain from the ports of Bombay and Karachi back to Punjab and was still raging a decade later. Plague mortality in Punjab province had reached the catastrophic level of 675,000 deaths in 1906–1907. Draconian attempts at containment had triggered extreme public opposition that was threatening to unseat imperial power.[32] By 1907, however, plague was a disease for which the imperial administration could at least point to some notional control measures in the form of rat destruction. By contrast, Mian Mir experience had shown that prospects were negligible for mosquito vector reduction sufficient to prevent 'fulminant' malaria epidemics in the vastness of rural India. After seven years of intensive mosquito 'extirpation' operations at Mian Mir, the cantonment was swept up in the autumn epidemic of 1908 as severely as most other regions of the province. Moreover, the costs of such rural operations on anything but a highly limited scale were fiscally ruinous. Thus, the 1908 malaria epidemic appeared in the midst of a dire crisis of public health legitimacy for the colonial regime. Dealing effectively with the latest 'pestilential' disease attracting public notoriety was imperative, all the more so in the context of Ross's acerbic critique.[33]

This political backdrop in itself, however, hardly explains why the Punjab malaria report with its incriminating economic conclusions would be formally published at this time, or indeed at all. Certainly, many imperatives underlay its commissioning. As will be argued in the course of this study, official publication of *Malaria in the Punjab* appears to have been a gamble in political manoeuvring, offered as a counterweight to the growing chorus of mosquito extirpation advocacy within the Indian sanitary and medical services. The need to understand, address, and deal with the underlying factors rendering malaria infection so highly lethal in years such as 1908 was inescapable, and urgent. Seen in this light, the content of Christophers's Punjab malaria report provided a scientific argument for explaining to puzzled sanitarians within the Indian Medical Service the inadequacy of anti-mosquito campaigns as a general approach to addressing the 'malaria problem' in the vast rural regions of the country. It amounted, in effect, to a confession: human destitution (starvation) was the key factor rendering malarial infection so destructive. In the political calculus of early 20th century colonial India, acknowledging and eradicating price famines had become an eminently more feasible option, technically and financially, than Sisyphean mosquito extirpation across the continent.

The Punjab study thus would become a platform for this admission, but also a stage for pointed critique of Ross's mosquito extirpation advocacy. In a rare moment of professional impatience, Christophers would urge, in the closing lines of the report's 'Human Factor' chapter,

> [t]hat at the back of such colossal manifestations as the epidemic of 1908 there should be profound and not easily averted natural influences at work is scarcely to be wondered at. When we approach the question of [malaria] prophylaxis, we shall do well to bear in mind the magnitude of the influences against which we are pitting ourselves and not be led in a foolish vein to reduce the remedy of the whole matter to trifling proportions.[34]

Malaria in the Punjab was directed, it would appear, as much to the advocates of mosquito eradication in the colonial sanitary service as to policy makers in the Government of India, and may also explain why the Punjab investigation and its economically incriminating results were published at all.

Modern critics of malaria control policy under colonial British rule who suggest layers of political subtext underlying Christophers's Punjab report thus are probably correct in viewing it as an effort to 'contain' prominent proponents of mosquito eradication such as Ross. They are correct as well in highlighting Christophers's enormous influence in shaping post-1900 malaria policy in India.[35] Published in the prominent series, *Scientific Memoirs by the Officers of the Medical and Sanitary Departments of the Government of India*, the 1911 version of his report, *Malaria in the Punjab*, was a more thorough, and more diplomatically cautious, draft of an initial report on the 1908 epidemic he presented two years earlier at the Imperial Malaria Conference at Simla in October 1909 more or less fresh from the Punjab plains.[36] The 1909 paper had formed the centrepiece to the Simla deliberations where future malaria policy was formulated that would inform public health decision-making for the remainder of the colonial period. Christophers's influence in the Indian Medical Service, therefore, is unquestionable. Yet rather than an apologist for imperial stringency and inaction, Christophers genuinely saw mosquito eradication as 'entirely chimerical' as a general policy for control of malaria transmission across rural India, and certainly not as a remedy for malaria in its epidemic 'fulminant' form.[37] The detailed body of epidemiological research from this period bears this out. While *Malaria in the Punjab* can be seen as a document which eased the government out of unlimited obligation for mosquito destruction, it was also one that argued irrefutably, if quietly, for fundamental shifts in famine and economic policy, its publication thus marking at once a political, demographic, and ideological watershed.

Malaria mortality after 1908

The 1908 regional epidemic analysed in such detail in *Malaria in the Punjab* would be one of the last to occur in the province.[38] With the exception of 1917 and 1942 under conditions of war-time hyper-inflation, malaria mortality in Punjab province would never again approach levels seen across the 1867–1908 period. Over the final three decades of colonial rule, autumn fever mortality declined markedly across a period that also saw overall death rates falling, in Punjab and elsewhere in India. By the time malaria transmission control programs based on residual insecticide mosquito control measures (DDT) became available in the early 1950s, mean autumn malaria mortality in the province had already fallen to less than one-third that of the pre-1920 period. 'Fulminant' epidemics had become a thing of the past, though seasonal transmission of malaria appears to have remained unchanged. By the late 1940s, life expectancy in some districts of Punjab had risen to over 50 years, a virtual doubling of 1910 levels.[39] Christophers's inquiry into the 1908 epidemic, then, lies at the temporal cusp of Punjab's epidemic and demographic transition.

Demographic analysis of this key period of South Asian mortality transition in the early 20th century is complicated by the fact that these years were marked by two epidemiologically exceptional diseases: plague beginning from the late 1890s, and in 1918, pandemic influenza. The extremely high death rates that prevailed between 1901 and 1918 reflected in considerable part epidemic mortality from these diseases,[40] mortality which has tended to obscure trends in death rates from endemic diseases across these early 20th century years. In this sense, the study of malaria is important not only because malaria contributed so largely to general death rates up to 1908, but also for the 'window' it provides on the behaviour of 'ordinary' (*viz.*, endemic) diseases across the critical period of mortality and demographic transition.

But the significance of the Punjab study extends beyond this northwest corner of the subcontinent. For if malaria took its most dramatic epidemic form in the plains of Punjab, it was considered a leading cause of death across much of India as well, historically designated in the Ayurvedic texts as the 'king of diseases.'[41] The size of this toll varied according to South Asian region, public health officials citing a range of between one-seventh and one-quarter of all deaths, amounting to well over 1 million deaths annually. Such estimates were, and remain, open to debate.[42] Yet there can be little doubt that malaria was a leading trigger of the high death rates *in general* prevailing across much of late 19th century South Asia, and in turn, little question about the central position the disease occupied in the landscape of the subcontinent's demographic and health history.[43]

Finally, and perhaps most remarkable of all, *Malaria in the Punjab* bears added historiographical significance, if paradoxically, because its conclusions regarding the role of hunger in the severe malaria epidemics of northwest India would soon fade from the pages of the expanding medical literature of the new sub-discipline of malariology. Through the 1910s and early 1920s, the importance of conditions of 'economic stress' in malaria lethality would continue to be cited in much of South Asian malaria research and public health writing, often explicitly articulated as hunger-induced compromised physiological *capacity* to produce an effective immunological response to malarial infection. Yet in the later inter-war years, academic attention to the human host was fading. By the late 1930s, the 'human factor' in international malaria analysis had come to be transformed, perhaps unconsciously, into a different concept, that of *acquired* immunity: decline or lack of malaria-specific antibodies – that is, a function of malaria transmission – rather than economic conditions of the human host.[44] In the early 1950s, Christophers's statistical 'correlations' from the 1911 Punjab study would be remembered as showing that 'the periodic epidemics were associated with certain rainfall characteristics and with an inadequate immunity in the local population.'[45] Here, 'inadequate immunity' implied 'non-immunes,' resulting in the 'human factor' being interpreted, in other words, not as a measure of hunger (semi- or frank starvation) but as simply another expression of malaria *transmission*.[46]

The transformation of the 'human factor' from an economic category reflecting hunger-induced immunosuppression, or immune *incapacity*, into one of insufficient *acquired* immunity is remarkable for how quickly it occurred, but also for how fully the 1911 study's central conclusions could be lost despite their analytic rigour and the scientific stature of their author. Increasingly, hunger was being interpreted not as a *cause* of the 'malaria problem' in imperial possessions, but as a *consequence*. This shift to an increasingly unidirectional paradigm was formalised in South Asia in J.A. Sinton's 1936 bibliographic monograph, 'What malaria costs India.'[47] But it was one presaged two decades earlier in Ross's calculations of the 'economical loss to the community caused by malaria.'[48] The view of malaria as a central cause of poverty and constraint on economic development has since come to be encapsulated in modern malaria thought in the concept of 'malaria as a block to development.'[49] Symptomatic of this conceptual inversion, *Malaria in the Punjab* would reappear fleetingly in a comprehensive major reference text on malaria published in 1988, now with its economic conclusions unwittingly turned upside down: 'Christophers, investigating the great cyclical epidemics of North-West India [Punjab], noted how adult mortality was so great that it interfered with the harvesting and distribution of food, *causing* serious shortages and inflating prices.'[50]

If puzzling to those familiar with Christophers's original study, this modern re-reading of the Punjab malaria report reflects a conceptual gulf already apparent half a century earlier in the 1930s, one that marks much larger shifts in medical and epidemiological concepts across the interval. Of any medical researcher in India, Christophers understood the potential for malaria to trigger economic havoc secondary to fever debility. Indeed, it was imperial concern over such economic disruption that underlay, in part, the Punjab malaria inquiry. Still, it is impossible to interpret his conclusions regarding the role of foodgrain prices in fulminant malaria in Punjab in any other way than as *preceding* and underlying epidemic occurrence. In effect, as microbiologic understanding expanded in the early 20th century, precision in epidemiological concepts and terms relating to the human host side of the epidemic equation simultaneously was being lost. The inversion in historical understanding speaks to the interpretative power of the paradigm shift that had taken place decades earlier.

Malaria, of course, was not the only disease subject to the increasingly reductive etiological framework of microbe transmission. Such a transformation reflects much broader developments in the history of medical thought. This narrowing in conceptual outlook was most prominently expressed in mid-19th-century sanitarianism in Britain, a trajectory given added force with subsequent identification of infection-specific microbes.[51] But the history of malaria in colonial Punjab offers an additional, and particularly transparent, window on the larger processes at play and their consequences.

In his efforts to convey the historical patterns of malaria mortality observed in Punjab, Christophers had found himself plumbing terminology belonging to a pre-sanitationist body of medical theory, epidemiological concepts that by the early 1900s had largely disappeared from Western medical discourse. In speaking of the 'human factor' as 'physiological poverty,' he was applying an earlier medical framework of epidemic causation in which the relationship between infection (exposure to a specific microbiologic disease agent) and disease (clinical illness, debility, and mortality) was understood as mediated by predisposing factors. Paramount among such factors were conditions of physical and metabolic exhaustion in the human host through insufficient food (energy): hunger.[52] *Malaria in the Punjab*, in effect, was quietly reinserting the human host back into the epidemic equation. But if reclaimed briefly in the Punjab study, application of that larger predispositionist framework would be unsustained in subsequent malaria research.[53]

Malaria in South Asian epidemic historiography

If the role of hunger in malaria history has largely been lost sight of in modern medical understanding, a parallel gap can be seen for South Asian malaria historiography as well. Relatively little quantitative analysis has been directed to the subject of malaria in the region's epidemic history, despite its widely acknowledged role as a leading trigger of mortality in the subcontinent. Reluctance on the part of historians to delve into the subject of South Asian malaria history no doubt stems in part from the biological complexities of malaria as a vector-borne infection. The intricate life cycle of the *Plasmodium* parasite is daunting in itself, but additionally so given that entomological conditions conducive to malaria transmission vary enormously across regions of the Indian subcontinent, often from one locality to the next within a single district.[54] At the same time, malaria mortality, unlike that for diseases such as cholera, plague, and smallpox, is less readily identifiable in the vital registrations records, and thus appears less amenable to quantitative analysis.

The first half of the colonial period – that period marked by recurring severe epidemics – saw relatively little investigation into malaria or malaria mortality by the colonial sanitary administration. For the British Raj, malaria neither posed a major military threat as did cholera,[55] nor did it jeopardise British Indian trade internationally as was the case with both plague and cholera, and to a lesser extent, smallpox.[56] Although malarial fever was a cause of considerable transient sickness in the military, by the second half of the 19th century, deaths were extremely few, and measures of control within the army and European administration, based on quinine and residential segregation, were straightforward and logistically feasible independent of the general ('native') population. To the extent malaria merited attention from late 19th century colonial administration at all, it did so incidentally as an economic 'nuisance': in areas where canal irrigation caused waterlogging and economic decline as in particular tracts bordering the West Jumna canal, in the 'dead river' tracts of Burdwan district in lower Bengal, and in railway construction through certain highly malarious tracts.[57] As with most other endemic causes of death among the Indian population, such as diarrhoea, pneumonia, dysentery, and tuberculosis, malaria was overshadowed in the earlier colonial sanitary reports by those diseases of special strategic or economic concern to the British colonial administration, what David Arnold has aptly referred to as 'political epidemiology.'[58]

The content of the 19th-century annual sanitary reports available to historians reflects these priorities. The Punjab sanitary reports of the 1870s and 1880s, for example, contained often 30 pages or more devoted to cholera, a disease that accounted for at most some 6,000 deaths per year in the province. By contrast, the 300,000 deaths attributed to fever each year, a large portion of which were considered malarial, often were accorded only a few lines of commentary. The Punjab Lieutenant-Governor in his review of the annual Sanitary Report for 1875 had at one point openly questioned this skewed response:

> The past year shows an enormous mortality from remittent fever. . . . The attention of the Sanitary Commissioner may with advantage be directed to this question, which in his report fills but one short paragraph while the bulk is devoted to cholera which seems to attract the attention disproportionate to its importance when it is considered that deaths from this disease ordinarily form an almost inappreciable proportion of the general mortality of the province.[59]

Nonetheless, the skewed attention continued. The 1879 Punjab Sanitary Commission report contained a 51-page account of cholera, for example, though the year was one of severe malaria mortality. Historical epidemic analysis, in turn, has generally been directed instead to those diseases for which abundant records exist – to cholera, to a lesser extent, smallpox, and later, to plague – but which together accounted for only a small proportion of annual deaths, generally less than 10 per cent.

From the early years of the 20th century, however, colonial sanitary (public health) attention swung dramatically away from cholera and smallpox and came to focus instead on malaria. This shift in interest was stimulated by Ross's 1897 confirmation of the role of mosquitoes in malaria transmission, work which appeared to offer the promise of feasible scientific methods of malaria control through vector 'extirpation,'[60] fostering, in turn, the rapid emergence in Britain of professional institutions of 'tropical medicine.'[61] But it was fuelled as well by cumulative documentation of the enormous role of malaria in famine mortality. Within a single decade, malaria had come to dominate the colonial public health research agenda, alongside plague, prompting research that has left a wealth of published and archival material at the disposal of historians. It would be a remarkable period in which a handful of medical researchers – initially British, but soon joined by Indian counterparts – would delve into the broader epidemiological dimensions of the disease alongside the entomological and microbiological. Appointed a member of the Malaria Committee of the Royal Society in 1898 at the age of 25, Christophers (1873–1978) was at the centre of this work.[62] Recognised early on as a brilliant scientist, he would join the Indian Medical Service in 1902 and soon became 'a legend in the IMS and in the larger sphere of medical parasitology,' leading and shaping medical and entomological research in India for the next 30 years.[63]

Malaria in the Punjab was only one of a number of exceptional epidemiological studies of malaria to be undertaken in the first several decades of the 20th century. Within only a decade and a half of the 1909 Simla conference, sufficient data on regional malaria vectors and transmission rates had been elucidated by medical researchers to allow construction of a 'Malaria Map' of British India detailing epidemic and endemicity patterns of malaria transmission across virtually the entire subcontinent.[64] In 1929, a bibliography of Indian malaria research was compiled by the Director of the Malaria Survey of India, J.A. Sinton, that contained over 2,200 entries of scientific articles, government reports, and texts.[65] Two years later, the Malaria Commission of the League of Nations Health Organization noted in a report of its study tour of India that much of the basic microbiological, entomological, and epidemiological understanding of malaria as a parasitic infection had come, up to that point, from research conducted in India.[66] This body of incomparably rich material remains largely unincorporated in the historiographic literature, the sheer volume of the post-1897 South Asian colonial malaria literature perhaps, paradoxically, deterring historians.[67]

Recently, some of this epidemiological legacy has begun to be explored in relation to South Asian famines, work that has confirmed the role of malaria as a leading trigger of famine mortality.[68] Analysis of the larger influence of malaria in the region's health history – malaria's general, or *endemic*, history – has yet to receive systematic, and quantitative, attention, however. Few monographs exist that are devoted specifically to South Asian malaria history,[69] although references to malaria frequently appear as incidental commentary within critiques of colonial irrigation, economic, or public health policies. Analysis specific to malaria appears instead in journal articles, a recent common theme being 'developogenic malaria': enhanced transmission associated with the vast expansion in canal irrigation under British rule and associated detrimental effects of 'untidy' irrigation and water-logging.[70] In recent decades, increasing medical interest in malaria history has led to a series of special issues published in the Italian medical journal *Parassitologia*, with considerable work directed to the South Asian colonial experience and research. William Bynum has provided an important thematic summary of the over 2,200 scientific articles, government reports, and texts on malaria published in British India between 1901 and the late 1920s,[71] research that encompasses both the pre-1920 period of extreme ('fulminant') malaria mortality, and the subsequent period of epidemic decline. Several studies in this collection have been highlighted in the earlier writing of Ira Klein, and more recently by Kohei Wakimura,[72] again with emphasis on the general 'malariogenic' effects of imperial infrastructure construction.

To date, however, much of the actual content of the colonial epidemiological research remains unincorporated within South Asian epidemic historiography. In the face of the failed 1902–1908 attempt at rural vector 'extirpation' at Mian Mir, negligible vector control post-1920 (beyond industrial enclaves), and continuing canal irrigation expansion, the 'malaria problem' has been assumed to have remained largely unchanged through the remainder of the colonial period.[73] Rarely defined, the term 'malaria control' appears to connote malaria *transmission*, of which quite correctly there is little evidence of decline pre-1947.[74] Yet in its general application, the term appears to imply malaria mortality as well.

What stands out in the thematic trajectory of this historiographic literature, then, is an inadvertent conflation of malaria infection (transmission) and malarial mortality. The distinction is an important one, and the case of Punjab is particularly instructive. While there is little question that irrigation channels offered highly favourable breeding sites for the primary rural malaria mosquito vector *(An. culicifacies)*, malaria was endemic, post-monsoon, to virtually all rural tracts of Punjab quite independent of the vast canal irrigation systems engineered under the British Raj. Moreover, as detailed in chapter 4, the western canal tracts were *less* affected generally by 'fulminant' malaria than elsewhere in the province.[75] As well, ongoing expansion of the canal networks in the final decades of the colonial period was associated not with heightened mortality but rather with declining crude death rates, again in step with trends in other regions of the province. Unfortunately, with attention directed primarily towards malaria *transmission*, patterns of actual *mortality* from the disease have remained generally unexamined, indeed largely invisible. In this sense, the conflation of malaria infection and malaria lethality has served to foreclose essential avenues for incorporating the overall impacts of colonial canal irrigation projects into analysis of historical mortality trends in the region.

There were, of course, serious ecological problems associated with canal irrigation. But where malaria developed as a severe health and mortality problem, this was associated with underlying decline in agricultural productivity consequent on waterlogging and soil salinization, changes triggered by canal irrigation in specific tracts. Often missing from historiographic accounts of canal irrigation impacts, in other words, is sufficient articulation of the temporal relationship of the entomological and economic effects, and their etiological chain of causation.

This observation does not imply that criticism of the colonial government's inaction on 'malaria control' is unwarranted. Even in highly localised urban areas where control of a specific vector was technically feasible, such as in the Bombay municipality, control efforts were underfunded, at best erratic, and frequently abandoned.[76] As for quinine provision, despite reliance on improved access to malaria treatment as one principal arm of malaria policy post-1908, *per capita* availability of the drug across the final decades of colonial rule increased only marginally relative to need in the years following the 1909 Simla malaria conference. The scope for criticism of 'malariogenic' rural development policies is similarly broad.[77] The ecological consequences of canal irrigation in Punjab for malaria transmission, and the detrimental effects, often preventable, of rail and canal embankments on rural drainage patterns, were real and extensive in terms of agricultural productivity and severity of malaria. The provincial government would quietly attend to the worst examples of blocked surface drainage where canal-induced waterlogging disrupted agricultural productivity most markedly. But there was little effort until the final years of the colonial period to address the general problem of seepage, local overusage of canal irrigation flows, and rising water tables. In large tracts of lower Bengal, similar effects of rail and road infrastructure construction were catastrophic. Here too, however, as will be argued, the underlying driver of heightened malaria intensity was primarily economic.[78]

Without in any way gainsaying the mortality risk inherent to malarial infection (falciparum malaria in particular), one can point, then, to limited appreciation within the historiographic literature of the immense range in disease lethality associated with seasonal malaria transmission: a spectrum varying from a week or so of recurring fever – 'ordinary' post-monsoon malarial fever with, in historical terms, a low mortality rate – on the one hand, to extreme prostration and death, on the other. In the absence of attention to coincident trends in malaria mortality, the critique of colonial malaria inaction, while apt in important ways, inevitably remains difficult to integrate effectively within malaria and epidemic history. Suffice to say, for South Asian malaria historiography, the failure to differentiate malaria fever (infection) from malaria mortality has left the discipline at an impasse, with seemingly little to study regarding the region's malaria burden under colonial rule until the arrival of the powerful residual insecticides in the 1950s period – and little also, it seems, thereafter. The seeming paradox of declining epidemic mortality in the face of limited – some would suggest dismal – commitment on the part of the British colonial government to malaria transmission control suggests that there is something incomplete with the existing paradigm.

A related consequence of inadequate attention to the infection: mortality distinction can be seen in relation to recent analysis of inter-war deliberations on malaria control policy within the League of Nations Malaria Commission (LNMC) where attention has been directed to the professional 'contest' between Commission members who saw malaria as largely a 'social' disease requiring broader economic measures for reducing its public health impact along with quinine access, and others, primarily U.S. malaria workers, who emphasised vector control.[79] Left largely unexplored to date in such accounts is the earlier epidemiological literature linking malaria intensity (the 'malaria burden') to human destitution, experience upon which the views of malaria as a 'social disease' were based.

Incorporating hunger in malaria history

If the conflation of infection (transmission) and disease (mortality) in epidemic historiography has held considerable consequences for South Asian malaria research, so too have conceptual gaps in understanding of hunger epidemiology. Until quite recently, approaches to human subsistence history have been constrained by a parallel conceptual narrowness, where investigation of the hunger-epidemic relationship is often limited to the most extreme form of hunger, overt famine, or to macroeconomic indices such as wage rates. At the same time, in recent European famine and demographic historiography, earlier understanding of famine-associated epidemics as mediated largely by hunger-induced immune suppression has increasingly been questioned with greater emphasis directed to famine-associated conditions conducive to infection transmission. The wandering of famine victims in their search for food and water and concomitant 'dysfunctional social behaviour' markedly enhanced exposure to disease agents, it is argued, a factor considered 'primarily responsible for allowing endemic infections to flare into regional and national epidemics.'[80]

This recent trend of according greater interpretative weight to the microbiologic realm in epidemic history analysis can be seen with respect to malaria historiography as well. In a prominent symposium on nutrition in history in the early 1980s, malaria came to be classified, alongside smallpox and plague, as an infection where the 'nutritional influence on outcome' was 'minimal,'[81] a categorisation that effectively relegates a very large part of human health history to the domain of inherently virulent microbes. In the case of South Asia, for example, where malaria was a leading trigger of mortality, this encompasses a period prevailing from the pre-modern era up to the early 20th century.[82]

The broader influence of the 1983 categorisation appears to have been substantial, with malaria frequently referred to in subsequent literature as an 'indiscriminate' epidemic disease, one that is 'insensitive to the nutritional status of the host.'[83] Moreover, a growing emphasis on microbial ecology is seen in current South Asian famine and epidemic historiography as well.[84] In the specific case of malaria, entomological hypotheses such as 'vector deviation' have been highlighted as likely important factors contributing to epidemic patterns in periods of famine: drought-induced mortality among livestock, it is argued, resulted in greater exposure to malaria as vector (mosquito) feeding shifted from cattle to humans.[85] A further variant of transmission-related explanations of malaria epidemicity emphasises immunological factors as determining epidemic vulnerability and patterns.[86] The Punjab region in modern medical thought has come to be seen as a quintessential example of 'unstable' malaria, where highly variable transmission year-to-year led to fluctuations in acquired immunity amongst the population, and, in turn, heightened vulnerability to epidemic conditions.[87] Generally missing, however, is accompanying empirical examination of the transmission-related theses that would account for post-1920 epidemic malaria decline in Punjab. Missing also is comparable attention to an epidemiology of acute and chronic hunger across the colonial period. Recent research in the field of South Asian health history has begun to break out of the analytic impasse resulting from the modern confla- tion of infection (transmission) and disease (mortality), and as well the relative invisibility of non-famine hunger in historiographical inves- tigation. In concert with European research,[88] nutritional anthropo- metric historiography has begun to shed light on South Asian patterns of undernourishment through trends in physical stature (nutritional stunting).[89] Equally important work by Sumit Guha and Christophe Guilmoto has highlighted the key distinction between *gaps* in food access and average *levels* of consumption, and the importance of this distinction for interpreting epidemic trends across the colonial period.[90] The need for a more comprehensive conceptualisation and tracking of historical hunger, however, remains. Indeed, this is a gap in epidemic and economic historiography more generally, and one that continues to present major challenges. In one notable attempt several decades ago to bring together a range of work on 'hunger in history,' Millman and Kates pithily observed that '[t]he history of hunger is for the most part unwritten. The hungry rarely write history, and histori- ans are rarely hungry.'[91]

A larger significance to Punjab malaria history

The history of Punjab epidemic malaria in relation to famine, and fam- ine control, offers an important setting to explore empirically many of the questions relating to the relative roles of economic and envi- ronmental factors underlying the famine-malaria relationship. As in all historical epidemiology analysis, questions of causation are often difficult to answer definitively in the manner of modern controlled epidemiological studies, for lack of reliable measures for key vari- ables. In the case of Punjab malaria history, the more readily identi- fiable character to malaria mortality in this region, and the relative wealth of vital registration and epidemiological data available, make it possible to transcend these archival limitations to a considerable extent. In addition to relatively complete vital registration data, Pun- jab province also was the site of much of the in-depth epidemiological and entomological malaria rural field research conducted under the auspices of the Malaria Survey of India in the final decades of the colonial period. These records shed light on seasonal and year-to-year patterns of malaria prevalence in the region and, in particular, falci-parum malaria, the more lethal form of the disease, across the second half of the colonial period. Public health and irrigation department records also make it possible to trace quinine availability and its dis-tribution in the province as well as malaria control efforts and trends in flooding.

As a major source of grain exports and land revenue, Punjab prov-ince was endowed also with an exceptional range of administrative records, explained by the importance of the region politically, eco-nomically, and militarily to the British colonial government. Taken together, these make possible reasonable inferences about trends both in malaria transmission in the province, in addition to mortality, and in access to treatment across the period of epidemic decline. In doing so, they offer a singular opportunity to assess, and to some extent 'control for,' levels of malaria infection in assessing the importance of acute hunger on lethality of malarial infection. It is this relative wealth of primary sources that allows exploration of the *general* relationship between epidemic disease (and endemic) and economic conditions over the colonial period as a whole, a level of understanding that is unavailable from accounts of individual famines.

At the core of Christophers's investigation of 'fulminant' malaria in pre-1920 British India lay the central question: what combination of forces episodically transformed a comparatively benign endemic dis-ease into its epidemic and dramatically more lethal form? '[T]hough malaria is always present and in a sense may be extremely intense,' Christophers observed, 'the disease is only associated with high epi-demic mortality under certain conditions.'[92] In his pursuit to compre-hend those 'certain conditions,' Christophers did not limit his powers of observation solely to heightened host susceptibility. Concerted attention would be directed to entomological and biomedical factors such as dose of infection and a range of hydrological and entomo-logical effects of rainfall and flooding specific to the region. In many respects, Christophers succeeded in his efforts to decipher the complex range of factors underlying such 'death storms.' In several aspects, his analysis fell short for lack of statistical capacity and the fact that he was working without the benefit of the key perspective provided by subsequent epidemic decline. In yet other areas, some conclusions were so politically guarded that they can be challenging to decipher in the pages of the official version of his published Punjab report.[93] Nevertheless, the study's framework for detailed spatial and tempo-ral mapping of malaria infection and mortality rates across the prov-ince in 1908, and for earlier major epidemics, presents an invaluable starting point for the investigation of malaria mortality history in the Punjab region and the subcontinent more widely.

Approaches to hunger in history

This study takes its cue in part from Christophers's exploration of the epidemiological form of hunger he considered to underlie 'exalted' malaria as seen in 1908 Punjab. In resurrecting the concept of 'physiological poverty,' he was attempting to assess the role of acute hunger (frank and semi- starvation) in both its epidemic and endemic forms, a distinction which by 1911 had been largely lost in medical analysis. What follows is a brief overview of the meaning and framework of 'hunger' explored in this study.

It is useful to distinguish three basic dimensions to hunger which, if self-evident, tend to become obscured or lost in modern usage of the terms 'malnutrition,' 'undernutrition,' or undernourishment. The first involves degree or severity of food (calorie) insufficiency; a second, extent or prevalence (proportion of a population affected at a given time); and a third, duration. As a mortality-enhancing physiological state, hunger encompasses a range of caloric levels of food consumption on a continuum of insufficiency: from slight and moderate inadequacy, at one end of the spectrum, to nothing at all to eat, on the other. In lay terms, these two general ranges might be termed 'not enough' to eat (undernourishment) versus 'not nearly enough' (semi- or frank starvation). The two can be distinguished, again in very general terms, in relation to basal metabolic rate, that level of energy required for all internal metabolic and physiological functions in a state of complete rest.[94] Severe food insufficiency (referred to as 'acute' hunger in this study) reflects caloric intake below basal metabolic rate, a level where weight loss is continuous and life cannot be supported beyond the short term. In contrast, undernourishment (often termed 'chronic' hunger) refers to food intake above basal metabolic requirement but below that required to meet all *external* energy demands (normal activity, and physical labour) as well as growth demands (in children and in pregnant or breastfeeding women). In both cases, duration of the two states largely determines mortality risk. The mortality risk with chronic hunger, though also associated elevated, related to weakened immunological competence, is less than absolute and less immediate compared with that for acute hunger (the term 'chronic' reflects this lower lethality, allowing for a longer duration unremedied). In the case of undernourishment, some physiological adaptation to calorie deficit is often possible through reduced physical activity (energy expenditure), or additionally in children, a reduction in physical growth rate (stunting). Both such states of 'adaptation,' however, entail immunological and cognitive costs as well as impairment of work capacity.

In young children, cumulative undernourishment is identified clinically by 'stunting' (low height-for-age), and acute hunger, by 'wasting' or emaciation (low weight-for-height). In many instances, both can be evident in the same child as levels of food inadequacy fluctuate over time.[95] In all states of caloric inadequacy, the added energy drain of concurrent infections further reduces the *net* calories physiologically available.

The conceptual distinction between acute and chronic hunger is important for historical analysis for several reasons. The most obvious relates to mortality risk. But another is methodological: the means by which the two states of hunger can be identified from historical records, and potentially measured, often differ markedly. Historical changes in mean physical stature in a population, for example, are likely to reflect change in chronic hunger prevalence (net undernourishment over time) more reliably than acute hunger,[96] whereas short-term fluctuations in foodgrain prices probably signal greater *relative* increases in acute hunger compared with chronic. At the macroeconomic level, the distinction between acute and chronic is important for interpreting the significance of various economic indices of human welfare grouped under the rubric of 'standard of living.' Finally, the conceptual distinction between acute and chronic hunger is particularly important in health and epidemic history because of potential differences in interaction between specific infectious diseases and type of hunger. In South Asia, the case fatality rate[97] for malaria appears to have been heightened, in particular, by acute hunger and less so by lesser degrees of undernourishment.

Towards an epidemiology of South Asian hunger

Prevalence of acute and chronic hunger cannot be traced in historical research with the precision expected in modern clinical research. Nevertheless, with a clearer conceptualisation of hunger, historical markers of hunger can be identified from a range of archival sources.[98] The two general categories of hunger, acute and chronic, can be identified in South Asian historical records, for example, in references to numbers of meals per day consumed: two meals a day considered 'enough to satisfy hunger.' Witnesses to the late 19th-century famine commissions in India often expressed hunger in exactly these terms, noting with alarm that even in years of good harvests, many landless households routinely had access to only a single meal each day – a single cereal-based meal likely implying considerable undernourishment (chronic hunger).[99] The categories of zero, one, and two meals per day encompass, albeit in very general form, the two central aspects of hunger in human history: on the one hand, reflecting (in)adequacy of levels of food (caloric) intake, and on the other, (ir)regularity of access to food, that is, the frequency with which subgroups of a population slip below one square meal into semi- or frank starvation (acute hunger). If one could graphically sketch acute and chronic hunger through history, one would be tracing, in effect, the relative prevalence in a population of persons with access to two square meals per day, one, or none over time – the term 'prevalence' here being used in its epidemiological sense of frequency, duration, and social extent.

Such a schematic framework requires qualification to take into account, for example, the exceptional needs of infants and young children who require far more than two meals a day because of their extremely high relative food requirements for growth, and their small stomach size. It is here, of course, where conditions of work for women, productive and reproductive, play such a large historical role. Attention has been directed recently to the nutritional drain of repeated infections, again of special relevance to young children. The concept of 'net' nutrition takes into account the potential additional impact on food sufficiency of transient illness-induced anorexia and added nutrient losses associated, in particular, with diarrheal episodes. In addition to questions of water supply, 'net nutrition' thus also reflects quite profoundly conditions of work: women's capacity to feed and care for young children to compensate for such recurring nutrient losses.[100]

One final comment on the relationship between hunger, epidemic lethality, and life expectancy in history. While the link between immune-suppression and both undernourishment and semi-/frank starvation is clear,[101] the contribution of subsistence insecurity to compromised immune capacity very probably embraces effects beyond the directly biological. A related, if ultimately unmeasurable, component derives from the immune-suppression effects of extreme psychological stress by way of heightened cortisol levels associated with food insecurity and acute hunger: the despair and human degradation accompanying the inability to protect oneself and family members, above all, one's children. Such despair was routinely expressed in the desperate resort to offering children into servitude for the price of their being fed, or the agony of watching them die in the streets and roadways absent of succour.[102] Separating the two sources of immune-suppression associated with acute hunger is an impossible – one might suggest, unnecessary – task. In this study, both are assumed to be at play.

Shifts in acute hunger prevalence

Changes in food (in)security – access to subsistence foodgrains – in India were bound up with broad shifts in the economy across the colonial period, a century that saw development of modern transportation and communications systems, and the rapid entry of South Asian foodgrains onto global markets in the second half of the 19th century. But the period also saw major changes in the response of the British Raj to food crises, policy shifts that bore directly on vulnerability to starvation and hunger prevalence. Here, the classic Indian famine studies by Bhatia and Srivastava offer invaluable documentation and analysis of specific relief policies and operations across the second half of the 19th century, the period of the 'great' famines. Relatively less attention, however, has been directed to subsequent developments in famine prevention over the first two decades of the 20th century.[103] These later changes have generally been seen as fine-tuning of the system of relief set out in the original 1880 Famine Commission Report. The revamping of government relief into effective famine prevention, it is generally assumed, awaited the post-Independence period and systematic public intervention in national food supply.[104]

Such a reading misses a great deal. Rather than minor adjustments, the approach to famine 'relief' initially set out in the 1883 provisional Indian Famine Code was fundamentally transformed in the years following the famine of 1899–1900. Relief measures post-1901 were not simply less punitive, but different in their basic framework, and also in their effectiveness. From palliative relief of 'established' famine, relief policy after the turn of the century shifted increasingly to early, pre-emptive support of the agricultural economy *before* frank famine 'had declared itself.' The significance of these changes has been documented by Arup Maharatna in his analysis of the 1907–1908 famine in the United Provinces.[105] However, the shift to more 'liberal and rational' relief as evidenced in 1907–1908 marked only the beginning of such policy changes. After 1908, drought relief increasingly became a policy of routine application in response to local harvest shortfall, in contrast to the 1880 policy which restricted relief to years of exceptional (catastrophic) and widespread harvest failure. From 1920 onward in Punjab province, relief also began to be sanctioned for other causes of crop failure such as flooding, and ultimately on the basis of 'scarcity' (high foodgrain prices) alone, without famine ever being declared. These were simple, one can say obvious and unremarkable, changes. But they held profound implications for human survival across periods of acute harvest failure.

The timing, extent, and potential impact of such changes have yet to be adequately traced but form a central aspect in the reconstruction of an epidemiology of acute hunger across the period of epidemic malaria decline.

Acute hunger was not limited, however, to episodic subsistence crises. The term 'famine' generally refers to a sudden and transient increase in acute hunger prevalence markedly *above that level normally prevailing* in a society: in epidemiological terms, an 'epidemic' of starvation (semi- and frank) in a population. Endemic starvation, by contrast, refers to a 'normal' prevalence of acute hunger in a population: at any one time, or season, a certain proportion of households or persons slipping from poverty (and often chronic hunger) into frank destitution due to local crop failure, loss of employment, illness, injury, or death of earning members, or specific conditions of work.[106] Given the large proportion of the South Asian population living at bare subsistence levels, and the virtual absence of social security measures in non-famine times, levels of endemic starvation unquestionably were high and possibly even increasing over the colonial period in those provinces such as Bengal where structural constraints made agricultural production especially unresponsive to population growth. Famine relief policies contained in the 1880 Indian Famine Commission Report addressed neither chronic hunger nor *endemic* acute hunger, but only the *epidemic* form of starvation – and indeed, as we will see, only a portion of that.

Endemic acute hunger, though far less visible in sociological or archival terms than epidemic destitution (famine), also bore important implications for the lethality burden of malaria across the subcontinent. Here, Christophers once again was at the forefront of exploring the magnitude of this relationship, analysing in collaboration with C.A. Bentley the causes of the peculiarly 'intense' (highly lethal) malaria observed in the labour camps of the northeastern Duars tea plantations, and coining the term 'tropical aggregation of labour' to refer to those conditions of work associated with destitution amongst subgroups of labourers, many working under 19th-century Indentured Labour Acts. Such conditions of semi-starvation were endemically present, and frequently underlay, they concluded, the 'exalted' form of malaria seen not just on the tea plantations, but in the vast industrial labour camps throughout India, including the slums of the industrialising small towns of Punjab.[107]

Assessing the impact of changes in both famine relief policy and labour conditions on food security, and in relation to broader shifts in the economy, is a complex task, to say the least.[108] Quantifying acute hunger prevalence presents obvious challenges for lack of direct measures. Nonetheless, the general contours of acute hunger risk, and prevalence, can be gauged through changes in famine relief policies and practice across the early decades of the 20th century; through trends in economic indices such as prices, harvest conditions, and wage levels; through incidental narrative accounts;[109] and, finally, through the timing of changes in the most extreme forms of labour exploitation brought about with changes in indentured and other labour laws. In the latter case, analysis will rely to a considerable extent on secondary literature.

'Nutrition' paradoxes

As noted earlier, important South Asian research has been undertaken recently in nutritional anthropometric history, historical trends in human stature in populations. As a biological gauge of subsistence (in)security, secular trends in adult height shed light on shifts in food access in terms of amount of food consumed (undernourishment) over time, as reflected in nutritional stunting. To date, this work suggests little improvement (increase in mean stature), and indeed, possibly slight decline in height amongst the poorer and most food-insecure subgroups across the colonial period.[110] In light of increasing life expectancy from the early decades of the 20th century, lack of improvement in adult stature appears paradoxical.[111] Yet seen from the context of both *gaps* in food access as well as *levels* of food intake, this pattern is perhaps less surprising.

It is unclear, for example, to what extent acute hunger is reflected in stature, in contrast to chronic undernourishment. Famine mortality could be expected to have been greatest among the most undernourished, those with least physiologic reserves.[112] More effective famine (acute hunger) control after 1901 likely meant proportionately greater improvement in survival chances among the chronically undernourished, possibly resulting, in turn, in a net increase in nutritionally stunted individuals within the post-famine population. Seemingly opposite trends – decreasing or stagnant mean stature levels and rising life expectancy – may not necessarily be inconsistent, then, with improving food security, when the distinction between acute and chronic hunger is taken into account. A similar explanation may also underlie to some extent the seeming paradox of post-1920 rising life expectancy despite decline in *per capita* foodgrain availability.[113]

Study framework

Two questions frame this study. First, was Christophers correct? Did acute hunger (starvation) play a central role in the regional epidemics that afflicted Punjab in the pre-1910 period? Second, to what extent did changes in food security – specifically, control of epidemic hunger – contribute to decline in malaria epidemicity, relative to improved access to treatment and possible changes in malaria transmission levels across the province?

Using *Malaria in the Punjab* as a point of departure (chapter 2), the study repeats Christophers's basic quantitative analysis of autumn fever mortality, rain, and grain prices, using modern statistical methods of multiple regression analysis (chapters 3–4). Unlike the 1911 inquiry, however, quantitative analysis is conducted at district level. Marked differences in ecology and agricultural conditions across the province underlay quite different relationships between harvest conditions and rainfall in Punjab, and, in turn, in the timing of acute hunger prevalence year to year. Major differences between districts, therefore, can be expected in the relationship between rainfall, acute hunger, and malaria mortality, differences that are likely to be obscured at the aggregate (province) level of analysis.

Statistical analysis begins with the 1868–1908 period of recurrent severe epidemics, the 41-year period of Christophers's analysis, exploring the relationship between annual malaria death rates in each of the 24 plains districts and those two factors most closely linked in the historical records with epidemic occurrence in Punjab: monsoon rainfall and associated flooding, on the one hand, and 'scarcity,' as reflected by local foodgrain prices, on the other. Similar quantitative and descriptive analysis is then extended to the post-1908 period of epidemic decline – that period (1909–1940) for which equivalent data are available: first, to identify regional timing and extent of epidemic decline across the province; then, through similar regression analysis, to explore the changing relationship between autumn fever mortality and rainfall and price levels across this later period. These quantitative results are then supplemented by narrative accounts of local economic and ecological conditions from the administrative records for each of the major epidemics of the period, in particular, for 'outlier' epidemics that do not conform to the rain-price epidemic model (chapter 5). Considering the quantitative results in relation to the narrative records, interpretation of the mechanism of 'intense' malaria is offered (chapter 6).

Part II of the study then turns to the question of why epidemic mortality declined after 1908. It begins by tracing the development of official malaria control policies leading up to, and in the aftermath of, the 1909 Imperial Malaria conference at Simla (chapters 7–8), outlining the political context to such policy shifts and distinguishing formal malaria policy statements from those policies actually pursued in practice in the years that followed. The institutional framework for malaria research and training is traced, along with specific vector control programs, flood control work undertaken post-1908, and trends in availability and access to quinine, and the likely impact of such programs on incidence and severity of malaria in the province is discussed (chapter 9).

In Part III of the study, observations on malaria incidence and treatment in Punjab are then set within the larger context of the changing nature of hunger and food (in)security across the period. An attempt is made to reconstruct broad outlines of an epidemiology of hunger across the 1868–1947 period, one that parallels that for malaria transmission (chapters 10–11). As in the case of malaria control policy, changes in famine policy and labour legislation at the all-India level are traced first, then examined specifically in the context of Punjab province.

The study concludes that Christophers was correct in identifying epidemic acute hunger, triggered by harvest failure (drought), agricultural paralysis (flooding), and famine-level grain prices as the key factor in the regional malaria epidemics of Punjab, and correct also in seeing this relationship mediated largely through compromised immune competence ('physiological poverty'). Heightened malaria lethality in years such as 1908 appears to have been largely a function of lack of physical resistance to malaria infection under conditions of widespread semi- and frank starvation: weakened capacity to initiate adequate immunological response to infection and quite possibly additional effects on ensuing dose of infection subsequently transmitted. The study concludes, in turn, that decline in epidemic starvation was the primary factor underlying decline in 'fulminant' malaria in the province. Such a finding is further supported by the return of severe malaria mortality with the re-emergence of famine conditions during World War II, in southeastern Punjab province in 1942, and in Bengal one year later. The primacy of acute hunger is further supported by the limited impact on general mortality levels of the rapid control of malaria transmission in (East) Punjab in the 1950s (chapter 12).

A central role for decline in destitution in post-1920 epidemic malaria decline offers indirect support for Thomas McKeown's view of the importance of increasing food security underlying 19th century mortality decline in England and Wales.[114] Although falciparum malaria is a very different infection from those endemic in 19th-century Britain, the history of its colonial mortality toll is a reminder of the wide variation in lethality of most common (endemic) infectious diseases, and the potential impact of improved access to food on that lethality. This study differs however from McKeown's work in several ways: first, in being able to distinguish more closely the contribution of hunger relative to exposure to infection in contributing to malaria mortality decline; and second, in demonstrating the importance of a clearer conceptualisation of 'nutrition' in historical health analysis, evident in the case of Punjab malaria history where the lethality-enhancing relationship appears to have been most pronounced for (semi-)starvation (acute hunger).

The conclusion that control of epidemic starvation was responsible for the dramatic decline in malaria lethality in Punjab after 1908 is, nevertheless, one at odds with modern medical understanding. The enduring attraction to immunological interpretations of epidemic history, as seen earlier, reflects the larger epistemic transformation that took place in Western medical thought with the identification of specific microbes and their modes of transmission. As powerful techniques of specific vaccines and water supply became available in the late 19th century, sanitary, and subsequently public health, practice increasingly was directed to interrupting microbe transmission. This trend was further reinforced during the inter-war and post-World War II years through the growing epistemic influence of emerging international health institutions and public health philanthropy of the metropoles.[115] Moreover, as biomedical developments in immunology were transforming perception of the 'human factor' in one medical sphere, changes in the conceptualisation of hunger also were taking shape in another, that of nutritional science. With the discovery of micronutrient deficiency states in the 1910s and 1920s, medical attention rapidly shifted in the later 1920s and 1930s to qualitative dietary issues of nutrient imbalance ('mal-nutrition') and away from caloric (in)adequacy – hunger.[116] Inevitably, the demise of the 'human factor' can be comprehended, therefore, only in the larger context of the history of modern scientific medicine and the profound influence of the emergence of medical sub-specialisms on medical thought.

The history of the modern public health movement has only recently begun to be re-examined and fully integrated within the socio-economic and political landscape from which it emerged. In his study of the early sanitary movement in 19th-century Britain, Hamlin has traced a similar process whereby a broader 'predispositionist' understanding of epidemic fever (in this case, typhus) was narrowed to an exclusive focus on an external agent – 'environmental' filth – and away from human destitution, the practical expression of which came to be manifest in the sewers and water-mains conception of sanitary hygiene championed by Edwin Chadwick. In the process, as Hamlin observes, understanding of the relationship between hunger and vulnerability to infective disease that was once commonplace, 'obvious, even truistic,' became a question, or obscured altogether.[117]

Many parallels exist in the conceptual shifts taking place in understanding of disease within the 19th-century English sanitary movement and the transformation in understanding of epidemic malaria in early 20th-century India. Both were periods of deep political and social crisis ushered in with the *laissez-faire* tenets of the new political economy. Both were periods of profound narrowing in medical thought and concepts of disease causation. And in both cases, a reductionist reading of epidemic causality would ultimately prevail within medical thinking – waning acquired immunity in the case of epidemic malaria on the plains of the Indian subcontinent, and 'bad air' (miasma) arising from environmental filth in the case of the fever epidemics in the slums of industrialising Britain – even though both 'diagnoses' were scientifically unfounded.[118] And each has received only limited modern historiographic attention.

In colonial South Asia, it was in the early years of the 20th century that the biomedical model of malaria confronted an earlier climatist understanding of fever that prominently encompassed predisposing subsistence conditions of the human host.[119] The so-called clash of medical paradigms unfolding on the stage of British India did not begin in 1908. Nor, indeed, even in 1897 with Ross's confirmation of mosquitoes as malaria vector. In the case of malarial fever, a process of conceptual narrowing was already underway as climatic theories of disease causation rapidly contracted to selective concern for environmental 'filth' (miasma) under the sway of the 19th-century European sanitary movement and subsequent entry of the new laboratory – and related 'tropical' – medicine.[120] That clash would come to a head at the turn of the century under the intense contradictions of colonial rule, heightened by confirmation of anopheline mosquitoes as malaria vector.

In reinserting the human host into malaria epidemiology, Christophers, in *Malaria in the Punjab*, was not rejecting modern scientific medicine. His entire professional life, on the contrary, remained devoted to it. He most certainly was not dismissing the value of access to curative anti-malaria treatment – much of the remainder of his scientific work after 1931 retirement to Britain was devoted to path-setting research in malaria chemotherapeutics. Rather, he was stepping back from an increasingly reductive view of the malaria problem and, thereby, from the false opposition of a germ 'versus' predisposition debate that had emerged and preoccupied the higher echelons of the colonial sanitary establishment from the final years of the 19th century[121] – and in the process, he was delicately implicating a market fundamentalism transported to the subcontinent, alongside a narrowed sanitationism, with the advent of imperial rule.

The history of malaria mortality in colonial South Asia thus adds an important chapter to the larger historiography of modern public health and disease theory by tracing the brief re-emergence in the Indian subcontinent of a broader understanding of the determinants of much epidemic disease. Precisely how the insights from this period came to be overshadowed in the ensuing decades is a question beyond the scope of the present study. However, by reclaiming human subsistence as a central historical subject, Punjab malaria history offers an important inroad into this larger epistemic question. Moreover, it helps to unlock key methodological avenues to analysis of South Asia's health and demographic history, and sheds light, in the process, on an embryonic moment in the evolution of South Asian food policy in the final decades of colonial rule. The history of epidemic malaria in Punjab province thus illuminates a still larger history relating to shifts in notions of social relationship and human obligation, encompassing a nascent loosening of the grip of classical political economy doctrine, and the Malthusian tenets underpinning it. For, even at the height of British imperial triumphalism, starvation, as Hamlin observes, 'was no mere diagnosis, . . . it was also an accusation of wrongful death.'[122]

Notes

1 Rural districts of upward of 1 million population were subdivided into three or four *thanas*, each under a sub-inspector of police.
2 Reporting of deaths was initiated in the mid- to late 1860s and extended to include births from 1881. The first annual sanitary report containing these data for Punjab province appeared in 1867. For detailed description of the vital registration system, see T. Dyson, 'Infant and Child Mortality in the Indian Subcontinent, 1881–1947,' in A. Bideau, B. Desjardins, H. Brignoli, eds., *Infant and Child Mortality in the Past* (Oxford: Clarendon Press, 1997), 109–135; T. Dyson, M. Das Gupta, 'Demographic Trends in Ludhiana District, Punjab, 1881–1981: An Exploration of Vital Registration Data in Colonial India,' in Ts'ui-jung Liu, et.al., eds., *Asian Population History* (Oxford: Oxford University Press, 2001), 79–104.

3 See, for example, T. Dyson, 'The Historical Demography of Berar, 1881–1980,' in T. Dyson, ed., *India's Historical Demography: Studies in Famine, Disease and Society* (London: Curzon, 1989), 150–196; A. Maharatna, *The Demography of Famines: An Indian Historical Perspective* (New Delhi: Oxford University Press, 1996); J.A. Ortega Osona, 'The Attenuation of Mortality Fluctuations in British Punjab and Bengal, 1870–1947,' in Ts'ui-jung Liu, ed., *Asian Population History*, 306–349; S. Guha, 'Mortality Decline in Early Twentieth Century India: A Preliminary Enquiry,' *Indian Economic and Social History Review*, 28, 4, 1991, 371–387 [hereafter *IESHR*]; C. Guilmoto, 'Towards a New Demographic Equilibrium: The Inception of Demographic Transition South India,' *IESHR, 28, 3,* 1992, 247–289.

4 The transition in general mortality levels may have begun a decade earlier, obscured by the exceptional mortality of the 1918 influenza epidemic and early 20th-century plague.

5 The 'paroxysmal fevers' were 'presumed to be putrescent, or at any rate, [caused by] decomposing vegetable matter derived from a moist and putrescent soil, which is carried into the body by the medium of water or of air'; E.A. Parkes, *A Manual of Practical Hygiene, Prepared Especially for Use in the Medical Service of the Army* (London: John Churchill, 1866), 444.

6 S.R. Christophers, 'Malaria in the Punjab,' *Scientific Memoirs by Officers of the Medical and Sanitary Departments of the Government of India* (New Series), 46 (Calcutta: Superintendent Government Printing Office, 1911), 109 [hereafter MP, and *Sci. Mem. Off. Med. San. Dep.*].

7 The term 'notorious' would be applied to Punjab malaria epidemicity by George Macdonald, Director of the Ross Institute, London School of Hygiene and Tropical Medicine; 'The Analysis of Malaria Epidemics,' in L. Bruce-Chwatt, V.J. Glanville, eds., *Dynamics of Tropical Diseases: The Late George Macdonald* (London: Oxford University Press, 1973), 146–160. Christophers termed Punjab malaria epidemics as 'disastrous,' MP, 127, 133.

8 MP, 127.

9 Ibid., 107 [emphasis in original].

10 The 1908 epidemic included much of eastern and central Punjab and the western districts of neighbouring United Provinces, affecting a population of some 30 million; S.R. Christophers, 'Endemic and Epidemic Prevalence,' in M.F. Boyd, ed., *Malariology* (Philadelphia: W.B. Saunders, 1949), 698–721, at 710.

11 For some time before 1897, the mosquito had been considered to play a role in malaria aetiology; M. Worboys, 'Germs, Malaria and the Invention of Mansonian Tropical Medicine: From 'Diseases in the Tropics' to "Tropical Diseases",' in D. Arnold, ed., *Warm Climates in Western Medicine: The Emergence of Tropical Medicine, 1500–1900* (Amsterdam: Redopi, 1996), 181–207.

12 S.R. Christophers, 'Suggestions on the Use of Available Statistics for Studying Malaria in India,' *Paludism,* 1, 1910, 16–32, at 16.

13 Dyson and Das Gupta, 'Demographic Trends in Ludhiana District,' 81–82.

14 S.R. Christophers, 'What Disease Costs India: Being a Statement of the Problem Before Medical Research in India,' Presidential Address at the

Medical Research Section of the Fifth Indian Science Congress, *Indian Medical Gazette*, Apr. 1924, 196–200, at 198 [hereafter *IMG*].

15 'Malaria especially gives a very characteristic curve rising sharply to its full height in October, remaining high for November and perhaps December, and falling gradually throughout the early months of the year'; 'A New Statistical Method of Mapping Epidemic Disease in India, with Special Reference to the Mapping of Epidemic Malaria'; *Proceedings of the Imperial Malaria Conference Held at Simla in October 1909* (Simla: Government Central Branch Press, 1910), 16–22, at 18 [hereafter Simla Conf.].

16 MP, 26.

17 Simla Conf., 34.

18 Christophers, 'Suggestions on the use of available statistics,' 28.

19 MP, 105.

20 On famine test works, see ch. 10.

21 MP, 26, 110, 112.

22 A brief period of *P. vivax* transmission often occurred in the spring months.

23 MP, 112. W.R. Cornish, Madras Sanitary Commissioner, earlier had documented also the close relationship between death rates and foodgrain prices across the 1876–1877 South Indian famine, work which at the time had met with markedly less enthusiasm from the British Raj; *Report of the Sanitary Commissioner for Madras for 1877* (Madras: Government Central Branch Press, 1878).

24 M. Davis, *Late Victorian Holocausts: El Niño Famines and the Making of the Third World* (London: Verso, 2001).

25 'Within Punjab, by 1928, the eight [canal] colony districts contributed more revenue than the remaining 21 districts put together'; I. Agnihotri 'Ecology, Land Use and Colonisation: The Canal Colonies of Punjab,' *IESHR*, 33, 1, 1996, 37–58, at 39.

26 Punjab grain exports in 1907–1908 reached 1.8 million tons, one-third diverted to the famine districts of U.P.; *Season and Crop Report* (Punjab), 1907–1908, 6.

27 *Paludism*, 4, 1912, 81.

28 N.G. Barrier, 'The Punjab Disturbances of 1907: The Response of the British Government in India to Agrarian Unrest,' *Modern Asian Studies*, 1, 4, 1967, 353–383 [hereafter *MAS*]; ———, *Banned: Controversial Literature and Political Control in British India, 1907–1947* (New Delhi: Manohar, 1976).

29 C. Hamlin, *Public Health and Social Justice in the Age of Chadwick* (Cambridge: Cambridge University Press, 1998).

30 Simla Conf., 66.

31 R. Ross, 'The Anti-Malarial Experiment at Mian Mir,' *British Medical Journal*, 1904, ii, 632–635 [hereafter *BMJ*].

32 I. Catanach, 'Plague and the Tensions of Empire: India, 1896–1918,' in D. Arnold, ed., *Imperial Medicine and Indigenous Societies* (Manchester: Manchester University Press, 1988), 149–171; R. Chandavarkar, 'Plague Panic and Epidemic Politics in India, 1896–1914,' in T. Ranger, P. Slack, eds., *Epidemics and Ideas* (Cambridge: Cambridge University Press, 1992), 203 240; F. Norman White, *Twenty Years of Plague in India*

with Special Reference to the Outbreak of 1917–1918 (Simla: Government Central Branch Press, 1929).

33 See ahead, chs. 7–8.

34 MP, 113.

35 S. Watts, 'British Development Policies and Malaria in India 1897-c.1929,' *Past and Present*, 165, 1999, 141–181.

36 S.R. Christophers, 'On Malaria in the Punjab'; Simla Conf., 29–44.

37 S.R. Christophers, C.A. Bentley, 'The Human Factor: An Extension of Our Knowledge Regarding the Epidemiology of Malarial Disease,' in W.E. Jennings, ed., *Transactions of the Bombay Medical Congress, 1909* (Bombay: Bennett, Coleman & Co., 1910), 78–83 at 83 [hereafter *Trans. Bombay Medical Congress*]. Watts's critique of Christophers's malaria research as a 'disingenuous' attempt to pre-empt calls for extensive investment in anti-mosquito campaigns and 'to fabricate information and to hoodwink potential critics' ironically dismisses those few official malaria studies that exposed the larger economic contradictions inherent to colonial rule; Watts, 'British development policies and malaria in India,' 176. See ch. 8.

38 Severe epidemics returned, in Punjab in 1942, and Bengal a year later, with war-time hyperinflation in the absence of the provincial Famine Codes being invoked. See ch. 12.

39 See ch. 12, and Dyson and Das Gupta, 'Demographic Trends in Ludhiana District,' 87, 89.

40 'Exceptional' here refers to their circumscribed contribution to mortality in the early 20th century, though 1918 influenza lethality itself appears influenced by prevailing famine conditions; I.D. Mills, 'The 1918–1918 Influenza Pandemic: The Indian Experience,' *IESHR*, 23, Mar. 1986, 1–40; *Twenty Years of Plague in India*.

41 Simla Conf., 95.

42 Between 1897 and 1906, the portion of deaths registered under the category of 'fever' by region varied from 68 per cent in Bengal, to 56 per cent in Punjab and 38 per cent in the Madras Presidency; *Statistical Abstract Relating to British India* (London: HMSO, 1840–1920). However, the seasonality of malaria transmission and mortality in much of the plains meant only a fraction of recorded 'fever' mortality was malarial. At the 1909 Imperial Malaria Conference at Simla, officials suggested an annual toll of five deaths per thousand; Simla Conf., 3–4.

43 'However inaccurate the diagnosis of "fever" may be, there is no doubt,' Christophers stressed, 'that excluding [recent] plague . . . the occurrence of a very healthy or a very unhealthy year as judged by total mortality returns depends almost entirely upon the excess of deaths from "fevers" which has gone to form the autumnal epidemic rise'; MP, 7.

44 The distinction contrasts immunological *capacity* to generate an effective response to *future* infection versus *presence* of specific anti-malarial antibodies (acquired immunity) induced by *past* infection.

45 G. Macdonald, 'The Analysis of Equilibrium in Malaria,' in Bruce-Chwatt and Glanville, eds., *Dynamics of Tropical Disease*.

46 In the absence of evidence for effective transmission control 'interventions,' immunological explanations of decline in infectious disease mortality continue to be turned to by default, both in general historical analysis and in relation to South Asian malaria; W. McNeill, *Plagues and Peoples*

(New York: Anchor Books, 1976), 197–203; Macdonald, 'Analysis of Equilibrium in Malaria,' 132; I. Klein, 'Development and death: Reinterpreting malaria, economics and ecology in British India,' *IESHR*, 38, 2, 2001, 147–179; Menno J. Bouma, H. van der Kaay, 'The El Niño Southern Oscillation and the Historical Malaria Epidemics on the Indian Subcontinent and Sri Lanka: An Early Warning System for Future Epidemics?' *Tropical Medicine and International Health*, 1, 1, Feb. 1996, 86–96.

47 Sinton's monograph published in three parts briefly cited Christophers's 1911 study. But the overriding emphasis was on malaria as impediment to agricultural and general development; J.A. Sinton, 'What malaria costs India, nationally, socially and economically,' *Records of the Malaria Survey of India*, 5, 3, Sept. 1935, 223–264; 4, 4, Dec. 1935, 413–489; 6, 1, Mar. 1936, 91–169 [hereafter *RMSI*].

48 R. Ross, *The Prevention of Malaria* (London: John Murray, 1910), viii; __, 'Introduction,' in W.H.S. Jones, ed., *Malaria, a Neglected Factor in the History of Greece and Rome* (Cambridge: Macmillan & Bowes, 1907).

49 For critique of the 'malaria blocks development' thesis, see P.J. Brown, 'Demographic and Socioeconomic Effects of Disease Control: The Case of Malaria Eradication in Sardinia,' *Medical Anthropology*, 7, 2, 1983, 63–87; __, 'Malaria, Miseria, and Underpopulation in Sardinia: The "Malaria Blocks Development" Cultural Model,' *Medical Anthropology*, 17, 1997, 239–254; J.A. Nájera, 'The control of tropical diseases and socioeconomic development, with special reference to malaria and its control,' *Parassitologia*, 36, 1–2, Aug. 1994, 17–33; R. Packard, ' "Roll Back Malaria, Roll in Development"? Reassessing the Economic Burden of Malaria,' *Population and Development Review*, 35, 1, 2009, 53–87.

50 I.A. McGregor, 'Malaria and Nutrition,' in W.H. Wernsdorfer, I.A. McGregor, eds., *Malaria: Principles and Practice of Malariology* (Edinburgh: Churchill Livingstone, 1988), 754–777, at 754 [emphasis added]. This reading of Christophers's 1911 Punjab report may well have been based on Paul Russell's interpretation; P. Russell, L.S. West, R.D. Manwell, *Practical Malariology* (Philadelphia: W.B. Saunders, 1946), 375.

51 Hamlin, *Public Health and Social Justice*.

52 'Physiological concepts of disease imply that a disease cannot be understood apart from a particular individual suffering from it. . . . [Whereas w]ithin the ontological tradition, disease is posited to be some sort of entity which befalls a previously healthy person'; W. Bynum, 'Nosology,' in W. Bynum, R. Porter, eds., *Companion Encyclopedia of the History of Medicine* (London: Routledge, 1993), 335–356.

53 In view of present-day policy debate over anti-malaria insecticide policy, it bears emphasising that this is not a blanket argument against insecticide use, but rather a reminder of the importance of the historical malaria experience in helping evaluate its appropriateness in specific circumstances.

54 For example, seasonal flooding in Bengal had an opposite entomological impact on malaria transmission to that of flooding in Punjab, such differences being a function of different mosquito vectors. If these complexities were perplexing to colonial sanitary officials, it is not surprising they remain a challenge for historical researchers.

55 On the importance of cholera and subsequently plague to colonial health policy, see R. Ramasubban, *Public Health and Medical Research in India: Their Origins under the Impact of British Colonial Policy*, SAREC report R4 (Stockholm: SIDA, 1982); __, 'Imperial health in British India, 1857–1900,' in R. Macleod, M. Lewis, eds., *Disease, Medicine and Empire* (London: Routledge, 1988), 38–60; M. Harrison, *Public Health in British India: Anglo-Indian Preventive Medicine 1859–1914* (Cambridge: Cambridge University Press, 1994), 61; J.C. Hume, Colonialism and sanitary medicine: The development of preventive health policy in the Punjab, 1860 to 1900, *Modern Asian Studies*, 20, 4, 1986, 703–724; D. Arnold, *Colonizing the Body: State Medicine and Epidemic Disease in Nineteenth-Century India* (Berkeley: University of California Press, 1993); D. Arnold, 'Crisis and Contradiction in India's Public Health,' in D. Porter, ed., *The History of Public Health and the Modern State* (Amsterdam: Rodopi, 1994), 335–355.

56 For an overview of the economic and political agendas underlying the International Sanitary Conferences in the later 19th century and importance accorded cholera, see for example, Ramasubban, 'Imperial health in British India'; J. Siddiqui, *World Health and World Politics: The World Health Organization and the UN System* (London: Hurst, 1995), ch. 3; Neville Goodman, *International Health Organizations and Their Works* (London: J & A Churchill, 1952).

57 See ch. 7. For discussion of the 'low priority attached to malaria by the colonial administration,' see also M. Harrison, ' "Hot Beds of Disease": Malaria and Civilization in Nineteenth-Century British India,' *Parassitologia*, 40, 1998, 11–18.

58 Arnold, *Colonizing the Body*, 202. See also A. Brownlea, 'From public health to political epidemiology,' *Social Science Medicine*, 15D, 1981, 57–67.

59 Proc. of the Lieutenant-Governor of the Punjab, in the Home Department (Sanitary) [hereafter PLGP], 3662, Nov. 4, 1876, in *Report on the Sanitary Administration of the Punjab*, (Lahore: Medical Department), 1875.

60 G. Harrison, *Mosquitoes, Malaria and Man*; W.F. Bynum, 'An Experiment that Failed: Malaria Control at Mian Mir,' *Parassitologia*, 36, 1994, 107–120.

61 Harrison, *Public Health in British India*, 164–165; M. Worboys, 'Germs, Malaria and the Invention of Mansonian Tropical Medicine'; __, 'Colonial Medicine,' 67–80, in R. Cooter, J. Pickstone, eds., *Medicine in the Twentieth Century* (Amsterdam: Harwood Academic Publishers, 2000).

62 Following medical studies and medical service on a British steamer in the Amazon, Samuel Rickard Christophers (1873–1978) was appointed in 1898 to the joint Malaria Committee of the Royal Society and Colonial Office to investigate malaria in central and west Africa, and in India in 1901, in 1902 joining the IMS. He assumed directorship of the King Institute of Preventive Medicine in Madras (1904), the Central Malaria Bureau (1910), and Central Research Institute of Kasauli (1920–1932).

63 'India in those years was a magnet for malariologists and Christophers was the star figure in the constellation'; C. Garnham, 'Christophers, Sir (Samuel) Rickard.' *Oxford Dictionary of National Biography*, doi:30928. '[O]n all scientific matters Christophers was the final court of

appeal and advice to the Indian Government'; 'Sir Rickard Christophers,' *BMJ*, Dec. 1, 1973, 506. Christophers later referred to these early years as the 'golden age' of malaria research in India; in 'Sydney Price James, 1870–1946,' *Obituary Notices of Fellows of the Royal Society*, 5, 1947, 507–523, at 512.

64 S.R. Christophers, J.A. Sinton, 'A malaria map of India,' *IJMR*, 1926, 14, 1, 173–178.

65 J.A. Sinton, 'A Bibliography of Malaria in India,' *RMSI*, 1, 1, Oct. 1929, 1–199. W. Bynum provides a detailed overview of the content of this body of research in ' "Reasons for Contentment": Malaria in India,' *Parassitologia*, 42, 1998, 19–27.

66 *Report of the Malaria Commission on its Study Tour of India* (Geneva: LN, 1930), 14. Among the 11 references, for example, listed in a 1978 WHO bibliography on the social and economic aspects of malaria under the heading of 'Drought, Crop Failure, Famine,' eight are South Asian colonial studies: five, British India; three, Ceylon (Sri Lanka). Under the category of 'Food Prices,' all five references are colonial India studies; J. Sotiroff-Junker, *Behavioural, Social and Economic Aspects of Malaria and its Control* (Geneva: World Health Organization, 1978).

67 For important exceptions, see W. Bynum's recent overview of the work of the Malaria Survey of India; 'Malaria in Inter-War British India,' *Parassitologia*, 42, 2000, 25–31; __, ' "Reasons for Contentment." See also, Klein, 'Development and Death'; __, 'Malaria and Mortality in Bengal, 1840–1921,' *IESHR*, 9, 2, 1972, 132–160; __, 'Death in India,' *Journal of Asian Studies*, Aug. 1973, 639–659.

68 A. Maharatna, 'The Demography of the Bengal Famine of 1943–1944: A Detailed Study,' *IESHR*, 31, 1994, 169–215; __, *The Demography of Famines*; __, ' Famines and Epidemics: An Historical Perspective,' in T. Dyson, C. Ó Gráda, eds., *Famine Demography: Perspective from the Past and Present* (Oxford: Oxford University Press, 2002), 113–141; Dyson, 'The Historical Demography of Berar, 1881–1980'; __, 'On the Demography of South Asian famines,' *Population Studies*, 45, 1991, 5–25; 279–297.

69 Two recent exceptions are texts on 19th-century malarial 'Burdwan fever' in lower Bengal, though the predisposing role of destitution is relatively unexplored; A. Samanta, *Malaria Fever in Colonial Bengal, 1820–1939: Social History of an Epidemic*, (Kolkata: Firma KLM, 2002); Ihtesham Kazi, *Historical Study of Malaria in Bengal, 1860–1920* (Dhaka: Pip International Publishers, 2004).

70 E. Whitcombe, 'The Environmental Costs of Irrigation in British India: Waterlogging, Salinity, Malaria,' in D. Arnold, R. Guha, eds., *Nature, Culture, Imperialism: Essays on the Environmental History of South Asia* (New Delhi: Oxford University Press, 1995), 237–259; K. Wakimura, 'Epidemic Malaria and "Colonial Development": Reconsidering the Cases of Northern and Western India,' Economic History Congress XIII, Buenos Aires, Argentina, July 2002, mimeo.

71 W. Bynum, ' "Reasons for Contentment." See also Bynum, 'Malaria in Inter-War British India,' 25–31.

72 Klein, 'Malaria and mortality in Bengal'; __, 'Death in India'; Wakimura, 'Epidemic Malaria and "Colonial Development." ' It was Ira Klein's 1973

'Death in India' article that first alerted me to the existence of the rigorous epidemiological studies of malaria by a handful of colonial researchers.

73 Arnold, 'Crisis and Contradiction in India's Public Health,' 352; Bynum, 'Malaria in inter-war British India,' 31; Harrison, '"Hot Beds of Disease",' 11–18, at 17; S. Polu, *Infectious Disease in India, 1892–1940: Policy-Making and the Perceptions of Risk* (London: Palgrave Macmillan, 2012); V.R. Muraleedharan, D. Veeraraghavan, 'Anti-Malaria Policy in the Madras Presidency: An Overview of the Early Decades of the Twentieth Century,' *Medical History*, 36, 1992, 290–305.

74 See chs. 4, 11.

75 It has been suggested that Amritsar district with its higher irrigated area was especially affected by the 1908 epidemic; Whitcombe, 'The Environmental Costs of Irrigation in British India,' 254. However, many other districts without substantial canal irrigation were also severely affected in 1908, and the western canal colonies were relatively spared. See chs. 2, 4, and 6.

76 See also Muraleedharan, Veeraraghavan, 'Anti-malaria policy in the Madras Presidency.'

77 See, for example, Agnihotri, 'Ecology, land use and colonisation'; I. Stone, *Canal Irrigation in British India: Perspectives on Technological Changes in a Peasant Economy* (Cambridge: Cambridge University Press, 1984); E. Whitcombe, *Agrarian Conditions in Northern India, I, The United Provinces Under British Rule, 1860–1900.* (Berkeley: University of California Press, 1972); __, 'The Environmental Costs of Irrigation in British India,' 237–259; Klein, 'Development and Death'; Wakimura, 'Epidemic Malaria and "Colonial Development"'.

78 Sunil Amrith highlights common village understanding of the primacy of economic conditions underlying Bengal malaria morbidity, expressed in the 1954 satirical novel *Maila Anchal* by Phanishwar Nath Renu, trans. as *The Soiled Border* (New Delhi: Chanakya Publications, 1991), in 'Political Culture of Health in India: A Historical Perspective,' *EPW*, Jan. 13, 2007, 114–121.

79 S. Litsios, 'Malaria Control, the Cold War, and the Postwar Reoganization of International Assistance,' *Medical Anthropology*, 17, 1997, 255–278; J. Farley, *Brock Chisholm, the World Health Organization, and the Cold War* (Vancouver: University of British Columbia Press, 2008); R.M. Packard, 'Malaria Dreams: Postwar Visions of Health and Development in the Third World,' *Medical Anthropology*, 17, 1997, 279–296; __, '"No Other Logical Choice": Global Malaria Eradication and the Politics of International Health in the Post-War Era,' *Parassitologia*, 40, 1998, 217–229; J.A. Gillespie, 'Social Medicine, Social Security and International Health, 1940–1960,' in E. Rodríguez-Ocaña, ed., *The Politics of the Healthy Life: An International Perspective* (Sheffield: European Association for the History of Medicine and Health, 2002), 219–239; S. Amrith. *Decolonizing International Health: India and Southeast Asia, 1930–1965* (Basingstoke: Palgrave Macmillan, 2006); Siddiqui, *World Health and World Politics*; H. Evans, 'European Malaria Policy in the 1920s and 1930s: The Epidemiology of Minutiae,' *Isis*, 80, 1989, 40–59.

80 J.D. Post, 'Nutritional Status and Mortality in Eighteenth-Century Europe,' in L.F. Newman, ed., *Hunger in History: Food Shortage, Poverty, and Deprivation* (Cambridge, MA: Basil Blackwell, 1990), 241–280 at 267; __, 'Climatic Variability and the European Mortality Wave of the Early 1740s,' *Journal of Interdisciplinary History*, 15, 1, 1984, 1–30. See also J. Walter, R. Schofield, eds., *Famine, Disease and the Social Order in Early Modern England* (Cambridge: Cambridge University Press, 1989), 17–21; M. Livi-Bacci, *Population and Nutrition: An Essay on European Demographic History* (Cambridge: Cambridge University Press, 1991); A. Hardy, *The Epidemic Streets: Infectious Disease and the Rise of Preventive Medicine, 1856–1900* (Oxford: Clarendon Press, 1993), 281. For a synthesis of broader famine experience, see Dyson and O'Grada, 'Introduction,' in *Famine Demography: Perspectives from the Past and Present* (Oxford: Oxford University Press, 2002), 1–18.

81 R.I. Rotberg, 'Nutrition and History,' *Journal of Interdisciplinary History*, 14, 3, 1983, 199–204 [hereafter *JIH*]. The classification of malaria was unaccompanied by empirical argument, except in passing reference to the recent medical thesis of 'refeeding malaria'; A.G. Carmichael, 'Infection, Hidden Hunger, and History,' *JIH*, 14, 3, 1983, 249–264, at 251. For analysis of the refeeding thesis, and broader conceptual difficulties underlying it, see S. Zurbrigg, 'Did Starvation Protect from Malaria? Distinguishing Between Severity and Lethality of Infectious Disease in Colonial India,' *Social Science History*, 21, 1, 1997, 27–58.

82 The 1983 categorisation coincided with a growing tendency in epidemic historiographical thought to view pre-modern health history as shaped largely by inherently virulent infectious diseases, in contrast to the early modern historical period that was largely spared such visitations; Carmichael, 'Infection, Hidden Hunger, and History,' 252; S.J. Kunitz, 'Mortality Since Malthus,' in R. Scofield, D. Coleman, eds., *The State of Population Theory: Forward from Malthus* (Oxford: Basil Blackwell, 1986), 279–302. One region where historical malaria transmission may well have held a marked determining demographic effect largely due to specific vector characteristics is holoendemic regions of sub-Saharan Africa where, Coluzzi suggests, the primary vector *(Anopheles gambiae)* combines anthropophilic characteristics – near-exclusive feeding on humans compared with livestock, leading to almost daily *falciparum* inoculation rates – with habitat preference specific to agricultural ecology, factors which together hindered emergence of intensive agricultural production; M. Coluzzi, 'Malaria and the Afrotropical Ecosystems: Impact of Man-Made Environmental Changes,' *Parassitologia*, 46, 1–2, 1994, 223–227; __, 'The Clay Feet of the Malaria Giant and its African Roots: Hypotheses and Inferences About Origin, Spread and Control of *Plasmodium falciparum*,' *Parassitologia*, 41, 1999, 277–283. For a detailed historical overview of the specific ecological conditions giving rise to holoendemic conditions in tropical Africa, see J.L.A. Webb, *Humanity's Burden: A Global History of Malaria* (New York: Cambridge University Press, 2009), 27–41.

83 P.G. Lunn, 'Nutrition, Immunity and Infection,' in R. Schofield, D. Reher, A. Bideau, eds., *Decline of Mortality in Europe* (Oxford: Clarendon Press,

1991), 131–145, 137; Livi-Bacci, *Population and Nutrition*; T. Bengtsson, C. Campbell, J.Z. Lee et al., *Life Under Pressure: Mortality and Living Standards in Europe and Asia, 1700–1900* (Cambridge MA: MIT Press, 2004), 42–44.

84 See, for example, E. Whitcombe, 'Famine Mortality,' *EPW*, 28, 1993, 169–179; D. Arnold, 'Social Crisis and Epidemic Disease in the Famines of the Nineteenth Century India,' *Social History of Medicine*, 6, 3, 1993, 385–404; B. Mohanty, 'Case Study of the Indian Famines of 1896–1897 and 1899–1900,' in S.N. Singh, M.K. Premi, P.S. Bhatia, A. Bose, eds., *Population Transition in India*, Vol. 2 (New Delhi: B. R. Publishing, 1989), 371–379, at 375.

85 Whitcombe, 'Famine Mortality.'

86 Klein, 'Development and Death,' 179.

87 G. Macdonald, 'The Analysis of Equilibrium in Malaria,' in Bruce-Chwatt and Glanville, eds., *Dynamics of Tropical Diseases*, 132.

88 R. Fogel, *Explaining Long-Term Trends in Health and Longevity* (New York: Cambridge University Press, 2012); R. Floud, R. Fogel, B. Harris, Sok Chul Hong, eds., *The Changing Body: Health, Nutrition, and Human Development in the Western World since 1700* (Cambridge: Cambridge University Press, 2011).

89 A.V. Guntupalli, J. Baten, 'The Development and Inequality of Heights in North, West, and East India 1915–1944,' *Explorations in Economic History*, 43, 2006, 578–608; L. Brennan, J. McDonald, R. Shlomowitz, 'The Heights and Economic Well-Being of North Indians under British Rule,' *Social Science History*, 18, 2, 1994, 271–307.

90 Both Guha and Guilmoto attribute 'crisis rarefaction' to the declining prevalence of acute starvation and point out the 'uncoupling' of price and epidemic mortality after 1920. Guilmoto questions whether the decline in subsistence crises was due simply to fortuitous weather, and points in addition to beginning rise in real wages, economic diversification and more effective drought relief; Guha, 'Mortality decline in early twentieth century India'; Guilmoto, 'Towards a New Demographic Equilibrium,' 284. See also S. Guha, *Health and Population in South Asia: From Earliest Times to the Present* (London: Hurst, 2001), ch. 2.

91 S. Millman, R.W. Kates, 'Toward Understanding Hunger,' in L. Newman, ed., *Hunger in History* (Cambridge, MA: Basil Blackwell, 1990), 3–24, at 22.

92 MP, 70.

93 On this, see ch. 2.

94 Average basal metabolic rate for an adult male, for example, is 1,500 kcal a day, but can range widely from 1,000 to over 2,000.

95 Weight-for-age ('underweight') may encompass both acute and chronic hunger but fails to indicate the relative contribution of each.

96 See, for example, R. Floud, 'The Heights of Europeans Since 1750: A New Source for European Economic History,' in J. Komlos, ed., *Stature, Living Standards, and Economic Development: Essays in Anthropometric History* (Chicago: University of Chicago Press, 1994), 12.

97 Case fatality rate is a measure of the lethality of a disease, the proportion of cases of a specified disease which are fatal over the course of the disease.

98 For an overview of archaeological markers of hunger among pre-historical populations, see M.N. Cohen, 'Prehistoric Patterns of Hunger,' in L.F. Newman, ed., *Hunger in History: : Food Shortage, Poverty, and Deprivation* (Cambridge, MA: Blackwell, 1990), 56–97.

99 See ch. 3 at note 49.
100 Floud et al., *The Changing Body*, 11.
101 See ch. 6, at note 22; also, N.S. Scrimshaw, 'The Phenomenon of Fam-ine,' *American Review of Nutrition*, 7, 1987, 1–21; N.S. Scrimshaw, C.E. Taylor, J.E. Gordon, *Interactions of Nutrition and Infection* (Geneva: World Health Organization, 1968).
102 W.R. Aykroyd, *The Conquest of Famine* (London: Chatto & Windus, 1974), 72 opp., Figure 3a.
103 B.M. Bhatia, *Famines in India* (Bombay: Asia Publishers House), 1963; H.S. Srivastava, *The History of Indian Famines, 1858–1918* (Agra: Sri Ram Mehra, 1968). Economists of modern India have given renewed emphasis to the role of public intervention in the control of famine in India; J. Drèze, 'Famine Prevention in India,' in J. Drèze, A. Sen, eds., *The Political Economy of Hunger*, Vol. 2 (Oxford: Clarendon Press, 1990), 13–122.
104 Drèze, 'Famine Prevention in India,' 35.
105 A. Maharatna, 'The Regional Variation in the Demographic Conse-quences of Famines in the Late Nineteenth Century,' *EPW*, 29, 23, 1994, 1399–1410; __, *The Demography of Famines*.
106 In English legal history, the term 'destitution' has been defined as 'those families who could not buy enough wheat over the year at the average price prevailing in that year, even if the entire family income was spent on wheat alone,' a state which barring outside charity suggests caloric consumption slipping from undernourishment to acute hunger, more col-loquially expressed as one where 'poverty became a desperate affliction rather than a customary privation'; D. Hay, 'War, Dearth and Theft in the Eighteenth Century: The Record of the English Courts,' *Past and Present*, 95, 117–160, at 131–132.
107 S.R. Christophers, C.A. Bentley, *Malaria in the Duars. Being the Second Report to the Advisory Committee Appointed by the Government of India to Conduct an Enquiry Regarding Blackwater and Other Fevers Prevalent in the Duars* (Simla: Government Monotype Press, 1909); 'The Human Factor,' *Trans. Bombay Medical Congress*.
108 N. Bhattacharya, 'Agricultural Labour and Production: Central and South-East Punjab, 1870–1940,' in K.N. Raj et al., eds., *Essays on the Commercialization of Indian Agriculture* (New Delhi: Oxford University Press, 1985), 105–152 at 146; T. Kessinger, *Vilyatpur 1848–1969, Social and Economic Change in a North Indian Village* (Berkeley: University of California Press, 1974); D. Kumar, *Land and Caste in South India: Agricultural Labour in the Madras Presidency during the 19th Century* (Cambridge: Cambridge University Press, 1965).
109 See, for example, the confidential 1888 Dufferin Enquiry, 'Conditions of the Lower Classes of People of India,' *Resolution of the Government of India*, 96-F/6–59 dated Oct. 19, 1888.
110 L. Brennan, J. McDonald, R. Shlomowitz, 'Long-Term Change in Indian Health,' *South Asia: Journal of South Asian Studies*, 26, 1, 2003, 51–69; Guntupalli and Baten, 'Inequality of Heights,' 592.
111 The seeming paradox has tended to redirect interpretation of South Asian mortality decline away from 'nutritional' explanations to instead immunological hypotheses; I. Klein, 'Population Growth and Mor-tality in British India Part I: The Climacteric of Death,' *IESHR*, 26, 4, 1989, 387–403, at 392; __, 'Population Growth and Mortality in

British India Part II: The Demographic Revolution,' *IESHR*, 27, 1, 1990, 33–63, at 60.

112 '[W]hile stunting measures the cumulative history of stress, wasting signals a deteriorating condition at the time of measurement. It is not surprising, therefore, that wasting appears to be more predictive of . . . mortality than stunting'; R. Martorell, 'Child Growth Retardation: A Discussion of its Causes and Its Relationship to Health,' in J.C. Waterlow, K.L. Blaxter, eds., *Nutritional Adaptation in Man* (London: John Libbey, 1985), 13–30, at 25.

113 See ch. 11, at note 135.

114 T. McKeown, *The Modern rise of Population* (London: Edward Arnold, 1976).

115 J. Farley, *To Cast Out Disease: A History of the International Health Division of the Rockefeller Foundation (1913–1951)* (New York: Oxford University Press, 2004); P. Weindling, 'Philanthropy and World Health: The Rockefeller Foundation and the League of Nations Health Organisation,' *Minerva*, 35, 3, 1997, 269–281.

116 N. Gangulee, *Health and Nutrition in India* (London: Faber and Faber, 1939); M. Worboys, 'The Discovery of Colonial Malnutrition Between the Wars,' in D. Arnold, ed., *Imperial Medicine and Indigenous Societies* (Manchester: Manchester University Press, 1988), 208–225; C. Petty, 'Food, Poverty and Growth: The Application of Nutrition Science, 1918–1939,' *Bulletin of the Society for the Social History of Medicine*, 40, 1987, 37–40 [hereafter *SHM*]; __, 'The Impact of the Newer Knowledge of Nutrition: Nutrition Science and Nutrition Policy, 1900–1939.' PhD thesis, London School of Hygiene and Tropical Medicine, 1987.

117 'Malthus,' Hamlin observes, 'saw no need to appeal to learned medicine to support these claims, for nothing he said about disease was controversial. It seemed obvious, even truistic, that disease was deadlier to the weak than to the strong'; *Public Health and Social Justice,* 26.

118 Hamlin, *Public Health and Social Justice,* 6.

119 S.J. Fayrer, *On the Climate and Fevers of India*, Croonian Lecture, Mar. 1882 (London: J&A Churchill, 1882); M. Harrison, *Climates and Constitutions: Health, Race Environment and British Imperialism in India* (New Delhi: Oxford University Press, 2002), 173–176.

120 Simla Conf., 2. The term 'zymotic' was first used by William Farr in the 19th century to classify diseases believed caused by miasma induced by atmospheric conditions conducive to fermentation and decay of environmental organic matter ('filth'). This broad spatial framework contrasted with diseases such as smallpox where transmission of particulate disease agents was traceable through patterns of direct contagion.

121 Here, again, it is important to distinguish the larger historical trajectory of disease lethality decline from the undisputed value of specific techniques in saving individual lives from infections that carry a substantial inherent case fatality rate. As Roy Macleod has stressed, 'It is clearly possible to examine the culture of western medicine without questioning the benefits of modern science'; Macleod and Lewis, *Disease, Medicine and Empire*, 12.

122 'Public Health and Social Justice,' 146.

Part I

Epidemic malaria in Punjab

The rain-'scarcity' model

2   Malaria in the Punjab
An overview

> To ascertain with any delicacy the distribution of these epidemics it is necessary . . . to resort to *thana* figures or even . . . to the returns of individual villages.
>
> – S.R. Christophers, Procs. Imperial Malaria
> Conference held at Simla in 1909, 21.

When in February 1909 Christophers began his investigation into the Punjab malaria epidemic of 1908, he was already acquainted with many aspects of the region's malaria epidemiology. In early investigations for the Malaria Committee of the Royal Society, Christophers, working with J.W.W. Stephens, had identified the chief anopheline vector in the region to be *An. culicifacies*.[1] Subsequent anti-mosquito efforts in 1902–1903 at the rural Mian Mir military cantonment in central Lahore district (Figure 2.1) had demonstrated the powerful influence of the semi-arid continental climate in circumscribing malaria transmission to the immediate post-monsoon period.[2] But the earlier work had not prepared him for the enormous lethality potential of malaria seen in 1908, an epidemic that swept through the Mian Mir cantonment along with much of the rest of the eastern and central regions of the province. That contrast, between the 'normal' (endemic) autumnal rise in malaria infection and mortality observed earlier, and the epidemic of death recorded in 1908, no doubt helped inform the scope of the inquiry. In the interval, observations from another assignment, a study of 'intense' malaria in the Duars tea plantations of northern Bengal undertaken the previous year,[3] had also brought heightened awareness of broader socio-economic factors shaping the epidemiology and endemiology of malarial disease in the subcontinent.[4] Christophers arrived in Punjab, in other words, primed by both the entomological and the economic complexities of 'the malaria problem' facing the British Raj.

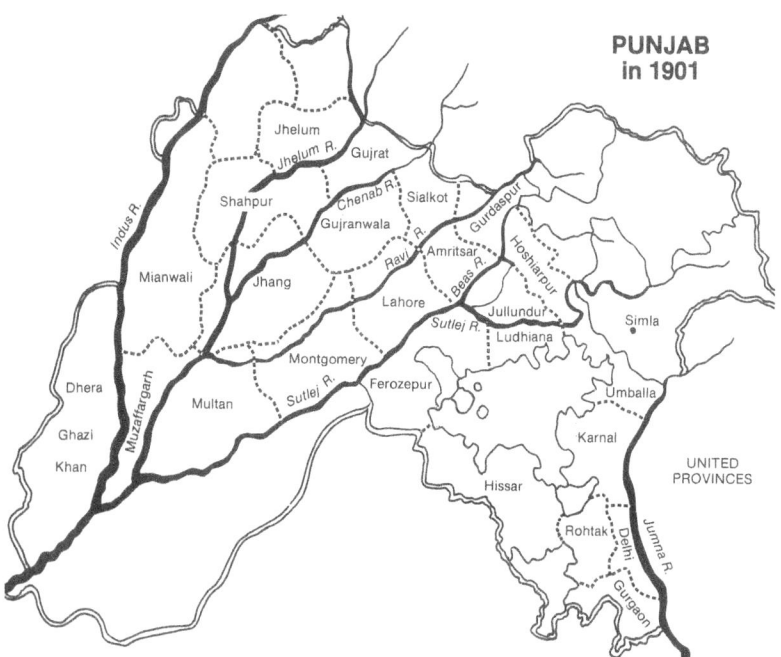

Figure 2.1 Punjab Province in 1901
Source: Author.

Eight months later, Christophers presented his preliminary Punjab findings at the Imperial malaria conference at Simla in October 1909, his analysis of the 1908 epidemic framing the proceedings.[5] An expanded version of his analysis, *Malaria in the Punjab*,[6] was published two years later. In addition to detailed mapping of the 1908 epidemic mortality patterns across the province, the 1911 report addressed two additional questions explored by him in the interval: analysis of the physical properties of the Punjab alluvial soils that underlay the region's propensity to flooding and the results of his laboratory research into the determinants of dose of malarial infection. The conclusions contained in this final report regarding epidemic causation, however, remained unchanged, if expressed in more nuanced fashion: above normal ('excess') monsoon rains and scarcity were the two key factors that underlay the 'disastrous' malaria epidemics of Punjab.

Detailed epidemiological malaria research into the biological and ecological mechanisms of malaria transmission in Punjab would continue to be conducted by members of the Indian Medical Service over subsequent decades, much of it undertaken at the Karnal Field Research Station in the southeast corner of the province. Yet the basic conclusions arrived at in *Malaria in the Punjab* with respect to the epidemic form of the disease would not be superseded in subsequent decades and continued to shape British Indian malaria policy for the remainder of the colonial period. If there had been any doubt remaining in advance of the Punjab inquiry, the 1911 report confirmed to the British Raj Christophers's stature as a consummate scientist and polymath with exceptional powers of observation and capacity for analytic synthesis.

The complexity of the factors – ecological, topographical, economic, entomological, and parasitological – encompassed in *Malaria in the Punjab* makes it a challenging document to comprehend fully on first reading. Adding to the task is Christophers's writing style, which combines exacting, voluminous descriptive detail with an exceedingly economical interpretative language. In pursuit of conceptual precision, Christophers at times resorts to neologisms to convey causal relationships, making paraphrasing that much more difficult. Moreover, as a loyal servant to the crown, observations in the economic realm are generally expressed obliquely, at times almost in code, making the fuller implications of his observations easy to overlook. What grounds the study amidst these complexities is Christophers's meticulous reconstruction, descriptive and quantitative, of the 1908 epidemic, and it is here that this study begins – prefaced with a brief sketch of the bionomics of malarial infection and its transmission by the principal anopheline vector of malaria in the northwest plains of Punjab.

Malaria transmission in Punjab

Malaria is caused by a single-cell protozoan parasite *(Plasmodium)*. Its transmission involves a complex life cycle with two separate stages of development. The first, asexual phase takes place in humans who form the 'reservoir' of infection; and the second, reproductive phase (sporogony), termed the 'extrinsic' cycle, occurs in particular species of *Anopheles* mosquitoes.

The asexual phase begins with transmission of malaria to the human host through the bite of an infected female mosquito, its blood meal required for egg production. Parasites ('sporozoites'), inoculated along with the insect's saliva that acts as an anticoagulant, are rapidly sequestered in the liver of the human host. After one to two weeks, large numbers of 'merozoites' are released into the bloodstream and infect red blood cells. Characteristic symptoms of episodic fever and chills begin to appear as successive batches of the parasite breakdown red blood cells, are released into the circulation, and infect further blood cells. Subsequently, some merozoites differentiate into male and female gametocytes, at which point the human host becomes infective to further feeding mosquitoes, initiating the second phase of the malarial parasite's life cycle. With fertilisation of the male and female gametes inside the insect gut, sporozoites develop in the stomach wall, multiply, and migrate to the mosquito's salivary glands where the cycle begins again.

Successful completion of the *Plasmodium* life cycle thus requires two blood meals by the vector mosquito a minimum of 10 days apart, an interval allowing sufficient time for development of the parasite inside the insect. Thus, transmission hinges upon anopheline lifespan, determined by both temperature and atmospheric humidity. Under ideal conditions (28°C and 60–80 per cent humidity), a single reproductive cycle for the *P. falciparum* parasite requires 30 to 35 days.

Subtropical in latitude but nestled within the Asian continental landmass, the Punjab plains are subject to enormous extremes in temperature and atmospheric humidity. With the exception of the Himalayan hill tracts, annual rainfall is low, in the western half of the province amounting to virtual desert conditions (Figure 2.2). For most of the year, low humidity reduces anopheline lifespan much below that required for development of the parasite. When the summer monsoon rains do fall, however, the region's flat topography and alluvial soils present entomological conditions favourable for malaria transmission. Initial rains quickly saturate the fine clay soil, causing subsequent rainfall to collect in countless pools suitable for larval development. Simultaneously, atmospheric humidity levels rise, extending mosquito longevity. In years of well-distributed rains, malaria infection rates in the population could soar exponentially from extremely low pre-monsoon levels to near-universal prevalence in the space of three reproductive cycles. With cessation of the rains in mid or late September, malaria transmission falls off abruptly, declining atmospheric humidity reducing mosquito longevity, and rapidly falling temperatures prolonging the maturation time of the malaria parasite inside them, such that by early or mid-October further transmission ceases. Thus, the entomological 'window' of sufficient humidity and conducive temperature was small. Adding further to the tenuousness of the vector-human transmission cycle was the fact that *An. culicifacies,*

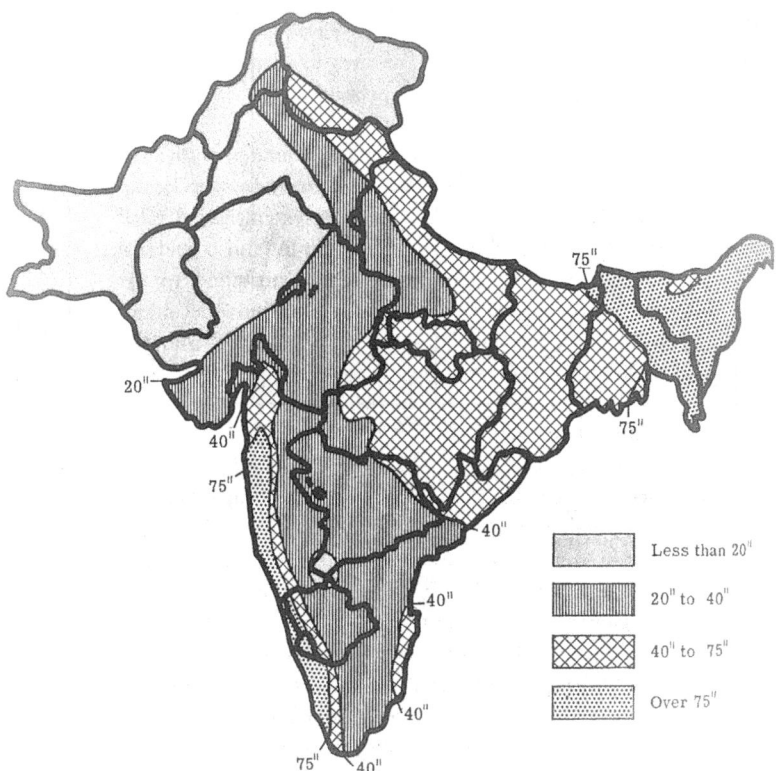

Figure 2.2 Mean annual rainfall, British India

Source: G. Blyn, *Agricultural Trends in India, 1891–1947* (Philadelphia: University of Pennsylvania Press, 1966), p. 136, Figure 6.2. Reprinted with permission of the University of Pennsylvania Press.

the primary vector of malaria in the region, was a zoophilic species, preferentially feeding on livestock rather than humans.[7] Still, even in years of average monsoon rainfall, malaria transmission rates in much of the province were quite high, vast numbers of mosquitoes making up for otherwise improbable conditions for maintaining the chain of transmission intact.

The two main malaria species transmitted in Punjab were *P. vivax* ('benign tertian') and *P. falciparum* ('malignant' or 'sub-tertian' malaria), the latter associated with greater morbidity and mortality related to proportionately greater parasitization of red blood cells. In the Punjab plains, the autumn rise in malarial fever typically appeared

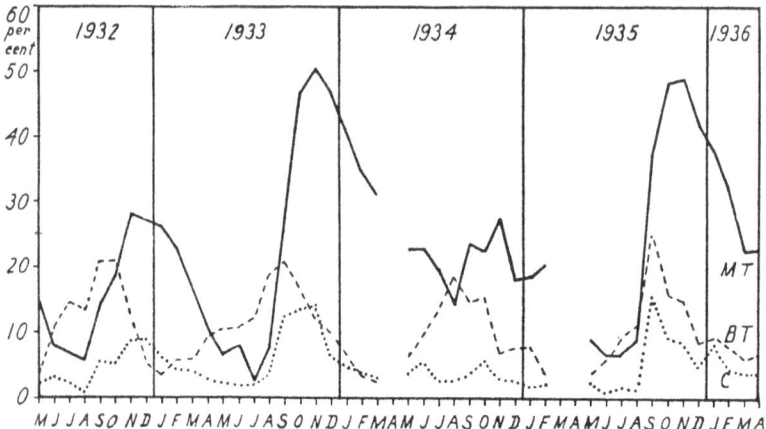

Figure 2.3 Monthly parasite rates for malignant tertian asexual forms (MT), crescents (C) and benign tertian, both forms (BT), in six villages, Karnal district, Punjab, 1932–1936

Source: E.P. Hicks, S. Abdul Majid, 'A Study of the Epidemiology of Malaria in a Punjab District,' *RMSI*, 7, 1, 1937, 1–43, Chart 2, p. 4.

in late August, initially consisting of vivax infection. In non-drought years, falciparum cases followed within two to four weeks, largely replacing vivax transmission by early October – its later timing related to the longer period (10 to 14 days) required for the appearance of gametocytes in the human host (Figure 2.3).[8]

Portrait of the 1908 epidemic

The 1908 malaria epidemic involved much of the eastern and north-central tracts of the province, involving an area of some 50,000 square miles.[9] Urban and rural populations were equally affected; in many areas, malarial fever often reaching near-universal levels. Between October and December, over 300,000 'excess' fever deaths were recorded in the province, in a population of 20 million. In Amritsar, a town of 160,000, over 6 per cent of the population succumbed. In many rural *thanas*, the October death rate reached 11 times the normal (June–July) death rate; in individual villages, up to 70 times.[10] Another 'remarkable feature' was its rapid onset, with Christophers describing the 1908 epidemic as 'a malaria cyclone . . . [with] places even hundreds of miles apart . . . affected simultaneously.'[11] For provincial officials, the mass debility and economic disruption was first brought to prominent attention 'by a sudden disorganisation of the train service due to "fever" among the employees at the large railway centre, Lahore. . . . With equal suddenness it made its presence felt through the whole Punjab.' At Amritsar, 'almost the entire population . . . [was] prostrated.'[12]

Conducting the study in early 1909, Christophers was working under a considerable handicap. Much of the detailed research into the role of humidity and temperature in malaria transmission would await confirmation through long-term field studies in the 1920s and 1930s.[13] From his work at Mian Mir, however, Christophers was aware of the value of the annual sanitary records in allowing identification of malaria mortality within the monthly death returns. The epidemic rise in fever mortality in the autumn months 'is extremely characteristic of death returns from the Punjab,' he observed.

> It is seen in the death curve of almost every town and thana except in . . . desert regions. . . . If we examine the mortality records of the Punjab we shall be struck by an almost exact repetition in most years of this curve, . . . the number of deaths lowest in June and July, rising in September, highest in October and November and falling again through the early months of the year.[14]

Each of the other major epidemic diseases, cholera, smallpox, and recently plague, generally displayed its own 'very distinctive' epidemic curve at other times in the year (Figure 2.4).[15] 'Even if one has no information regarding the disease concerned in the epidemic, it is possible nearly always to make a correct diagnosis from this seasonal occurrence and other features of the curve, just as one may diagnose some diseases by means of a temperature chart.'[16] On this basis, he offered, one can in fact study a death curve with its periodical epidemic rises as dispassionately as we could the record of a seismography or other recording instrument.'[17]

Initial plotting of 1908 monthly death rates revealed that the timing of epidemic mortality followed closely that of the ordinary autumnal pattern of malarial deaths in non-epidemic years (Figure 2.5), simply greatly exaggerated in height and duration. Such extended mortality through November and December was considered the result of lingering illness from earlier infection, active transmission having ceased months before. Provincial dispensary records in 1908 also showed a typical autumnal increase in admissions for fever and splenic enlargement, but again greatly amplified, illness which through the autumn

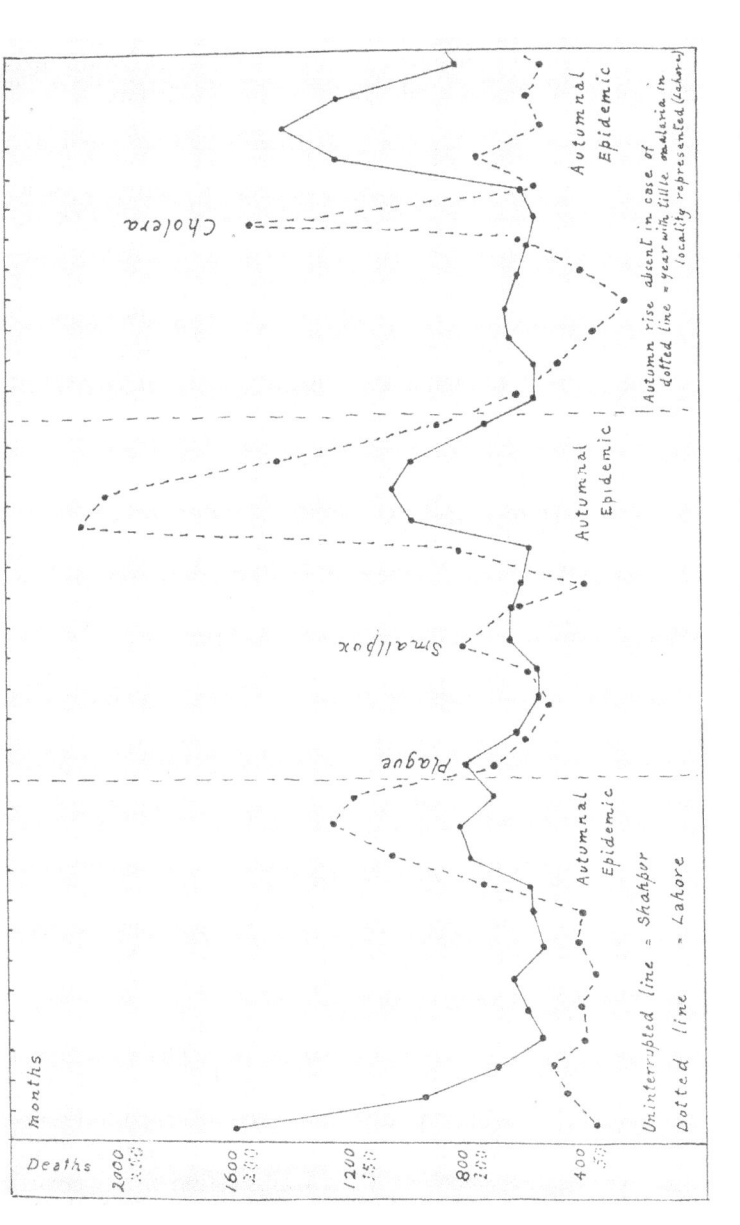

Figure 2.4 Seasonal distribution of epidemic mortality, Shahpur and Lahore districts, Punjab, early 20th century

Source: S.R. Christophers, 'Malaria in the Punjab,' *Sci. Mem. Off. Med. San. Dep.*, 46, 1911, Chart 1.

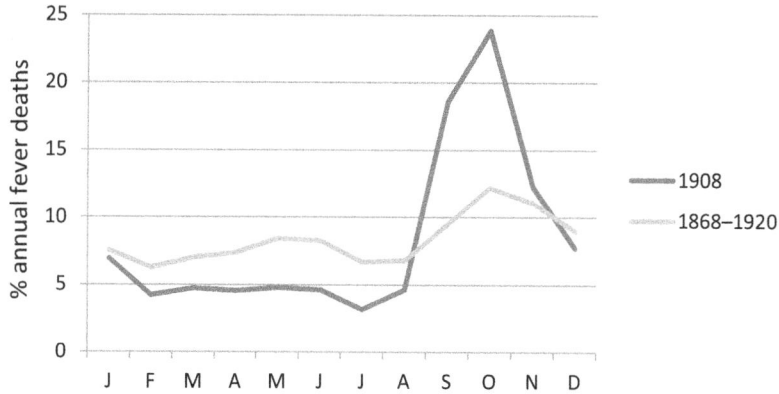

Figure 2.5 Per cent distribution monthly fever deaths, Hissar district, Punjab, 1908, mean 1868–1920

Source: *Report on the Sanitary Administration of the Punjab*, 1868–1920.

was everywhere 'popularly . . . attributed without hesitation to malaria.'[18]

Because of the severity of the fever cases observed in 1908, many colonial officers initially had doubted its malarial nature.[19] No blood smears were available from the urban hospitals or dispensaries to confirm microscopically the malarial diagnosis. However, the illness was popularly recognised as malarial and widely referred to colloquially as spleen fever (*'tilli tap'*). When Christophers began his investigation the following February, severely affected villages still showed 'almost universal' malaria parasite rates and splenic enlargement.[20] The only other significant infectious disease associated with splenomegaly in the subcontinent was Kala Azar, a disease virtually unknown in Punjab. Christophers, nevertheless, undertook a series of spleen smears (cadaver biopsies) to rule out the possibility.[21]

While the vital registration records allowed a general tracing of the epidemic across the province, closer analysis of its progression required more temporally detailed data. For this, Christophers turned to the weekly urban dispensary and burial records. Both indicated that fever incidence appeared with 'extreme suddenness,' an 'almost simultaneous onset of the epidemic throughout the Punjab.'[22] For the town of Bhera, fever admissions initially began to increase at the end of August and rose rapidly to peak in the final week of September, with a second peak one month later (Figure 2.6, 'Chart 2').

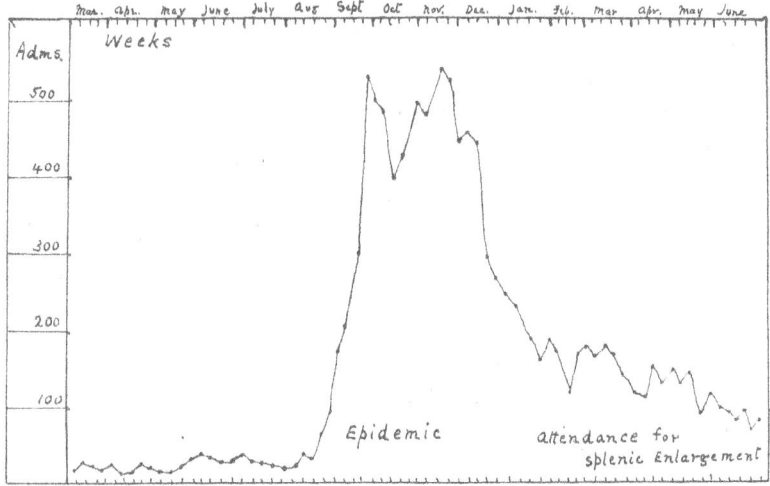

Figure 2.6 Weekly fever admissions for malaria, Bhera Dispensary, March 1908–June 1909

Source: Christophers, 'Malaria in the Punjab,' Chart 2.

In addition to the rapid increase of infection, malaria cases in 1908 were distinguished by the clinical severity of the disease. In non-epidemic times, malaria fever was more typically 'intermittent,' the term applied to the clinical profile of malaria or 'ague' as observed among troops or in Europe in previous centuries: soaring fever that classically 'broke' after a number of hours, with body temperature returning to normal between recurring paroxysms. In 1908 Punjab, fever by contrast was generally 'remittent,' failing to return to normal between paroxysms, suggesting reduced physiological capacity to control the infection. In severe cases, fever was continuous, a pattern more typical of typhus. Dysentery or diarrhoea often accompanied or followed the febrile attacks, the Punjab Sanitary Commissioner noted, and 'contributed largely to their fatality.'[23]

This virulent character was apparent from the earliest stages of the epidemic. Plotting weekly 1908 mortality data for the towns of Amritsar, Bhera, and Palwal (Figure 2.7), Christophers showed that the death rate rose 'almost sheer' in the final weeks of September and early October in 1908, a rise which followed the

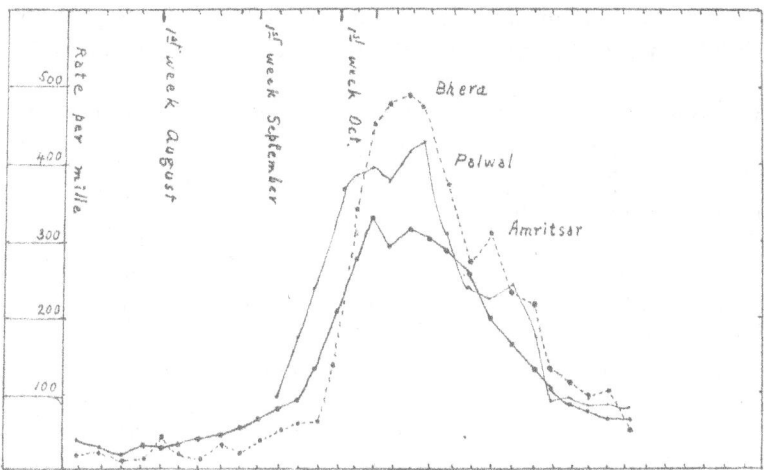

Figure 2.7 Weekly mortality Bhera, Palwal, Amritsar towns, July 1908–January 1909

Source: Christophers, 'Malaria in the Punjab,' Chart 3.

increase in sickness by a period of two to three weeks.[24] A 'peculiar' feature of the 1908 epidemic, he stressed,

> was that the increase in admissions to dispensaries for fever only very slightly preceded the increase in general mortality showing that deaths were not the result of protracted sickness but apparently of the intensity of the infection. . . . At Miani sickness and mortality appeared almost coincidentally.[25]

C.A. Gill, at the time an officer with the Inspector-General of Civil Hospitals, Punjab, described the 'most strikingly obvious feature' of the epidemic as 'the change in the clinical picture associated with [its] onset.'

> In place of mild attacks of intermittent fever, a remittent fever often attended by bilious vomiting and purging is a common occurrence, whilst graver forms of malaria, in which hyperpyrexia [extreme fever], coma, and convulsions are conspicuous, are by no means rare. During the early stage of an epidemic the course of the

disease is extremely rapid, and deaths (especially of infants) often takes place within twenty-four hours of the onset of illness. Many children also succumb to the effects of diarrhea and dysentery.[26]

This profile of 'enhanced toxicity'[27] appears to have marked the entire course of the epidemic. Weekly fever death rates remained extremely high until late November and on into December, though rates of new infection fell quickly following their peak in October.

For determining the age profile of deaths in the epidemic, Christophers turned again to the urban Amritsar burial records. Of a total of 10,202 deaths registered in the autumn of 1908, he estimated 'more than 7,000 must have been directly due to the epidemic.' Forty-seven per cent were recorded among children under the age of 5 years (Table 2.1), with children under 3 years accounting for three-quarters of these deaths.[28] A further 18 per cent of deaths occurred among the elderly, above the age of 60 years.[29] This age profile of mortality mirrored that of non-epidemic years. 'In so severe an epidemic mortality it is surprising to find so few distinctive features,' Christophers would remark, 'the ratios suggesting only a great exaggeration of normal stress.'[30] He noted two exceptional aspects, however: 'an extraordinary increase' in stillbirths, 568 reported in Amritsar; and

Table 2.1 1908 Amritsar city burials 'during the epidemic,'* by age group

		% of total deaths
Stillbirths	568	
0–12 months	1,389	14.4
13–24 months	1,253	13.0
25–36 months	958	9.9
37–48 months	576	6.0
49–60 months	352	3.7
0–4 years		47.0
5–9 years	795	8.3
10–15 years	310	3.2
15–20 years	225	2.3
20–30 years	518	5.4
30–40 years	403	4.2
40–50 years	502	5.2
50–60 years	605	6.3
>60 years	1,748	18.1
Total deaths	9,634	

* Deaths reported as occurring 'during the epidemic,' appear to be Oct.–Dec. 1908.
Source: S.R. Christophers, 'Malaria in the Punjab,' p. 12.

second, a proportionately greater increase in deaths in children aged 1–2 years.[31] Although the largest increase in excess deaths in absolute numbers occurred in children under 12 months of age – the infant mortality rate increasing from 206 deaths per 1,000 to 412 per 1,000 live born in 1908 – the actual number of deaths (1,253) registered between 1 and 2 years of age was almost equal to that recorded for infants (1,389).

The relatively heightened vulnerability to malaria among children 12 to 24 months of age likely reflects the greater risk of undernourishment in this age group relative to infancy, a pattern generally found in impoverished populations where sole breastfeeding is increasingly insufficient to meet caloric needs after the age of 6 months. However, some of the 568 stillbirths reported likely were neonatal deaths, leading to downward bias in recorded infant deaths. Christophers himself considered that reported stillbirths included 'children dying within the first day or so of birth.'[32]

The Amritsar burial records also made it possible to compare the weekly progression of mortality by age group. 'The mortality curve for children under two years of age,' Christophers describes,

> was found to rise almost sheer [in mid- to late September] reaching its maximum in the second and third week of October, but at once falling rapidly. The curve of children under 10 rises more slowly and reaches its maximum in the first week in November. The curve of adult deaths rises still more gradually and reaches its maximum only in the last week in November. The curve of old people resembles that of children under 10.[33]

While most of these data apply only to Amritsar city, they nevertheless support the general view as to the proportionately large toll of malaria on young children. They shed light also on the immediacy of this effect, above all for infants. They thus accord with the general observation that fulminant epidemics were marked by a 'sudden rise in the intensity of infections [at] the onset of the epidemic . . . accompanied, but at a slower pace, by the diffusion of infection amongst the community.'[34] The question was 'why.' What made malarial infection in 1908 so much more lethal, seemingly from the outset of the epidemic?

Deciphering the roles of rainfall

With heavy monsoon rains throughout the eastern and central divisions of the province and widespread flooding, entomological conditions for malaria transmission in 1908 no doubt had been highly favourable. For the 24 plains districts as a whole, rainfall had reached near-record levels, 23.7 inches compared with a mean of 13.9 inches. Mapping July–September rain data, Christophers was able to show a westerly movement of the 20-inch (heavy) rainfall line,[35] conditions that expanded the area subject to flooding.

In earlier survey work in 1902–1903 at the rural Mian Mir cantonment in Lahore district, immense numbers of *An. culicifacies* larvae had been found in irrigation channels, and it was assumed that they formed the main breeding site.[36] However, autumn fever mortality appeared to be as great in non-canal tracts as in canal areas.[37] Thus Christophers's attention increasingly turned to the enabling role played by post-monsoon surface water collections as prime vector breeding site. Returning to Punjab to observe more closely conditions across the 1909 monsoon period, he observed vast 'sheets of water . . . in some cases . . . stretching for miles,' despite rainfall only slightly above average levels.

> I was greatly struck with the numbers of anopheles such sheets must give rise to. . . . The larvae of *M. culicifacies* . . . were in immense number everywhere. . . . In other cases very extensive sheets of water may be hidden in the grass and vegetation, and may escape notice . . . or acres of land may be covered with small puddles lying in furrows and invisible even a few yards off.[38]

He went on to distinguish between 'permanent' (year-round) and 'temporary' breeding places, suggesting the latter, the 'shallow accumulations of rain water' created with monsoon rains, were 'the most interesting' as bountiful sources of *An. culicifacies*.

> [W]ithin a few weeks of the first fall of rain anopheles are again found breeding in the utmost profusion everywhere . . . [I]nstead of larvae being chiefly confined to large collections of water, such as tanks and sluggish weed grown channels, they are now found in every situation where water remains any length of time.[39]

The flatness of the Punjab plains – with a slope of scarcely one foot per mile – inevitably left the region flood prone.[40] But the region's propensity to flooding was also related to the character of the soil itself. The fine alluvial silt was 'peculiarly impervious' to water, a state compounded by the 'tendency to the formation of a concretionary layer of so-called "Kunker," hardened salts, a few feet beneath the surface.'[41] Collections of water thus often remained for extended periods, weeks, even months, and Christophers concluded, on the basis of his hydrological studies, that flood waters abated more by surface evaporation than by subsoil capillary vertical drainage.[42]

The entomological implications were obvious. As flood waters evaporated, countless small pools would be formed, ideal for larval development of *An. culcifacies*. But an even more critical effect of surface waters was their influence on atmospheric humidity, raising levels conducive to extended mosquito lifespan. The importance of flood conditions was confirmed by Christophers's initial mapping of several local areas of extreme epidemic intensity. 'When epidemic areas are examined in detail,' he observed, 'villages are found to have suffered almost exactly in proportion as they have been flooded.'[43]

Yet as prominent as the influence of flooding appeared to be within specific epidemic tracts, could flooding explain 1908 fever mortality for the province as a whole? From his work at Mian Mir, Christophers was also aware that even in average rainfall years, *An. culcifacies* mosquitoes were prodigious in number and autumnal malarial infection widespread.[44] The distinction, he urged, was not between malarial and non-malarial years, but between 'endemic' autumnal malaria and what he referred to as 'the "mortality-causing" or . . . "virulent" type of malaria.'[45]

> [I]n the investigation of malaria in the Punjab, we have to consider not only the conditions associated with mere transmission of malaria, but even more urgently to ascertain what are the causes of the peculiar epidemics. . . . [T]hough malaria is always present and in a sense may be extremely intense, the disease is only associated with high epidemic mortality under certain conditions.[46]

Christophers's notion of 'high' malaria mortality was, of course, one taken in historical context: for him, it meant lethality leading to stagnant or even negative population growth rate, a definition that left room for considerable malaria mortality in non-epidemic years. Nonetheless, the mortality differential between epidemic and non-epidemic years was large even in the context of a relatively high baseline 'non-epidemic' toll. It was determining those 'certain conditions' giving rise to soaring mortality that lay at the heart of his investigation. Detailed accounts of local flood conditions were not available in the administrative records, so the question of the overall role of flood waters in 1908 was one that could not be answered directly. However, it was possible, Christophers surmised, to approach the question indirectly, by tracing epidemic mortality patterns spatially across the province.

Mapping malaria mortality

In his initial local surveys of severely affected epidemic tracts, Christophers had calculated October 1908 fever death rates for individual villages. Such detailed study, however, was not possible for the 50,000 villages across the province. Mortality data available in the annual sanitary reports, on the other hand, provided only summarised district-level statistics, each district covering an expanse of some 3,000 square miles. For purposes of spatial mapping, a much finer resolution of malaria mortality was required, and here Christophers sought out the original unpublished sub-district mortality records from the province's 500 *thana* (police station) registration units.[47]

Use of the absolute autumn death rates calculated from these *thana*-level records posed a problem however for comparing epidemic intensity across the province due to differences in deaths registration completeness among districts. For the purposes of mapping comparative levels of epidemic intensity in 1908, Christophers devised a ratio measure of autumn malaria mortality to take into account these limitations. For each *thana*, he calculated what he termed an 'epidemic figure,' derived by dividing the number of deaths recorded in October by the average non-epidemic monthly death rate. The latter was calculated as the previous five-year average of June and July deaths, 'avoiding those years in which plague or cholera disturbed the figures.' Epidemic tracts were considered those where October deaths were five, seven, or 10 times the 'non-epidemic' (June–July) levels (Figure 2.8). As such, the map delineates only those regions most severely affected.[48]

The resulting map confirmed what had been evident from the narrative and dispensary records: that virtually all regions of central and eastern Punjab experienced increased malaria mortality in 1908. It also confirmed a general correspondence between heavy rainfall and epidemic severity. But the relationship was not exact (Figure 2.8, inset). Tracing what Christophers termed lines of 'equi-mortality,' it became apparent that within the general increase in mortality in 1908, there existed two large epidemic areas where mortality had risen to extraordinary heights, one in the north-central region of the province and another in the southeast. These epidemic foci were remarkable not just for their size, but also in the way they 'exhibit[ed] a regular increase of epidemic intensity as we pass from the periphery to the centre of the area,' fever mortality reaching levels of 20 to 30 times the normal non-malaria death rate at the nucleus core.[49] 'Their distribution,' he suggested, 'vividly calls to mind such phenomena

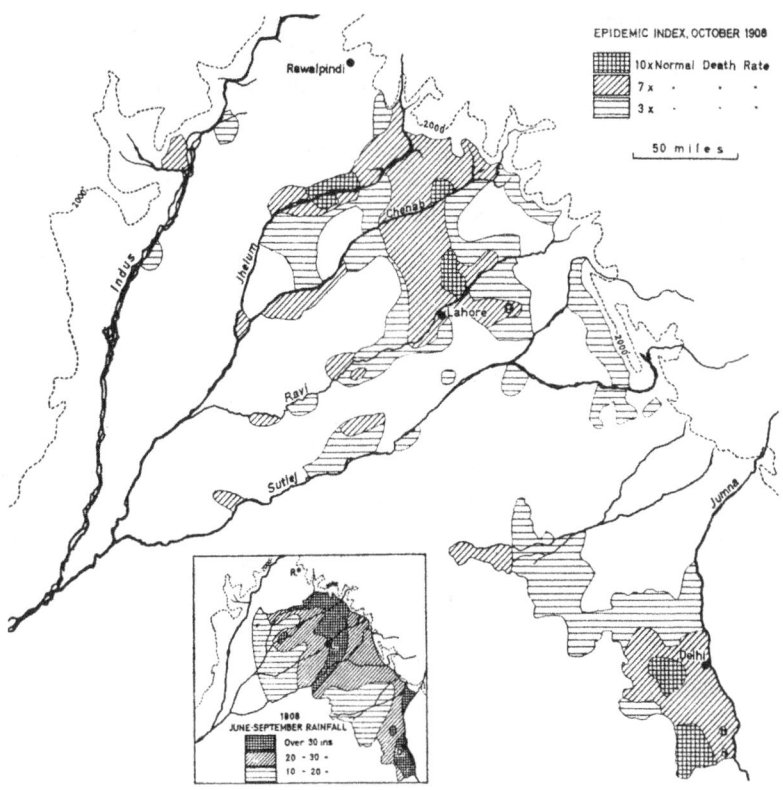

Figure 2.8 1908 Epidemic malaria mortality, June–Sept. rain (inches) [inset], Punjab

Note: Epidemic index should read: 5, 7, and 10 ×Normal Death Rate.

Source: Christophers, 'Malaria in the Punjab,' No. 46, 1911, Map I; adapted by A.T.A. Learmonth, 'Some Contrasts in the Regional Geography of Malaria in India and Pakistan,' *Transactions and Papers* (Institute of British Geographers), 23, 1957, 37–59, at 47. Reprinted with permission of Wiley & Sons Ltd.

as areas of low or high barometric pressure and not at all that of a disease following lines of communication or even local peculiarities of the ground.'[50]

In the north districts, 'certain tongues of epidemic' severity extended away from the main nucleus of mortality, following the course of rivers. Here, lack of geographic congruence between rainfall and epidemic intensity could perhaps be explained by flooding along rivers downstream of heavier rainfall. But elsewhere, including in much of the southeastern epidemic nucleus, 'though the fringes of the epidemic show a relation to rivers, etc, the main epidemic areas show relatively little relation to any physical features and affect without exception the thanas over a very wide extent of country.'[51] It was unlikely, he concluded, that even downstream flooding could fully explain the general pattern of epidemic mortality. What the map of malaria mortality in 1908 revealed instead was a distinctly non-haphazard distribution of mortality.

> Had the malaria of 1908 depended on merely local causes, the number of pools about a village and so on, we should have expected to obtain a map covered with confused figures indicating haphazard variations, as the intensity of the disease rose and fell from thana to thana. There would be no reason why numbers of severely affected thanas should form as it were a nucleus to epidemic areas or that the intensity of the disease should show a more or less regular decline as we pass outwards from these foci. . . . [T]he map alone is sufficient to show that there was in the epidemic of 1908 some general determining influence over and above merely local conditions which acted much as an area of low or high atmospheric pressure might have acted, supposing this to affect the mortality.[52]

Something beyond rainfall and local flooding, in other words, appeared to underlie the overall pattern of mortality observed in 1908.

So struck was Christophers by the focal character of mortality in 1908 that he went on to map mortality patterns for earlier major epidemics as well. Applying the same measure of epidemic intensity, he identified 11 additional epidemic years between 1867 and 1908. Some epidemics appeared to show only a single focus, such as that in 1892 (Figure 2.9),[53] whereas others demonstrated several broad foci, as in the case of the 1908 epidemic.[54] He concluded that

> in the Punjab we have malaria normally exhibiting itself in a very peculiar and definite way, one of the characters of which is the formation over some part or other of the Punjab of what might almost be called a malaria cyclone. . . . [The] peculiar increase of intensity as the [mortality] nucleus was approached . . . enables one to map out these Punjab epidemics as one might do the varying levels of land by contour lines or the differences of atmospheric pressure by isobars.[55]

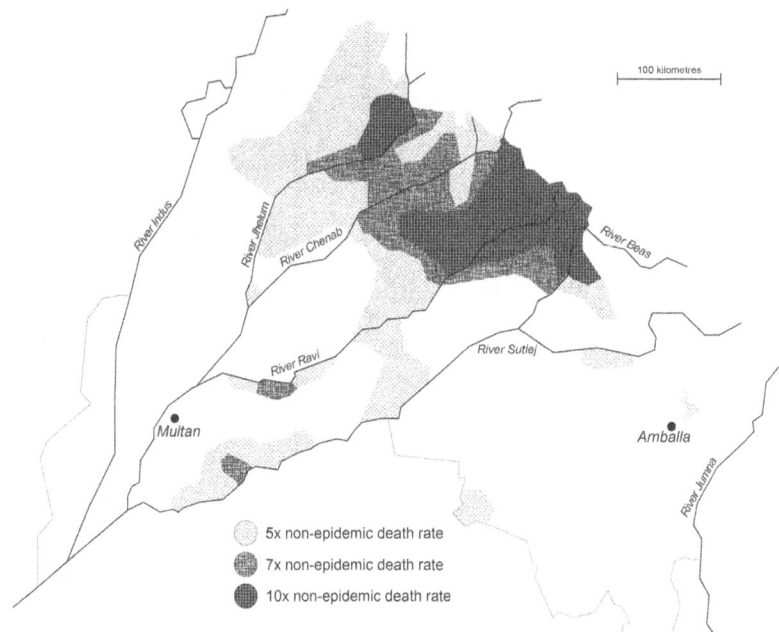

Figure 2.9 1892 Epidemic malaria mortality, Punjab

Legend: Light to dark shading represents 'Epidemic Figures' 5×, 7×, and 10× non-epidemic levels.

Source: By the author, adapted from S.R. Christophers, 'Malaria in the Punjab,' 1911, Map 3.

Such epidemics affecting broad geographical areas 'might well be called "fulminant" malaria,' he suggested, a term that would remain in the lexicon of malariologists throughout the remainder of the colonial period.[56] Elsewhere, Christophers would describe them as 'death storms . . . displayed as a pestilence,' what would also, in time, come to be termed 'regional' epidemics.[57]

Broadening the pestilential framework

In an effort to depict the propensity for 'fulminant' epidemics in the province, Christophers identified *thanas* where October mortality over the preceding 40-year period had 'at least once' reached 'over 5 (7, or 10) times the normal.' The resulting map (Figure 2.10)[58] showed that 'the western half or comparatively rainless portion of the Punjab [was]

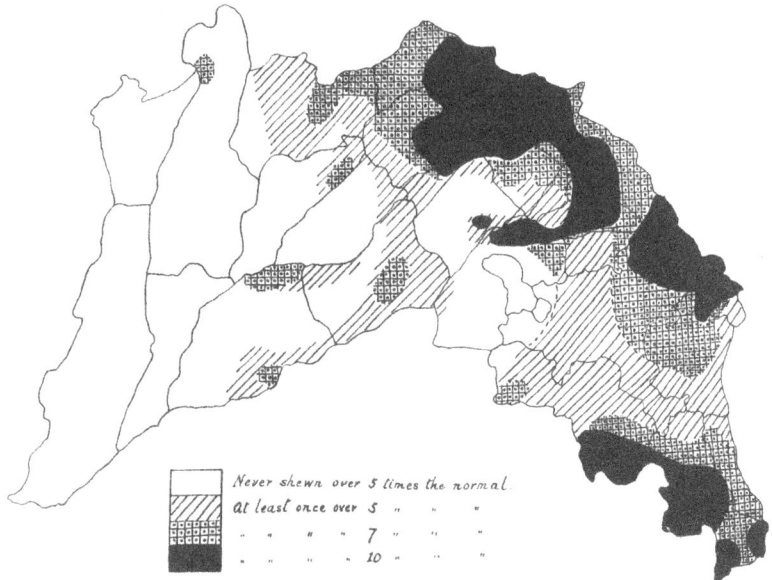

Never shewn over 5 times the normal
At least once over 5 „ „ „
„ „ „ „ 7 „ „ „
„ „ „ „ 10 „ „ „

Figure 2.10 Epidemic [malaria] frequency, Punjab, 1868–1908
Source: Christophers, 'Malaria in the Punjab,' Map 9.

relatively unaffected.'[59] But it also showed that epidemics were not confined to high water-table areas or overtly waterlogged tracts: fulminant malaria over the preceding four decades had 'descend[ed] as if capriciously' across much of the eastern and north-central portion of the province.[60]

In his efforts to convey the scale and etiological character of fulminant malaria in the province, Christophers found himself looking back to earlier concepts of epidemic disease. 'The word epidemic, applied as it is to outbreaks of disease on a small scale, does not sufficiently characterise such vast exhibitions of the power of zymotic disease,' he observed in later writing, 'and I propose to call such phenomena *zymonic* from their likeness in distribution to cyclonic disturbances in the atmosphere.'[61] The 19th-century term 'zymotic' referred to diseases believed to be caused by a fermentative process and resulting 'miasma,' and connoted a general factor affecting large areas simultaneously, the result of broad atmospheric conditions conducive to decay of organic matter (or 'filth'). This contrasted with diseases such as smallpox where localised transmission of a particular agent was generally traceable through patterns of direct person-to-person contagion. Here, however, Christophers was choosing to adapt the term zymotic to convey a different 'atmospheric' agent at play, while still retaining the sense of the broad spatial character observed with the malarial 'death storms' in Punjab. Hence, the neologism, 'zymonic.' He went on to designate lines of equi-mortality as 'isothans' from the Greek, *thanos*, or death.

If we were to prepare and examine the thanatographs of a large number of registration units

> lying near one of these death storms we should find that practically all shewed simultaneous rises . . . those situated towards the centre . . . [reaching] sometimes 10, 20 or even 30 times the normal. . . . [H]ad we some method of photographing mortality telescopically from the moon, we should find that these various epidemics appeared as great splashes of abnormal mortality, often shewing a focus of special intensity covering hundreds of miles of country.[62]

What, then, was the 'general determining influence' suggested by the focal character of epidemic mortality? Christophers's reluctance to go beyond empirical evidence meant his published conclusions remained understated though they point clearly to economic hardship: harvest failure. In extending the analysis to the entire 41-year period, it had become evident that most of the visitations of fulminant malaria had occurred during periods of 'scarcity'-level foodgrain prices. '[A]nnual average [foodgrain] prices,' he pointed out,

> have risen and fallen in the course of years almost in a rhythmical manner. . . . [W]e cannot help being struck by the fact that if we take the summit of the [price] curve in each case it will be found to coincide with an epidemic . . . [T]hat the epidemics should always occur at the culminating point strongly suggests that it occurred when in a period of drought and scarcity a heavy monsoon fell.[63]

As to why harvest failure in the province manifested in relatively distinct regional foci, Christophers offered a characteristically indirect explanation:

> [W]hilst there are three types of epidemics, northern, central and southern, and that these rarely occur together in the same year, there are also three main types of agricultural areas, namely a

wheat area in the north dependent mainly on the spring crop, a maize area in the central districts and a gram and millet area in the south, both dependent mainly on the autumn crop.[64]

Full stop. Differences in cropping patterns, he appears to have been suggesting, reflected differences in vulnerability to drought and crop failure across the province. Harvest failure was rarely experienced uniformly across the province because of marked variation in availability of irrigation (well, inundation, or canal) and crop requirements, and yearly distribution of rainfall. Such differences determined which region in a given agricultural year would experience crop failure and economic hardship, differences he had come to conclude were expressed in turn in broad focal patterns of epidemic mortality. '[W]e may say,' Christophers concluded, 'that periods characterized by high prices are likely to be followed at the first heavy monsoon by an epidemic and that particular *areas subject to adversity are likely to be picked out* by the epidemics if the other factors are favourable to this result' – 'adversity' that he designated as the 'human factor.'[65]

The primacy of general economic conditions was evident, moreover, in the fact that heavy rainfall, on its own, was not associated with the most severe epidemics. Adequate rainfall was essential for malaria transmission to occur.[66] But there were 'very interesting' years where severe flooding was not accompanied by fulminant malaria.

> In 1875, the rainfall is the heaviest recorded in the Punjab not even excluding the rainfall for 1908. . . . But the epidemic increase in deaths is small. In 1894, another very heavy year, the mortality we have seen was not at all in proportion to the precipitation. . . . This want of relation is brought out quite as prominently by a study of the figures for different areas and is not due, as one might think, to the average figure employed, giving faulty impression of the conditions.[67]

To highlight such rain-anomalous years, Christophers plotted epidemic mortality and rain-price coefficients for the 41-year period, a graph that revealed a cluster of heavy rainfall years in the quadrant of low mortality (Figure 2.11).[68] This 'illustrates very clearly that heaviness of the rainfall is not the only factor at work,' he observed, adding

> whilst the epidemic years are seen to follow the correlation line, a very interesting group of non-epidemic years characterised by heavy rainfall are seen markedly diverging from this. The group

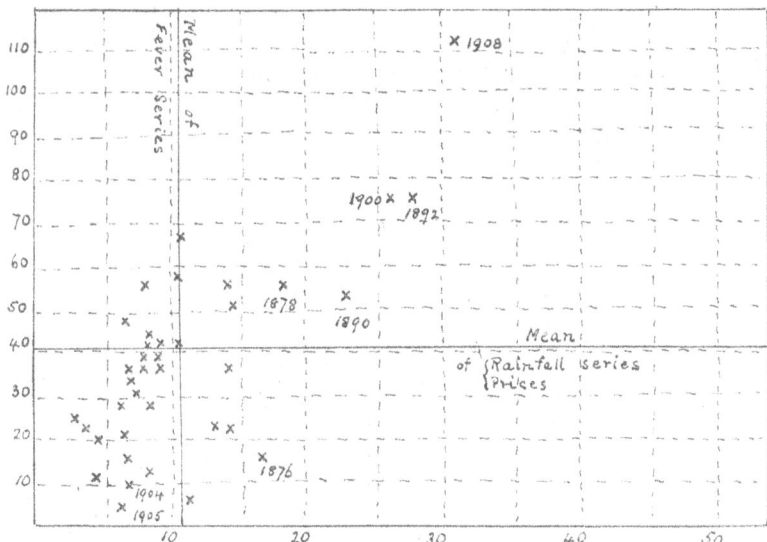

Figure 2.11 Correlation between 'fever mortality' and rainfall × prices
* X-axis = 'fever mortality'; Y-axis = rainfall × wheat price.
Source: Christophers, 'Malaria in the Punjab,' Chart 7.

illustrates very clearly the fact that heaviness of the rainfall is not the only factor at work. It is significant that all these years are years of low prices. . . . [W]e cannot predict in any particular year what a heavy rainfall will bring about, . . . [b]ut if heavy rain were to fall upon a famine-stricken district, we might then reasonably expect this to be followed by severe epidemic conditions.[69]

Rainfall was a necessary factor in the aetiology of severe epidemics. But it was not, it appeared, a sufficient one.

[W]e should not expect to find [scarcity] acting in the absence of the necessary factor of rainfall. We must not look also for the effect of famine in this respect in the famine districts at the time of the famine, for at this time the essential, excess of rainfall, is absent.[70]

It was favourable entomological conditions superimposed upon pre-existing 'economic hardship' that allowed malaria to take on fulminant form.

The importance of economic hardship in 'fulminant' malaria in Punjab was suggested also by observations on class profile of mortality. In Amritsar, 'the increased rate [of deaths] among the Mohamedans who form the bulk of the poorer classes is very noticeable,' the October death rate calculated as 390 per mille as against 203 among Hindus. '[I]n arriving at an estimate of the effects of malaria in different towns and villages, it is necessary,' Christophers urged, 'to recognise and allow for this class coefficient.'[71]

To what extent could class mortality differentials be explained by differences in exposure to malarial infection? It was a question Christophers considered in some detail. In the largest towns, such as Amritsar, it was likely that the more peripheral wards were more exposed to malaria infection due to less dense build-up and proximity to neighbouring agricultural fields and irrigation channels. But the outer wards also housed a disproportionate number of the very poor and destitute.[72] Thus, it was difficult to differentiate between the effects of poverty and those of greater exposure.

For much of the rural population, however, large class differences in exposure to malaria were less likely. Village communities were built up from the surrounding plains as clusters of contiguous mud houses. *An. culicifacies* breeding occurred mainly in accumulations of standing water in adjacent fields, irrigation channels, and waste tracts. The size and physical compactness of villages meant that substantial differences in exposure from surrounding mosquito breeding sites were unlikely.

> Palwal [town] as compared with the villages around shows a greater mortality rate. The malaria conditions in both are identical or slightly more adverse in the villages; but whilst Palwal has a large population of dependent classes living in great squalor and poverty, the villages have a population consisting for the most part of well-to-do cultivators with a small proportion only of dependents.[73]

'One may say,' he concluded, 'that the amount of mortality in any town or village will be determined very largely by the relative proportion of well-to-do to partially poverty stricken dependant classes.'[74]

Rain-price-fever mortality correlations

It was the recurring association of epidemics with famine-level prices that led Christophers to attempt a quantitative analysis of the relationships between malaria mortality, rainfall and foodgrain prices, and of the 'general determining influence' that he was observing geographically. Modern methods of multiple regression analysis were not available to him in 1909. However, using October and November fever deaths as an index of annual malaria mortality, he calculated correlation coefficients between malaria mortality, monsoon rainfall, and wheat prices for the 41-year period for which data were available. The mathematical calculations employed are not fully explained in his report. Nor is it clear how he arrived at some of the aggregate data summarised in the Appendix to the 1911 report. What is of interest here, however, are the concepts he was pursuing in these quantitative efforts.

Initial calculations showed a correlation coefficient of .67 between mortality and monsoon rainfall, and one of .61 between wheat prices and mortality for this period. He then calculated a composite correlation coefficient of .80 for the three variables together. In an attempt to better capture the association with preceding drought he went on to construct what he termed a 'rain coefficient,' a measure of the differential between rainfall in a given epidemic year and that of the preceding year of drought, derived by dividing current rainfall by the previous year's rain.

> If, instead of merely looking for an association of high rainfall with epidemics, we take also in consideration the previous year . . . by dividing the average rainfall of each year by that for the previous year. . . [we] bring into proportionate prominence years of heavy rainfall following years of deficient rainfall.[75]

The correlation coefficient between fever deaths, prices, and the rain coefficient thus calculated was .83. '[T]he process,' he concluded, 'not only picks out most of the epidemic years but in any particular year even approximates in value to the number of deaths from fever.'[76]

A link between harvest failure, famine, and epidemic malaria was hardly new, Christophers stressed. 'That the most severe epidemics follow very frequently this [scarcity] sequence is apparently the general experience of all who have had intimate acquaintance with the Punjab.'[77] What *was* new, however, and set *Malaria in the Punjab* apart from earlier accounts, was extension of this relationship beyond official (frank) famine. Christophers identified additional epidemics associated with famine-level foodgrain prices but where famine had not been formally declared, as was indeed the case for 1908 as well.[78]

Turning to the epidemics of 1878 and 1879, he quoted the Gurgaon district *Gazetteer*:

> [T]he scarcity caused by the failure of harvests [in 1877] hardly deepened into actual famine, although there were some deaths from starvation, and a large portion of the population was greatly weakened by want; *but it was followed in 1878 and 1879 by a dreadful epidemic of fever, and in those two years 103,000 persons or more than a seventh of the total population died.*[79]

Such periods of not 'actual famine,' where high foodgrain prices ('scarcity') were accompanied by soaring epidemic mortality, would certainly be considered famine in the modern context. However, in the 19th century only the most severe and advanced stages of mass destitution were officially recognised and designated as such, and thus as meriting public relief. In other words, 'scarcity' could entail very substantial harvest failure and starvation, as in 1878, though not appearing either sociologically (with classic markers of 'famine wandering' or abandonment of dependents) or administratively as established 'famine.'[80] Again, in relation to the 1879 epidemic, he observed that 'mortality is very much increased even *if the epidemic is not strong* by a condition of stress among the people in the previous year,' adding that if two consecutive crops 'fail there comes a condition of stress, almost of famine, and the people are in a very bad way indeed and this seems to be one of the important causes of the epidemic.'[81]

Scarcity-flooding interaction

In this attention to economic hardship, Christophers was not dismissing a role for excess rain and flooding in epidemic causation.[82] *Within* the broad foci of epidemic intensity, he pointed out, the worst affected tracts were those affected by prolonged flooding: 'the higher epidemic figures seem to depend entirely upon floods and *fulminant malaria of a certain intensity is almost synonymous with malaria of diluvial origin.*'[83] Yet neither heavy rainfall nor waterlogging could explain the location of the epidemic nucleus itself, nor its focal character. While '[p]hysical features influence epidemics and low water-logged areas are especially susceptible to epidemic conditions. . . . these differences,' Christophers added, 'are often lost when a district becomes involved in the nucleus of an epidemic area.'[84]

Flooding and surface flood waters undoubtedly enhanced entomological conditions by ensuring continuous elevated atmospheric humidity and thus exponential increase in levels of malaria transmission. But alongside their entomological effects, surface flood waters held profound economic consequences as well, destroying standing crops and remaining stores of grain, and blocking agricultural recovery, thus prolonging and deepening the economic paralysis triggered initially by preceding drought. At the same time, local rural roads were submerged, physically isolating village communities for extended periods and making access to outside food and work through trade or migration difficult. In his introductory comments at the Imperial malaria conference at Simla in October 1909, the Sanitary Commissioner for the GOI, J.T.W. Leslie, had explicitly linked the economic consequences of flooding to malaria lethality, describing how

> when large tracts of country are submerged, houses collapse, harvests are destroyed and the poorer classes of the peasantry are not only thrown out of employment, but are exposed to great privation and hardship. It is then that the mortality among children and the aged is so high – malaria, owing to the simultaneous occurrence of exposure and privation, has become a very fatal disease.[85]

Contained within the factor of 'excess rain,' in other words, there was an additional powerful dimension of compounded human destitution.

Direct reference to the economic implications of flooding, curiously enough, does not appear in the text of *Malaria in the Punjab*. Here, Christophers perhaps defers to the Simla conference testimony of Leslie, as the highest official in the sanitary administration. Yet there can be little doubt that he was deeply aware of the economic paralysis that flooding induced, having personally found many villages in the early months of 1909 still unreachable for surrounding expanses of flood waters.[86] Several times he hints in the closing pages of his report at the larger non-entomological impacts of flooding: first, in a seemingly offhand remark that 'the close association of fulminant malaria with actual flooding suggests something more than the ordinary reproduction of the [anopheline] genus in pools, etc.,' and second, prefacing his discussion of the urgent need for flood control measures with an uncharacteristically casual side comment, that '[w]hat the action of flood waters may be does not at present concern us.'[87] Coming from perhaps the foremost entomologist of the period, this remark is more than a little curious. It was followed by the simple recommendation: that '[i]n the controlling of floods we have then one very clear objective and one which is within some measure of possible attainment.'

But the significance of flooding merited emphasis for a further reason, one central to understanding malaria fulminancy in the region. Through detailed soil drainage experiments conducted in subsequent visits to the province, Christophers had come to appreciate that flood propensity in the province was not limited to waterlogged tracts or areas subject to peri-riverain overflows. In years of above normal rainfall, surface pooling of rainwater could occur almost anywhere, a consequence of the impervious nature of the soils in general of the northwest plains. In years of heavy rains, '*something very like flooding* occurs in so far as extensive sheets are formed.'[88] Indeed, the provincial sanitary commissioner had described flooding in 1908 as 'almost universal' across the province.[89]

This near-ubiquitous 'flood' potential meant that in heavy rainfall years, a flood-'scarcity' synergism could potentially be expressed anywhere pre-existing harvest failure prevailed. In effect, the soils and topography of Punjab rendered the monsoon rains highly efficient in realising malaria's fulminant potential. Few of the drought-debilitated would escape infection, with continuing economic paralysis unrelieved by return of the rains. And yet, on their own, heavy rains failed to trigger fulminant conditions.

Dose of infection

Christophers clearly saw hunger-induced immunosuppression as a major factor underlying epidemic malaria in the province, citing previous officials' description of epidemic malaria victims as 'weakened by want.' Yet he was reluctant to assume that epidemic lethality was related to immunosuppression alone. Accounts of fever prostration from the outset of the 1908 epidemic suggested that clinically severe infection was a more generalised phenomenon in the population, even though actual mortality appeared to be concentrated amongst the destitute. It was here that he turned to investigate microbiologic dimensions to fulminancy.

The possibility of new, potentially more virulent strains of the malaria parasites explaining this intensity was unlikely, given the near-simultaneous appearance of epidemic mortality across the province. Another theoretical explanation was a relative shift in *plasmodium* species: an increase in the proportion of falciparum infection compared with vivax malaria under more entomologically conducive conditions. In the absence of blood smear data, there was no record of malaria species over the course of the 1908 epidemic. This seemed unlikely, however, given that intensity of malarial fever was marked from the earliest days of the epidemic when the normally milder vivax form of the disease would be more common. Moreover, it was already clear from surveys among troops stationed at Mian Mir and among jail populations that *P. falciparum* transmission was the predominant form of post-monsoon malaria even in non-epidemic years.[90]

Christophers hypothesised instead that the clinical severity of malaria infection in 1908 might reflect a shift in the amount ('dose') of malarial infection being transmitted in individual cycles of mosquito-man transmission. In the absence of any specific data on parasite counts, he took on the question himself, conducting a series of experiments on avian malaria to explore the effect of both numbers of infective bites and dose of infection (sporozoites) inoculated, on subsequent infection parasite levels. 'When commencing the experiments,' he wrote, 'I had thought only of the "number" of infected mosquitoes concerned.'

> But it is obvious that there is another matter to be considered. . . . [I]n mosquitoes fed on a bird whose blood contains very numerous gametes, the mid-gut is studded with hundreds of zygotes and when the sporozoites have reached the glands these become swollen with innumerable multitudes of sporozoites. Such a mosquito must inject a dose perhaps a hundred times greater than one of the slightly infected mosquitoes. . . . Using scantily infected mosquitoes even in great numbers it is difficult to get a severe infection; single heavily infected mosquitoes on the other hand often give quite severe infections. But by using a number of heavily infected mosquitoes not only was the incubation period reduced from nine days to as little as five days, but the resulting infections were much more severe and death in every case occurred.[91]

Severity of infection in avian malaria, he concluded, was 'largely dependent on the dose inoculated. . . . It is easy therefore to see,' he concluded, 'that in malaria everything may depend upon the existence of heavy gamete carriers; and if these are present upon the number of anopheles.'[92] Extrapolation from avian malaria to human, admittedly, was a large leap. Christophers, nevertheless, believed the results suggested a possible additional mechanism involved in human malaria in its fulminant form and devoted an entire chapter of his study to this experimental work.

Still, the question remained: where did heavy doses originate from in epidemic years? In the 1911 report, Christophers refrained from explicitly linking dose of malarial infection and human destitution, leaving the hypothesis at the level of inference. It was a question, however, that delegates at the Simla conference had raised openly earlier, in response to Christophers's Punjab presentation in October 1909. '[T]he fact that epidemics appeared so suddenly,' he had responded then, 'suggested that many heavy gamete carriers existed previously. These were largely found among poor and squalid communities in Indian towns and villages.'[93] Left unarticulated was the inference that with greater numbers of the 'poor and squalid' in times of scarcity and famine, there would be proportionately greater numbers of heavy gamete carriers.

How did Christophers *know* this? No data on gametocyte counts by social class appeared in the 1911 report, although spleen rates were documented as higher amongst the poor and lower caste groups.[94] The question of dose of infection, however, was one he had been grappling with even before taking on the Punjab inquiry. One year earlier, he and colleague C.A. Bentley had investigated malarial conditions in the Duars tea plantations in the northeastern Himalayan hills, concluding that the 'virulent and intense' form of malaria observed was largely a function of residual infection amongst destitute labourers, rather than driven primarily by hyperendemic entomological conditions on the hill estates. Villages adjacent to the tea estates, where transmission conditions were similar, or even more favourable with widespread rice cultivation, did not exhibit the same fever lethality.[95]

> [Where] natives often originally possessed of poor physique and little stamina [are] living under conditions of depression, privation and hardship pushed to their extreme, it is obvious that these will form a soil far more suitable for the continued existence of malaria. . . . [I]nfection diminishes very slowly even in the absence of anopheles, and the presence of even a very small number of anopheles appears to be quite sufficient to keep up the maximum degree of parasitic infestation. This factor of Residual Infection may thus convert a whole community into a reservoir of infection, ever ready to involve its neighbourhood in epidemic sickness, and . . . diffusing malarial infection far and wide.[96]

Entomological and economic conditions in Punjab differed from those in the Duars tea estates.[97] Yet in relation to a major epidemic in Amritsar city in 1881, Christophers would make a direct link between endemic destitution and enhanced transmission analogous to that in the Duars. Economic hardship in the province that year, he pointed out, was not limited only to harvest failure and high grain prices. Economic downturns in urban industries brought cycles of destitution quite independent of rural agricultural conditions, and heightened vulnerability to epidemic disease in turn.

> Epidemic conditions in the Punjab generally were not very severe in this year (1881) and even in Amritsar District the mortality bore no relation to that in the city. It seems very probable that the severity of the outbreak was associated with economic conditions affecting the large bodies of Kashmiri workers who about this time were adversely affected by the decay of the shawl trade in Amritsar. . . . [I]t was clear that there were all the possibilities of an exaggerated human factor. . . . [A]mong the labouring and artizan classes in Amritsar City, especially among the Kashmiris, the pinch of poverty is severely felt . . . living under conditions which favour the continuance of residual infection.[98]

The term 'residual' infection connotes delayed recovery, inability to throw off malarial infection. But residual infection was not necessarily the same as dose of infection. The former referred to prolonged presence of malarial parasites in the human host. Dose referred to the *amount* of infection (number of sporozoites) transmitted to the human host in a single bite by an infected mosquito. Yet if not the same, were they related? Did the compromised immune capacity associated with residual infection also lead to greater parasite loads being transmitted to the vector mosquito, and, in turn, heavier doses of the parasite (sporozoites) transmitted to the human host in subsequent cycles?

Christophers does not argue this explicitly. But it is clear he considered the heightened general clinical intensity of malaria observed in epidemic years as possibly contributing secondarily to the fulminant death toll. Indeed, he concluded the 1911 report, as he had at Simla, by urging much further investigation into 'quantitative questions': 'the whole subject of endemic malaria which by supplying the gamete carriers may be an underlying cause of epidemic conditions.'[99] What was being suggested was both a direct and an indirect impact of economic hardship on case fatality rates. Moreover, in raising general questions of recovery rate and dose of infection, Christophers was implicitly extending the implications of his study beyond Punjab. For the endemic destitution evident in Amritsar or Palwal was not limited to the northwest corner of the subcontinent. In his earlier Simla presentation Christophers had included, in addition to a section on 'scarcity,' a separate portion that explicitly addressed 'the influence of squalor and poverty' in contributing to general malaria intensity.[100] Though less visible in sociological or archival terms than overt famine, endemic acute hunger, he was implying, bore important implications for the lethality burden of malaria in the larger subcontinent.

Deciphering Christophers's conclusions

Amidst the complex array of ecological, entomological, and economic observations, what conclusions emerged from the Punjab inquiry? The epidemic form of the disease, Christophers stressed, was distinct from that of the 'normal' seasonal autumnal fever mortality in the province.

> The terrible effects of an epidemic are greatly in excess of anything that results from the normal endemic conditions. And even though the death rate is raised by endemic malaria, the effect of epidemic conditions is vastly larger and more important, . . . a form of malaria which alone forces itself upon the public notice, so as to cause comment and alarm.[101]

Nor was vulnerability to such epidemics, he concluded, related to varying endemic levels within the province: 'this liability of the Punjab to epidemic malaria is not simply due to the fact that its inhabitants are less protected by immunity than are those of some other areas.' The northern submontane districts with generally higher endemic levels of transmission were at least as prone to fulminant epidemics as the north-central and southeast districts (Figure 2.10).[102] Nor was fulminancy related geographically to canal irrigation. 'The canal tracts of the Punjab for the most part irrigate high lands unsuitable for epidemic malaria, and, in spite of irrigation and a certain amount of endemic malaria,' he observed, they 'stand out in relief as areas of low epidemic mortality,' adding that the phenomenon of fulminant epidemics clearly predated construction of the vast irrigation canal systems in the central-western region of the province.[103] The primary driver and underlying cause of the fulminant form of malaria in the region appeared to be neither ecological nor immunological, but related to economic conditions: acute hardship triggered by harvest failure and exacerbated by flood-induced economic paralysis. Underlying this dynamic, he concluded,

> malaria . . . [was] the main agent which brought to a head in actual mortality the effects produced by the great economic

stresses. . . . [T]he effects of scarcity are to a large extent held over until the appearance of the first heavy monsoon. Then though the effect of the rain is to reap a harvest of deaths, the period of stress is brought to an end.[104]

Articulation of such a politically incriminating finding was phrased, not surprisingly, sparely in the concluding pages of the report. The 'determining causes' of fulminant malaria, the report read, was 'excessive rainfall and scarcity; the former is an essential whilst the latter is an almost equally powerful influencing factor.'[105] Nor would economic measures appear in the report's ensuing recommendations on preventive measures. Policy discussion was directed instead to flood control, and to the equally challenging task of convincing a sanitary establishment, groomed in the sanitationist principles of mosquito 'extirpation,' of the rationale behind policies that largely ignored vector control. '[T]he immediate removal or prevention of flood water,' Christophers advised,

> *should be the first step in the sanitation of a rural tract.* [emphasis in original] . . . What the action of flood waters may be does not at present concern us. . . . In the controlling of floods we have then one very clear objective and one which is within some measure of possible attainment.[106]

Here, Christophers was quick to rule out subsoil drainage, urging that

> [surface] drainage must not be confused with drainage of the soil . . . Under the circumstances present in India it [the latter] can only be carried out in a limited manner. If we seek to avert epidemic malaria by such means we have 50,000 square miles to treat before we have the zone of epidemics under control.[107]

At the Simla conference, he had also made clear that the goal was not *general* surface drainage, explaining that

> epidemics are not confined to any given tract and may attack almost any part of the submontane or southeastern Punjab. . . . Under such circumstances drainage would mean that we should have to do what nature has failed to do, namely provide a drainage that will carry off excessive monsoon rain from the Punjab.[108]

The key need was to ensure unimpeded flow of rainwater. This meant identifying local drainage patterns and eliminating obstructions to them wherever feasible. Even here, he warned, flood control required detailed local analysis and engineering work.

> [I]f we carry out large hydraulic measures, we have to calculate on the conditions which produce epidemics, not on those in a normal year when there is no question of flooding. A case in point is the town of Bhera, which it is proposed to drain by a dyke into the Jhelum. Such a drain in the very year of need will be found wanting, for under such circumstances the Jhelum itself is likely to be in flood, and in one year actually was the cause of the flooding of Bhera.[109]

But dealing with flooding also required immediate support of affected populations with food relief through the period of economic paralysis. Specific policies in this regard, however, appear nowhere in the text of the 1911 report. Yet, as will be traced in subsequent chapters, government relief obligations would soon include – for the first time – direct flood relief measures, along with fundamental changes in the character of famine and drought relief.

Least of all did the rural 'drainage' envisaged by Christophers encompass anti-larval brigades. Anopheline vectors were plentiful even in non-epidemic years of normal rainfall. Mosquito breeding during the monsoon rains was not limited to localised pools or irrigation channels but was near-ubiquitous across the rural plains.[110] Under such conditions, it was impossible to eliminate or even substantially reduce rural anopheles numbers during the monsoon rains.

> [I]f we seek by mosquito destruction to diminish epidemics under the peculiar conditions of the Punjab, we must be able to control the breeding of anopheles not during the non-essential ten months of the year, but during the two months or so in which the whole mischief is done, the two months when flood rains fall and water is everywhere, when anopheles are breeding in the furrows of ploughed fields and in innumerable situations where owing to the impervious and sodden soil the tiniest collections of water can rest.[111]

In such circumstances, 'the most energetic anti-mosquito campaign,' he warned, 'can influence but little the vast mortality which may occur in any year in almost any district.'[112]

Despite the emphasis on flood control, specific recommendations were surprisingly few, however. The single example offered was that for Gujrat district, where 'flooding is largely a matter of overflow of rivers and here extensive bunds are called for.'[113] Moreover, flooding was not always related to river overflow or even obstructed drainage but amounted simply to vast expanses of surface rainwater collection, for which there was little immediate remedy. It was this hydrological reality that led Christophers to turn to quinine as interim 'prophylactic' measure. '[U]ntil drainage can be instituted, the use of quinine . . . as a means of saving the life of actual sufferers must be pushed to the utmost. . . . [I]t is not quinine prophylaxis but quinine treatment we are in need of.'[114]

What then are historians to make of *Malaria in the Punjab* and its conclusions? Christophers's report was a scientific document, directed to determining the causes underlying the 'disastrous' epidemics of malaria mortality in the region. Only secondarily was it a policy report – though its conclusion bore profound policy implications. As a medical researcher, Christophers was exploring dimensions to epidemic causation essential to arriving at an understanding of what preventive measures might realisitically pre-empt 'fulminancy.' The report at times shows Christophers carrying on a conversation as much with himself as with the reader as he navigated through highly complex biological relationships. With regard to flood propensity, his discussion of soil porosity was labyrinthine.[115] Yet an understanding of the intricacies involved was essential for arriving at effective policy. In its exacting thoroughness – at once cryptic and convoluted – *Malaria in the Punjab* is a challenging document to comprehend. The myriad details can at times be overwhelming when it is unclear where Christophers's arguments are heading. His was a mind that could function on many dimensions simultaneously, and this is how the report reads as well.

Complicating comprehension further, all reference to economic dimensions in the concluding section of the report was addressed in oblique form: the determinants of fulminant malaria expressed simply as 'excessive rainfall and scarcity; the former is an essential whilst the latter is an almost equally powerful influencing factor' – wording that conveyed little of the key distinction between 'exciting' and 'predisposing' causes in epidemic aetiology. 'Excessive rain' was left undefined, no doubt because what constituted 'normal' varied so enormously across the province; but also because heavy rains on their own, did not trigger the most severe epidemics. Nor did the report's 'excessive rainfall and scarcity' conclusion hint at the economic dimensions to excess rainfall. Arguably, as written, it was perhaps inevitable that the role of 'excessive rainfall' would often be interpreted in subsequent years primarily in entomological terms.

This muted reference to the economic dimensions elucidated in the 1911 report's conclusions contrast sharply with that expressed at the Simla conference two years earlier. There, of the three factors cited as responsible for fulminant malaria in Punjab, Christophers had listed 'scarcity and high prices' first; 'physical features, waterlogging, large sheets of water,' second; and rainfall, third.[116] It seems likely the later more muted wording reflected diplomatic reticence to highlight the politically charged issue of starvation in a document destined for broad dissemination in the *Scientific Memoirs* series. Certainly, the two-year interval between his Simla presentation and publication of *Malaria in the Punjab* in late 1911 suggests behind-the-scenes deliberation over releasing the report at all. Hesitation is hardly surprising on the part of a colonial government that was facing, at the time, international obloquy for recurring famines, a plague hecatomb viewed as threatening metropolitan shores and global trade, and a surging nationalist movement. For in pointing to foodgrain prices, 'squalor,' and poverty, Christophers was implicitly linking the phenomenon of Punjab's fulminant epidemics to the larger dimensions of hunger prevailing across the subcontinent and thus opening up the larger imperial economic project to scrutiny and challenge. Christophers's findings, in other words, held profound implications far beyond public health policy. Clearer articulation of 'scarcity,' moreover, was unnecessary, for he clearly had the attentive ear of the GOI and would already have been aware of fundamental changes in famine relief policy unfolding behind the scenes.

Response and misreadings

As for members of the sanitary administration, *Malaria in the Punjab* was greeted by some with puzzlement and undisguised frustration. With rural anti-mosquito measures ruled out, the uncertainties of flood control self-evident, and economic remedies scarcely visible, the report was viewed as recommending 'quinine alone,' policy which amounted, in effect, to simply 'more of the same.' A similar reading of the Punjab malaria inquiry has appeared in recent South Asian malaria historiography as well, the report interpreted by some as largely a sop to deflect criticism away from the 'malariogenic' effects of canal irrigation, and Christophers himself as an apologist for GOI inaction on mosquito sanitation.[117]

Unquestionably, the inquiry into the 1908 epidemic, and its presentation, were shaped by imperial interests. For the British Raj, the report's conclusion regarding the geography of the 'disastrous' epidemics in the province helped shift the spotlight away from the myriad hydrological problems associated with the massive canal irrigation schemes and their continued expansion through the early decades of the 20th century. Yet, as will become apparent, Christophers was correct in concluding that heightened malarial endemicity associated with perennial canal irrigation was a very different issue than the recurring visitations of fulminant malaria. Epidemic mortality was neither spatially nor temporally correlated with canal irrigation. He was correct also in suggesting that epidemic (fulminant) malaria was the more important form of malaria affecting public health in the region. At the same time, Christophers did not entirely ignore the detrimental effects of canal irrigation, citing, if not elaborating upon, the 'very serious effects' of canal infrastructure where it interfered with surface drainage, effects that exacerbated epidemic severity in the northern region of the province in the tracts where canal system off-take from the major rivers originated.[118]

It is difficult, then, to see the Punjab inquiry itself as a whitewash of imperial economic policy 'sins,' above all where epidemic hunger was at least as incriminating an indictment of colonial governance as canal irrigation malaria. For by this point, the term 'scarcity' was no longer one implying 'natural' causes, its meaning by the early 20th century now tied intimately to colonial trade, taxation, and agricultural policies – which is to say, to issues where imperial economic theory and governance was increasingly under siege.

A further aspect contributing to the relative historiographic neglect of the 1911 inquiry report quite likely relates to the delicacy with which the economic conclusions in its final pages are phrased. Scarcity designated as 'an almost equally powerful factor' can be cursorily read as suggesting a secondary role for the 'human factor.' A modern reader, unfamiliar with the multidimensional relationship between rainfall, topography, soils, and the Punjab economy, is likely to assume primarily an entomological role for rain. Hunger, in this context, tends to appear as something of a 'side-bar,' taking on a casual character of 'making a bad situation worse' but leaving core causality in the entomologic realm. If so, this is a very different conclusion than that conveyed in the main body of the 1911 report where Christophers was at pains to point out that 'excess rainfall' generally did not, on its own, predict fulminant malaria.

More unfortunate than the report's historiographic dismissal as simply politically motivated, however, is the limited attention *in general* that historians have accorded to the study and the colonial malaria literature of which it forms a part. *Malaria in the Punjab* is cited not infrequently in modern malaria literature, but largely in passing. The range of empirical observations and insights contained in its 135 pages remains unexplored, leaving their implications yet to be integrated within the region's malaria historiography, and broader demographic analysis. Arguably this reflects a more general predicament within South Asian malaria historiography, where the actual *content* of much of the colonial epidemiological literature on malaria has been overshadowed by the drama of intra-professional personality conflict associated with the Mian Mir 'debate.' That contest – between high-profile advocates of mosquito extirpation led by Nobel laureate Ronald Ross on the one hand, and malaria researchers such as Christophers attempting to understand the broader determinants of the 'malaria problem' in India, on the other – is understandably riveting, but ultimately difficult to interpret without a full understanding of the questions being grappled with in *Malaria in the Punjab*.

Yet if misread by many at the time, and since, the basic content and analysis presented in the 1911 report would stand unrefuted in subsequent field research for the duration of the colonial period.

Questions remaining

From the perspective of modern historical methods, the more prominent questions in Christophers's study relate to his quantitative analysis. Some of the report's calculations are unclear, as are the sources of the data upon which they are based. More problematic, his use of aggregate provincial-level data on rainfall, prices and fever death rate inevitably obscures major differences in agricultural economies and impacts of rainfall across the province. (Christophers was certainly aware of this and that these differences meant substantial variation in the relationship between rainfall, grain prices and malaria transmission and mortality among regions.) Nonetheless, when the report's province-level 1868–1908 data are submitted to modern methods of regression analysis, the results lend support to his general conclusions.[119] Rain and foodgrain prices are both significant predictors of epidemic malaria in the province, and thus indicate the importance of pursuing a similar analysis at district level.

A related question is that of 'outlier' epidemics. Christophers noted several major epidemics which did not fit the rain-price model of malaria epidemicity but offered only limited discussion of their interpretive significance.[120] There are, in fact, a number of 'anomalous' epidemics that oblige greater exploration to assess the extent to which they undermine, or support, the study's conclusions.

Beyond inherent limitations to quantitative analysis, the report inevitably also left important interpretative questions unresolved, or unaddressed. Christophers was working at a time when there was only beginning appreciation, for example, of differing vector feeding habits and the role such bionomics could potentially play in patterns of malaria transmission. Other questions relate to the possible roles of infective dose and acquired immunity in malaria fulminancy. Christophers emphasised there was little evidence that differences in exposure to malarial infection could explain epidemic patterns in the province in 1908. But in later years, malaria workers would return to the question of the impact of fluctuating immunity levels on epidemic patterns.

From the vantage point of 1909, it was difficult for Christophers to delineate any more precisely than he did the contribution of economic factors (acute hunger) to epidemicity relative to factors influencing malaria transmission. The subsequent four decades of marked decline in epidemic mortality, by contrast, offer a key opportunity to do so. Indeed, it is through analysis of post-1908 epidemic patterns that many of the outstanding questions can begin to be addressed. It is to these questions that this study is directed, re-examining the analysis and conclusions offered in *Malaria in the Punjab*, and placing them analytically in the context of subsequent malaria research and post-1908 patterns of epidemic decline. In this expanded task, Christophers's original study provides essential tools and concepts with which to do so.

Notes

1 J.W.W. Stephens, S.R. Christophers, 'The Relation of Species of Anopheles to Malaria Endemicity,' *Report to the Malarial Committee of the Royal Society*, VII, Feb. 1902, 15–19 [hereafter *RMCRS*]; J.W.W. Stephens, S.R. Christophers, 'Relation Between 'Species' of Anopheles and the Endemicity of Malaria,' in *Transactions of the Malaria Conference held at Nagpur in January 1902* (Nagpur: Nagpur Central Jail Press, 1902), 85–88, at 86. In larger urban areas such as Delhi an additional vector was *An. stephensi*.

2 S.R. Christophers, 'Second Report of the Anti-Malarial Operations in Mian Mir, 1901–1903,' *Sci. Mem. Off. Med. San. Dep.*, 9, 1904.

3 S.R. Christophers, C.A. Bentley, *Malaria in the Duars: Being the Second Report to the Advisory Committee Appointed by the Government of India to Conduct an Enquiry Regarding Blackwater and Other Fevers Prevalent in the Duars* (Simla: Government Monotype Press, 1911).

4 The term 'endemiology' appears to be a neologism coined by Christophers to distinguish 'normal' (endemic) levels of malaria mortality from that of exceptional 'epidemics,' hence to highlight the large range in clinical morbidity and mortality related to malaria transmission but determined by conditions of the human host. For further discussion, see ch. 13, pp. 408, 410, 414n.3.

5 'On Malaria in the Punjab,' *Proceedings of the Imperial Malaria Conference Held at Simla in October 1909* (Simla: Government Central Branch Press, 1910), 29–47 [hereafter Simla Conf.].

6 S.R. Christophers, 'Malaria in the Punjab,' *Sci. Mem. Off. Med. San. Dep.*, 46 (Calcutta: Superintendent Government Printing Office, 1911) [hereafter MP].

7 T. Ramachandra Rao, *Anophelines of India*, 1st ed. (New Delhi: Malaria Research Centre, ICMR, 1984), 374, 407.

8 E.P. Hicks, S. Abdul Majid, 'A Study of the Epidemiology of Malaria in a Punjab District,' *Records of the Malaria Survey of India*, 7, 1, 1937, 1–43, Chart 2, 4 [hereafter *RMSI*]. See also, 'Directorate of the National Malaria Eradication Programme,' *Malaria and Its Control in India*, Vol. 1 (New Delhi: Ministry of Family Welfare, 1986), 295.

9 MP, 132.

10 Ibid., 18, 21, 62.

11 Ibid., 26, 9, 11; Simla Conf., 30. The single exception in 1908 was the southeast region where fever deaths rose 'about a fortnight earlier,' timing which paralleled an earlier onset of the monsoon rains in this region.

12 MP, 9.

13 For a review of this research, see B. Mayne, 'The Influence of Relative Humidity on the Presence of Parasites in the Insect Carrier and the Initial Seasonal Appearance of Malaria in a Selected Area in India,' *IJMR*, 15, 4, 1928, 1073–1084; for Punjab, Hicks and Majid, 'Study of the Epidemiology of Malaria'; C.A. Gill, *The Genesis of Epidemics and Natural History of Disease* (London: Bailliere, Tindall & Cox, 1928), 151, Chart XI.

14 MP, 5–6.

15 S.R. Christophers, 'A New Statistical Method of Mapping Epidemic Disease in India, with Special Reference to the Mapping of Epidemic Malaria'; Simla Conf., 16–22, 18.

16 Ibid.

17 MP, 6. See also, S.R. Christophers, 'What Disease Costs India: Being a Statement of the Problem Before Medical Research in India,' *Indian Medical Gazette*, Apr. 1924, 196–200, at 198 [hereafter *IMG*].

18 MP, 10, 7.

19 Ibid., 10.

20 Ibid., 17–18.

21 Ibid., 17.

22 Simla Conf., 30; MP, 96.

23 Simla Conf., 30; *Report on the Sanitary Administration of the Punjab, 1908* (Lahore: Medical Department, Punjab), 13 [hereafter *PSCR*].

24 MP, Chart 3; *Gill Genesis of Epidemics*, 64. A similar picture of early intensity of infection is apparent in the severe 1929 epidemic in Sind; G. Covell, J.D. Baily, 'The Study of a Regional Epidemic of Malaria in Northern Sind,' *RMSI*, 3, 2, Dec. 1932, 279–321.

25 MP, 14, 11.; MP, Chart 2: Admission for Malaria, Bhera Dispensary; Simla Conf., 30.

26 Gill, *Genesis of Epidemics*, 69–70.

27 Ibid.

28 MP, 12.

29 Ibid., 12. In smaller towns where age distribution was likely to be less influenced by selective adult male migration, the predominance of deaths in children under 10 years of age was even more pronounced; ibid., 13.

30 Ibid., 13.

31 Ibid., 13, 14; Chart 4.

32 Ibid., 14.

33 Ibid.

34 Gill, *Genesis of Epidemics*, 107. Christophers would later describe a similar sequence in the 1934–1935 Ceylon malaria epidemic, a 'rapid increase in parasite density and later . . . [the] parasite rate'; 'Endemic and Epidemic Prevalence,' in M.F. Boyd, ed., *Malariology* (Philadelphia: W.B. Saunders, 1949), ch. 27, 698–721.

35 MP, 93.

36 S.P James, 'Malaria in India,' *Sci. Mem. Off. Med. San. Dep.*, 2, 1902, 81.

37 MP, 84; The discrepancy had prompted convoluted explanatory hypotheses by military officers involved in the Mian Mir anti-malaria operations; E.P. Sewell, 'Anti-Malarial Operations at Mian Mir,' *Journal of the Royal Army Medical Corps*, 5, 1905, 132–134.

38 MP, 83–84.

39 Ibid., 78, 80.

40 G. Macdonald, J. Abdul Majid, 'Report on an Intensive Malaria Survey in the Karnal District, Punjab,' *RMSI*, 2, 3, Sept. 1931, 423–477, 424–425.

41 MP, 2.

42 Ibid.

43 Ibid., 128.

44 Despite below-average rainfall, 1904 malarial fever hospitalisation rates among troops at Mian Mir were almost as high as in 1908; S.P. James, 'Malaria in Mian Mir,' in W.E. Jennings, ed., *Transactions of the Bombay Medical Congress, 1909* (Bombay: Bennett, Coleman & Co., 1910), 84–93, at 87 [hereafter *Trans. Bombay Med. Congress*].

45 MP, 71.

46 Ibid., 70–71.

47 Simla Conf., 21.

48 MP, 19. A reproduction by Learmonth of Christophers's original colour map of the 1908 epidemic is given here, for purposes of clarity. Note: the legend of Figure 2.8 is incorrectly labelled as "3X" rather than "5X" normal death rate.

49 Ibid., 20.

50 Ibid., 127.

51 Ibid., 21.

52 Ibid., 20.

53 Later, Christophers reproduced simplified versions of his 1911 maps that convey more clearly the focal spatial character; S.R. Christophers, 'Endemic and Epidemic Prevalence,' *Malariology*, 698–721, Figure 211.

54 A.T.A. Learmonth, 'Some Contrasts in the Regional Geography of Malaria in India and Pakistan,' *Transactions and Paper* (Institute of British Geographers), 23, 1957, 37–59, at 47.

55 MP, 26, 24; Christophers, 'What Disease Costs India,' 197.

56 MP, 26; Simla Conf., 32; C.A. Gill, 'Epidemic or Fulminant Malaria Together with a Preliminary Study of the Part Played by Immunity in Malaria,' *IJMR*, 2, 1, July 1914, 268–314.

57 Christophers, 'Endemic and Epidemic Prevalence,' 707; Gill, *Genesis of Epidemics*, 49, 52.

58 MP, Map 9 (in the text, referred to as 'Map 11'); ibid., 96–97.

59 Ibid., 71.

60 S.R. Christophers, 'Epidemic Malaria of the Punjab, with a Note on a Method of Predicting Epidemic Years,' *Paludism*, 2, 1911, 17–26.

61 Christophers, What Disease Costs India,' 197–199.

62 Ibid.

63 MP, 110.

64 Simla Conf., 39.

65 Ibid. [emphasis added].

66 MP, 107.

67 Ibid., 112, 95.

68 Ibid., Chart 6.

69 Ibid., 112, 107–108.

70 Ibid., 107.

71 'On Malaria in the Punjab'; Simla Conf., 38–39; MP, 105, 106. These monthly figures are calculated as an annualised rate, derived by multiplying a monthly death rate by 12, a technique common at the time for conveying short-term epidemic mortality severity, similar to monthly tracking of modern inflation levels expressed as an annualised inflation rate. See, for example, *PSCR* 1890, 4, 6.

72 MP, 105, 29–33; Simla Conf., 38–39.

73 Simla Conf., 38.

74 Ibid., 39. Christophers did not record class differentials in mortality except by broad religious group, but did note a consistent pattern of greater prevalence of splenomegaly, and greater size of spleen, amongst rural lower caste groups; MP, 106. The impact of hunger and 'physiological poverty' was already detailed in a paper presented at the Bombay Medical Congress in Feb. 1909; S.R. Christophers, C.A. Bentley, 'The Human Factor: An Extension of our Knowledge Regarding the Epidemiology of Malarial Disease,' in W.E. Jennings, ed., *Transactions of the Bombay Medical Congress* (Bombay: Bennett, Coleman & Co., 1910), 78–83 [hereafter 'The Human Factor'].

75 MP, 95.

76 Ibid.

77 Ibid., 108.

78 Ibid., 110.

79 Ibid., 108 [emphasis in original].

80 The term indicated a rise in staple foodgrain prices of more than 40 percent, a level at which, under the Famine Code, districts officials were required to 'test' for famine conditions by offering work on terms more punitive than those met with even on the large famine relief works. See ch. 10 at note 37.

81 *Proceedings of the Imperial Malaria Committee Held in Bombay on 16th and 17th November 1911* (Simla: Government Central Branch Press, 1912), reprinted in *Paludism*, 4, 1911, 1–129, at 82 [emphasis added] [hereafter Bombay Malaria Conf., 1911].

82 Christophers, 'Epidemic malaria of the Punjab, with a Note,' 22.

83 MP, 128 [emphasis in original].

84 Ibid., 129.

85 Simla Conf., 5.

86 Christophers calculated the 'extraordinary epidemic figure of 70' for Darawala village in Gujrat district, unreachable by him in early 1909 'for the flooded condition of the country'; MP, 62.

87 Ibid., 129, 132.

88 Ibid., 128 [emphasis added].

89 PSCR 1908, 13.

90 Simla Conf., 30–31; Gill, 'Epidemic or fulminant malaria,' 299 (Chart III); Gill, Genesis of Epidemics, 106.

91 MP, 124–125.

92 Ibid., 125, 129.

93 Simla Conf., 45.

94 MP, 106.

95 Christophers and Bentley, Malaria in the Duars, 62; Christophers and Bentley, 'The Human Factor,' 78.

96 Christophers and Bentley, 'The Human Factor,' 78–79.

97 The main Duars vector, An. minimus, is a highly anthropophilic species (feeding primarily on humans) in contrast to An. culicifacies, that feeds preferentially on livestock. Christophers's earlier Duars study had revealed extreme sporozoite rates of 6 to 25 per cent; W.W. Stephens, S.R. Christophers, 'Blackwater Fever: Summary and Conclusions,' RMCRS, 5, 1901, 12–27, at 20.

98 MP, 30.

99 MP, 128; Simla Conf., 43.

100 Ibid., 38–39.

101 MP, 131, 71.

102 Ibid., 73.

103 Simla Conf., 38.

104 MP, 112.

105 Ibid., 127.

106 Ibid., 132.

107 Ibid.

108 Simla Conf., 43.

109 Ibid.

110 MP, 83–84, 26.

111 Ibid., 43.

112 Ibid., 132.

113 Ibid.

114 Ibid.

115 Ibid., 98–102.

116 Simla Conf., 40.

117 S. Watts, 'British Development Policies and Malaria in India 1897-c.1929,' Past and Present, 165, 1999, 141–181.

118 MP, 129, 102–103.

119 See ch. 4.

120 MP, 110.

3 Theoretical and methodological issues

> The exceptional mortality of the year began just when the famine ended [and] the scourge of the times was 'fever.'
> – W.R. Cornish, *MSCR* 1877, Appendix 1, xxviii–xxix.

This study of epidemic malaria in Punjab takes as its point of departure Christophers's 1911 analysis based on the insights and tools it offers historians for estimating annual malaria mortality in the region and for analysing its determinants. Here, as a first step in testing his conclusions, we look at each of the three variables employed in the original study (Oct.–Dec. death rate, July–Sept. rainfall, and annual wheat price) to consider how well they can be expected to reflect malaria mortality in Punjab across the colonial period and those factors considered key determinants of malaria epidemicity: malaria transmission and acute hunger.

Punjab province in the late 19th century encompassed 29 districts: twenty-four in the alluvial plains of the northern Indus and Jumna river systems; two Himalayan hill districts of Simla and Kangra; and the northwestern hill tracts of Rawalpindi, Bannu, and the Peshawar division (Figure 2.1). Christophers's 1911 malaria study was based on observations from the 24 plains districts where malaria manifested a sharply seasonal and identifiable pattern of autumn transmission, and where the fulminant form of the disease appeared most prominently.[1] The statistical analysis that follows is based upon these 24 plains districts, incorporating several minor district boundary changes in the later years of colonial rule.[2] The present study extends the analysis to the 1908–1940 period and includes only 23 districts: with the 1911 transfer of the imperial seat of government from Calcutta to the city of Delhi, Delhi district no longer remained within the administrative jurisdiction of Punjab province.

Much of the routine statistical and administrative reporting was interrupted in the final years of colonial rule with the severe food crisis and famine conditions associated with World War II, the abrupt handover of political power in 1947, and socio-administrative dislocation with ensuing Partition. The last year a regular annual public health report was published for the province was 1940. Due to these exceptional circumstances, regression analysis of the rain-price-epidemic mortality relationship has been limited to the 1868–1940 period. Village-level vital registration data continued to be collected, and were later published in various summary volumes after 1940. However, only those volumes relating to the 11 eastern districts constituting the post-Partition Indian state of (East) Punjab are considered in the present study. They nonetheless make possible quantitative tracking of autumn (malaria) mortality trends in the eastern half of the former colonial province of Punjab across the late pre- and early post-Independence years, a period that encompasses abrupt decline in malaria transmission in the state under the 1950s DDT-based malaria eradication program.[3] These 1941–1960 results are presented separately in chapter 12.

Land and livelihood: the Punjab agricultural economy

The dramatic contrast in the character of malaria between its 'ordinary' and its 'fulminant' forms in colonial Punjab was a function, Christophers concluded, not simply of yearly fluctuations in malaria transmission in the province, but also of equally wide fluctuations in the region's agricultural economy from year to year – heavy monsoon rains, drought, and foodgrain price swings that undermined access to subsistence food for considerable portions of the population. So it is here, with the land and its people, that we begin in assessing the 1911 inquiry's conclusions.

Forming the most westerly portion of the fertile Indo-Gangetic plains of the Indian subcontinent, the Punjab region historically was defined geographically and economically by the five rivers from which this northwest corner of the Indian subcontinent derives its name (*punj*, five; *ab*, water) (Figure 2.1). Landlocked, the region is subject to climatic extremes, experiencing freezing temperatures in winter and dry heat of 45–50°C. degrees in the pre-monsoon months of May and June. As in much of the rest of the subcontinent, the yearly agricultural cycles of Punjab were shaped by rainfall patterns: the southwest monsoon rains (July–September), and scantier winter showers. Total annual rainfall in much of the region was low, declining in relation to distance from the Himalayan mountain range in the north (Figure 2.2). From a mean of over 30 inches in the submontane districts, average rainfall fell to 10 to 20 inches in the central and southeastern Hissar Division (now Haryana), and to less than five inches in the desert southwest. Hence the key historical role played by the region's silt-laden rivers in cultivation and human settlement.

The late June to September rains provided 75 to 90 per cent of the annual rainwater potential over most of the northern subcontinent,[4] a seasonality even more pronounced in the drier northwest. Moreover, the rain that does arrive in this region is highly variable from year to year, characteristic of all low rainfall regions.[5] In 1903, the Irrigation Commission estimated that in central and southeast Punjab, one in four years were 'dry' years, and one in 10 were years of severe drought (deficiency of 40 per cent), comparable variability seen only in parts of the Madras Deccan.[6]

With the exception of the northern submontane districts, agriculture in much of the Punjab region historically depended largely on naturally occurring inundation irrigation of fields bordering its major rivers. Flowing southward from the Himalayan foothills, the region's five rivers cross 200,000 square kilometres of alluvial plains, converging in the southwest to form the Indus River system. Autumn *(kharif)* crops were sown with the monsoon rains and irrigated by flood waters derived from summer rainfall catchment in the Himalayan foothills above the plains. Winter-spring *(rabi)* crops depended on light winter rains and inundation flows derived from melting snow in the same mountains.

The degree of dependence upon rainfall and inundation flooding for cultivation varied across the province. In the near-desert southwest, agriculture depended on riverain inundation and canal irrigation. In the northern districts, natural river inundation flows were supplemented by rainfall, and to a varying extent by well irrigation. In the north-central districts of Jullundur, Hoshiarpur, and Amritsar, for example, where ground-water was only 10 to 20 feet below the surface, well irrigation was used extensively (Table 3.1), leaving production relatively insulated from the vagaries of the monsoon, and here population density was high.[7] The rural economy of the southeastern region of the province, by contrast, was much more dependent on the vicissitudes of the summer monsoon rains. Only a single perennial river, the Jumna, traversed the southeast, a tributary of the Ganges further east, and rather than transecting the region, it formed the eastern border of the province. In Hissar district, now western Haryana, inundation waters came from the hills to the south, and flowed only

Table 3.1 Per cent area irrigated (acres), by well, govt canals, 1903–1904, 24 plains districts, Punjab

	Total cropped area (acres)	% area irrigated		
		Govt canals	Wells	Total
Southeast:				
Hissar	1,866,161	11.3	0.1	11.7
Rohtak	830,342	16.4	2.7	19.1
Gurgaon	801,546	9.3	10.4	19.8
Delhi	478,469	13.4	18.9	32.3
Karnal	971,018	14.4	10.0	26.1
Amballa	782,370	0.2	2.5	4.1
Central:				
Hoshiarpur	845,048	1.1	4.1	7.0
Jullundur	803,105	0.0	46.7	**47.0**
Ludhiana	794,452	6.3	20.6	27.0
Ferozepur	1,838,277	26.0	7.7	**42.3**
Lahore	1,227,575	49.4	22.2	**76.7**
Amritsar	928,133	30.2	25.3	**55.8**
North:				
Gurdaspur	951,623	4.7	10.9	19.0
Sialkot	1,024,652	0.0	37.6	**42.6**
Gujrat	855,855	0.0	19.2	19.2
Gujranwala	1,067,181	39.2	27.3	**66.8**
Jhelum	632,867	0.1	4.9	5.4
West/Southwest:				
Shahpur	811,044	34.3	18.0	**58.8**
Jhang	1,856,999	79.2	13.2	**92.8**
Multan	784,211	70.9	10.3	**83.7**
Montgomery	535,967	32.0	40.5	**75.1**
Dhera Ismail Khan	620,826	0.0	17.3	19.9
Muzaffargarh	478,118	62.3	10.5	**77.7**
Dhera Ghazi Khan	668,850	32.8	6.1	**42.9**

Note: Total irrigated area >40% in bold.

Source: *Season and Crops Report*, Punjab, 1903–1904.

briefly during the summer monsoon. Moreover, with a water table often below 150 feet, well irrigation was impractical. Here, harvest failure, Bhattacharya observes, was 'an integral part of the life of the region.'[8]

Regional differences in rainfall and irrigation potential across the province meant major differences in timing and patterns of foodgrains cultivation. In much of the north-central and western regions, the spring *rabi* harvest was more important for food crops, with wheat and gram nourished by winter rains and the spring run-off from melting snows in the Himalayan foothills; 'dry' millet crops were sown with the monsoon rains on unirrigated, higher land. In the dry southwest, wheat also predominated in the riverain tracts dependent on inundation irrigation, its cultivation much expanded with a vast expansion in canal irrigation in the second half of the 19th century. Cultivation in the southeast, in contrast, was limited largely to a single monsoon-dependent *kharif* crop, the population depending on unirrigated 'dry' crops as staple foodgrains: bajra (spiked millet), gram (chickpea), and jowar (sorghum).

Historically, the southeastern region made up by Hissar and Rohtak districts was primarily pastoralist. Its agricultural economy was closely interdependent, however, with that of north-central Punjab, the latter representing the main market for cattle reared in the southeast. Jullundur district alone imported over 10,000 bullocks annually, whereas in years of drought, a 'reverse flow of foodgrain and fodder' took place.[9] 'Pastoral and agricultural zones experience food and bad years in different ways,' Bhattacharya observes. '[W]hen Hissar lost its herds, Jullundur did not.' By the turn of the 20th century, several branches of the West Jumna Canal reached into Hissar district and its cultivated area modestly expanded, yet agriculture remained precarious relative to other regions of the province.

Thus, failure of the monsoon rains had quite different effects across the Province depending on the area, crop patterns, and availability of ground well and inundation irrigation. In much of central and southeastern Punjab, drought and reduced inundation flows affected both 'dry' and riverain crops. Loss of a single season's harvest might not trigger disastrous declines in food accessibility where some field work was still available in anticipation of adequate rains for the subsequent season. However, consecutive seasons of drought, especially those spanning more than a single year, would almost certainly trigger massive declines in employment in addition to crop losses, triggering sell-off of livestock at distress price levels and soaring acute hunger.

By contrast, flood-triggered harvest failure was common to all regions of the province. The line between beneficial inundation and destructive floods was a fine one, the extreme flatness of the plains rendering much of the region prone to extensive flooding. Given historical peri-riverain human settlement, heavy rains upstream meant a large proportion of the population of some districts, and standing crops, were subject to potentially destructive flood action. In addition, the extremely gradual slope of the land meant that the river beds were constantly shifting, leaving many deserted riverains as depressed areas 'peculiarly liable to flooding.'[10]

Thus, although a region of great agricultural productivity by virtue of its river-borne alluvial soils, Punjab was also subject to wide fluctuations in harvests and prosperity. Historically, that vulnerability was further heightened by geography. Forming the corridor between central and western Asia and the Indian subcontinent, Punjab was also a region of enormous strategic importance, subject through the millennia to invading armies. Thus, superimposed upon general climatic vulnerabilities were the recurring famine-triggering depredations of warfare.

Following the decline of the Mughal empire in the 18th century, Sikh military dominance gradually extended outward from the Amritsar area. Most of Punjab, however, had come under British control by 1849 following costly wars across the first half of the 19th century. The new colonial administration soon embarked upon construction of a vast network of irrigation canals in the province. Tapping the waters of the five major rivers as they emerged from the northern hills, canals diverted irrigation water along the watersheds of the *doabs*, the bands of slightly higher land between the rivers unreached by the seasonal inundation flows (Figure 3.1). '[T]he Punjab offered,' Paustian observed with characteristic imperial enthusiasm, 'an almost ideal base for the development of irrigation schemes. The Himalayas provided a natural reservoir of water which flowed down the rivers during the very portion of the year when moisture was most needed on the parched plains.'[11] The canal system made possible perennial irrigation of millions of hectares of land primarily in the dry central and western districts of the province, the canal-irrigated area quadrupling from 943,043 acres in the early 1880s to 4,123,548 acres by the turn of the century. Overnight, much of the region was transformed into a wheat export market economy as well as a crucial source of taxation and irrigation revenues for the British Raj.

This hydrological transformation was not without major ecological impacts. The vast network of canals and rail transportation affected surface water drainage, triggering waterlogging in many local areas, including in the northern submontane districts from which the canal headwaters emerged. Constructed without lining of channel beds, a large portion of the irrigation waters was lost to subsoil percolation, raising subsoil water levels. An even more serious problem was increasing alkalinisation of canal-irrigated soils. Together, these processes undermined productivity in affected tracts, and remained largely uncorrected, and in the latter case, unhalted, through the colonial period.[12]

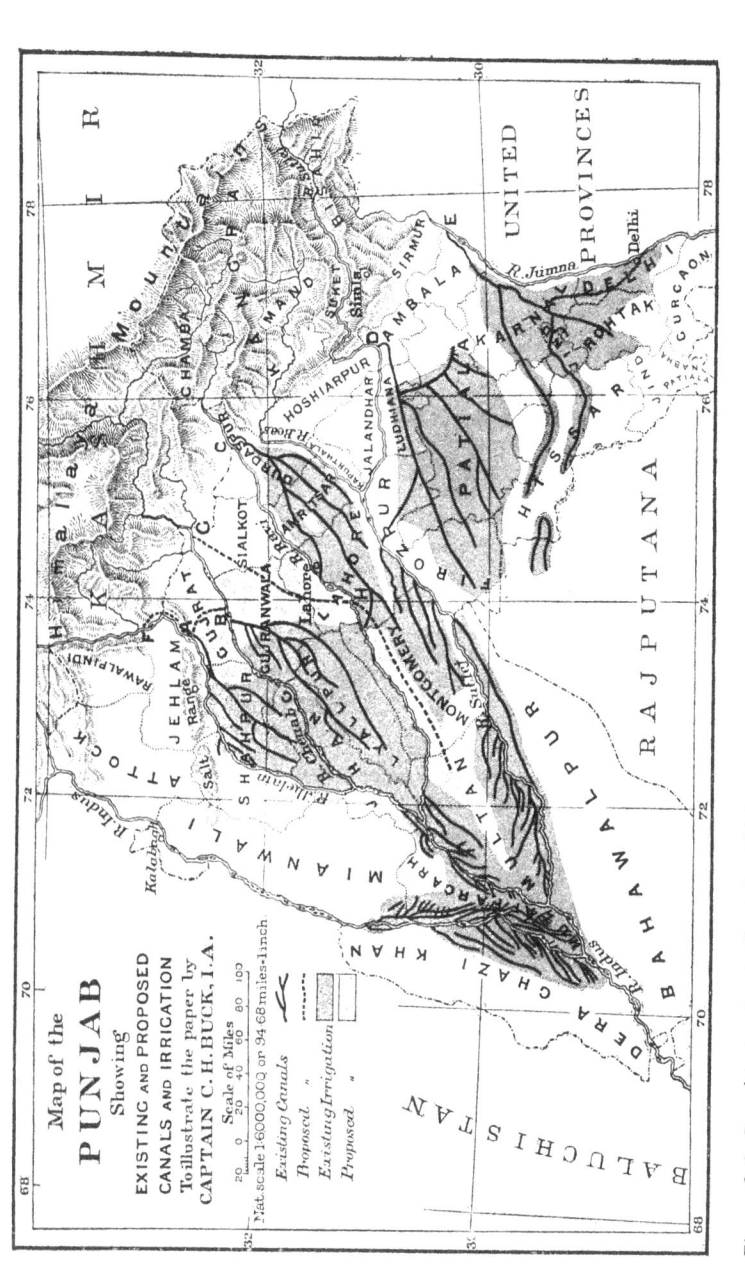

Figure 3.1 Canal irrigation in Punjab, 1906

Source: C.H. Buck, 'Canal Irrigation in Punjab,' *Geographical Journal*, 27, 1, Jan. 1906, p. 61.

But the commercialisation of agriculture also brought changes in land tenure and foodgrain price behaviour, affecting food security more broadly, shifts that would be reflected in patterns of malaria mortality across the colonial period. It is this period of profound ecological and socio-economic change which forms the backdrop to Christophers's 1911 study of epidemic malaria in the region.

Estimating malaria transmission

In his study, Christophers traced malaria transmission rates in 1908 Punjab through dispensary records, fever cases rising in mid- to late September, peaking in early October, then rapidly falling off thereafter as humidity and temperature levels fell. Subsequent researchers confirmed this general timing in the build-up in malaria incidence in relation to elevated atmospheric humidity levels over the course of summer monsoon season. They confirmed, further, that total July–September monsoon rainfall largely predicted the crucial factor of rainfall continuity in maintaining adequate atmospheric humidity.[13] It was on this basis that malaria workers considered July–September rainfall levels as predictive of autumn malaria incidence, a measure employed in the present study as well.

Spleen enlargement (splenomegaly) was also considered a general indicator of malaria prevalence in a region, following mid-19th-century investigations by Dempster and Baker of malarial fever in southeastern Punjab.[14] As the principal organ that breaks down damaged red blood cells, the spleen typically enlarges over a period of several months following malaria infection, becoming readily palpable on abdominal examination: the 'spleen rate' is typically defined as the per cent of children under the age of 10 years in which the spleen is palpable below the left rib cage. Twice yearly spleen rate surveys were conducted on Punjab school children between 1914 and 1943.

As a measure of year-to-year malaria transmission in the province, however, these data are of limited value since they are available only after 1913. Moreover, spleen enlargement is not necessarily specific to a given year. Following the 1908 epidemic, spleen rates were high across much of eastern Punjab, subsequently declining over several years. In addition, poverty was repeatedly observed to prolong recovery rate and increase relapses, affecting both spleen size and rate, thus limiting further its value as a measure of current malaria transmission.[15] Their value in historical analysis lies primarily in qualitive terms, indicating presence and very general levels of malaria in a population.

The parasite rate, that proportion of persons found with microscopically confirmed malaria parasites in the bloodstream (parasitaemia), is a more direct measure of transmission levels,[16] but time-series data are even more limited, and relate only to very local conditions rather than entire regions. By contrast, rainfall data, though an indirect measure, indicate likely transmission levels in Punjab over entire regions and extended time periods.

No single source of district-level monthly rainfall data is available for the entire 73-year study period (1868–1940) for Punjab province. For the period 1868–1899, district monthly rainfall data appear in the annual provincial sanitary reports. For the years 1901 through to 1940, data from the *Season and Crop Reports* series are employed.[17] For the remaining year, 1900, district rain figures are computed from fortnightly data available in the 1900–1901 Punjab Land Revenue Administration report.

Measuring malaria mortality

Malaria in the Punjab also demonstrated that malaria mortality rates in the province followed transmission rates by two to three weeks, peaking in mid- to late October, with excess fever mortality continuing into the months of November and December in epidemic years (Figure 2.5). In his quantitative analysis, Christophers employed October–November fever deaths as an estimate of annual province-level malaria mortality.[18] In the current study, district Oct.–Dec. fever death rate (per mille) figures are used, as was employed in subsequent analysis in the province,[19] and a detrended series is constructed as a means of adjusting for changes in levels of reporting over time.

Inevitably, some of the deaths recorded under the fever category for these months were non-malarial.[20] But in the absence of other major autumn epidemic diseases, the detrended Oct.–Dec. fever death rate data set provides annual fluctuations from trend that can be considered principally malarial, and thus an estimate of yearly *epidemic* malaria mortality intensity. One exception to this was influenza. However, there appears to be no reference to influenza recorded in the colonial sanitary reports, with the single exception of 1918.[21] Influenza mortality was enormous in Punjab in war-time 1918, a year also of undeclared famine across the region,[22] and most of these deaths were recorded under the 'fever' category in the months of November and December. In this case, because those deaths are indistinguishable from malarial fever deaths, the year 1918 has been omitted from statistical analysis of post-1908 malaria trends.

One source of potential *under*-registration of malaria deaths relates to the clinical symptoms predominant in epidemic (fulminant) years. In its non-famine 'intermittent' form, episodic fever was followed by intervals of normal body temperature. In epidemic years, this profile altered considerably, with fever taking a 'remittent' form more characteristic of relapsing fever, or a 'continuous' fever typical of typhoid and typhus fevers.[23] And among the famished, gastrointestinal symptoms frequently predominated alongside fever, with sanitary officials repeatedly remarking on the difficulty of distinguishing between cholera and malarial fever.[24]

Certainly, much of famine-related 'choleraic fever' was actual cholera. In the case of the 1877 Madras famine, a severe cholera epidemic broke out among the starvation victims herded into hastily constructed famine relief camps at a point well before the return of the rains and active malaria transmission. A similar outbreak occurred during the 1899–1900 famine in Punjab among 11,000 relief workers transported by rail to work on new canal irrigation sites in western tracts of the province, also well before the monsoon rains.[25]

Deaths reported as cholera in Punjab between 1867 and 1896 show a bimodal pattern: the first, smaller peak appearing in the months of extreme heat and dryness of May–June, and a larger, second peak in August–September.[26] Between 1897 and 1921, a period of recurring famines, reported cholera deaths in the August–September period were three times the level recorded in May–June. Among these late- and post-monsoon cholera deaths, some may well have been due to malaria that was 'choleraic in severity.'[27]

Finally, as seen in chapter 2, Christophers, in mapping comparative epidemic intensity levels across the province in given epidemic years, devised a second measure, an 'Epidemic Figure,' as a way of adjusting for temporal and inter-district differences in completeness of vital registration. As a ratio measure, however, it introduces problems of its own. In the famine-prone districts, early summer death rates leading up to the monsoon period tended to be higher than in districts with greater access to well irrigation. As a ratio of autumn to summer mortality, the Epidemic Figure thus introduces an under-estimation bias in such districts.[28] In the present study, modern methods of detrending are employed instead to adjust for changes in completeness of vital registration in the earlier years and inter-district differences in reporting and measuring malarial fever deaths.

Estimating acute hunger

The word 'starvation' does not appear in *Malaria in the Punjab*. Though his entire 'Human Factor' chapter was devoted to the subject, only once does Christophers point to acute hunger directly, the reference repeated here because of its import: that 'a full dietary . . . falls to the lot of but few of the poorer classes, and . . . in times of scarcity these are accustomed to adapt themselves to circumstances *by proportionately restricting the amount of the food they take.*'[29] Despite its clinical reserve, this single sentence encapsulates the two central dimensions to historical hunger: not enough to eat ('chronic' undernourishment), and episodically not nearly enough to eat, semi- or frank starvation. It was to the latter that *Malaria in the Punjab* was addressed.

How can acute hunger trends be assessed? Christophers's decision in 1909 to employ market foodgrain price levels as a quantitative gauge of famishment no doubt reflected the colonial administration's assiduous attention to foodgrain prices levels as a predictor of economic stress and social unrest, and is one followed in the present study.[30] The decision is based on two different aspects of starvation vulnerability. The first, self-evident, reflects the cost of food *per se*. For those already at bare subsistence levels, a 40 per cent price rise meant a 30 per cent reduction in caloric consumption. The second aspect is as a signal of collapse in agricultural production, rural employment, and livelihood. Poor harvests drove prices up, but also meant contraction of the entire local rural economy. To a major extent, then, the hunger implication of rising prices was indirect, as a signal of widespread loss of earnings – in Amartya Sen's terms, a loss of 'exchange entitlements.'[31] Lost livelihood meant little access to food *regardless of its price*. Indeed, it was recognition of the importance of unemployment that informed colonial efforts at famine relief which were directed to employment generation. Though prevalence of both hungers would increase under such conditions,[32] what distinguished periods of 'scarcity' was the much greater *relative* increase in acute hunger: semi- and frank starvation.

The dual character to high prices ('scarcity') is particularly important with regard to district-level Punjab analysis because of marked regional differences in rural agricultural economies. In the southeast, with little secure irrigation, agricultural collapse was triggered primarily by drought, as was the case also for much of the Indian subcontinent. Here, prices reflected both prohibitive cost as well as plummeting employment and income. By contrast, in much of the north-central and submontane tracts of Punjab, where natural inundation flows were supplemented by well irrigation (Table 3.1), collapse in agricultural production was triggered more severely by *excess* rainfall, through flooding. As one official remarked,

> [Amritsar] district as a whole is probably as well protected from the effects of drought as any in the Province. A failure of the summer rains may mean a shortage of fodder and pulse crops, but in the greater part of the district an excess monsoon . . . causes more extensive loss and suffering. . . . [t]he evil effects of [which] . . . may last for years.[33]

Heavier rainfall, however, meant bountiful harvests *in general* for the province and northern subcontinent as a whole and thus was associated with downward pressure on grain prices. Thus, periods of agricultural paralysis in the well-irrigated districts were associated often with low foodgrain prices rather than high, and the dual character of prices as hunger indicator did not apply.

This regional dichotomy in drought impact on food insecurity was not absolute. Low rainfall would limit the acreage sown even in many of the north-central districts in areas where cultivation of non-wheat crops extended to higher tracts beyond the reach of irrigation systems. Also, high foodgrain prices, regardless of cause, would affect those landless households forced to purchase staple grains on the open market for any portion of the year. Price vulnerability was especially acute in the towns where urban artisans and other wage labour households were dependent on the market throughout the year.

In reading the provincial sanitary reports from the late 19th century, it is difficult not to be struck by the importance accorded foodgrain prices as a predictor of the state of public health (mortality levels). The annual reports were prefaced by detailed data on prevailing foodgrain prices, wage rates, rainfall, and harvest conditions, information considered essential for interpreting health and mortality levels in a given year. From the earliest days of 19th-century official famine relief efforts, rising grain prices were the primary warning sign of impending famine. For the colonial administration, tracking price levels was of vital interest in anticipating social unrest. The importance of foodgrain prices, then, as a general *signal* of acute hunger for this period is less disputable than the methodological question as to how closely yearly price data can be expected to 'pinpoint' and *measure* shifts in food access.[34]

Limitations of foodgrain price data

Limitations to foodgrain price data as a measure of acute hunger relate to issues of both sensitivity and specificity. Official price data represent retail prices at major district markets, not rates paid by villagers in remote rural areas buying in small quantities from local dealers. But district market price reports themselves were subject to considerable inaccuracy. Explained one official, district data 'do not sufficiently represent the oscillations' in price levels. 'Extreme abnormalities are generally smoothed away by the clerks and *(horresco referens)* the officials concerned who fear they may be called upon to explain them.'[35]

Beyond questions of accuracy, prices were an imprecise indicator of starvation prevalence across a scarcity period extending several years. Typically, a single episode of high prices triggered by drought would overlap two, often three, calendar years. Grain prices would begin to rise immediately following failure of the monsoon rains. Levels of acute hunger and frank starvation, however, would peak only a year later, at the point where return of the rains finally brought the drought and famine to an end. Market prices, however, generally remained elevated well into the post-famine year, as surplus peasant producers tended to hold on to grain as they replenished household stores.[36] This three-year pattern can readily be seen in the behaviour of Punjab wheat prices for the 1869–1908 period (Figure 3.2). Episodes of above normal grain prices generally were associated first with a year of negligible malaria transmission (drought); a second year in

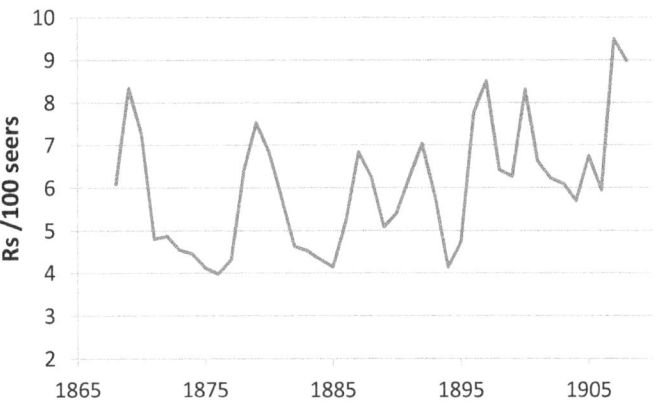

Figure 3.2 Mean annual nominal wheat price (Rs/100 seers), 1868–1908, 24 plains districts, Punjab

Source: See Table 4.1.

which hunger reached its peak; and a third year in which agricultural conditions, and starvation, were returning to normal levels. Of the three, only in the middle year would epidemic starvation coincide with malaria transmission (normal or above normal depending on the character of the monsoon rains), and therefore only in this one year could one expect to see, and measure, a relationship between malaria and acute hunger.

Beyond methodological limitations, use of market grain prices as a measure of acute hunger is further complicated by the fact that the first half of the colonial period saw a fundamental transformation in the rural economy of Punjab brought about by the commercialisation of much of the South Asian agricultural economy. These changes profoundly altered the behaviour of foodgrain prices in relation to local harvest conditions. Before development of the railways that began in 1853, the cost of transporting bulk goods overland was prohibitive. With the exception of limited river transport, foodgrain surpluses were marketed mainly locally[37] and regional foodgrain prices bore a fairly simple relationship to local harvest conditions. Bountiful crops brought prices down and poor conditions pushed them up.[38] Moreover, in years of good harvests, surplus producers tended to store grain rather than sell it at very low prices, a form of food security insurance that also tended to moderate price fluctuations, a buffering effect, however, that was limited in the case of consecutive poor harvests.[39]

This relationship was transformed after 1860 with developments in rail transportation in Punjab and across the subcontinent. In 1870, construction was completed on a railway which joined the seven major cities of the province (Figure 3.3). By 1878, this system extended to Karachi on the Arabian Sea, the port from which Punjab wheat was exported to Europe and other international markets. In years of good harvests, it became increasingly possible for larger landowners and traders to market surplus grain rather than keeping stores within the village, a development which quickly undermined the traditional practice of rural grain storage. With extension of rail links across the subcontinent by the 1870s, local foodgrain prices in Punjab very quickly came to be influenced by harvest conditions prevailing in other parts of the subcontinent, as seen in the case of the drought-triggered south Indian famine of 1876–1877.[40] A decade later, Punjab wheat and other grains were often selling at near-famine-level prices in spite of generally good harvests across the province, due to a dramatic increase in exports to Britain in response to high international prices.[41]

In a remarkably short period of time, access to staple foodgrains for those groups with little or no land of their own had become

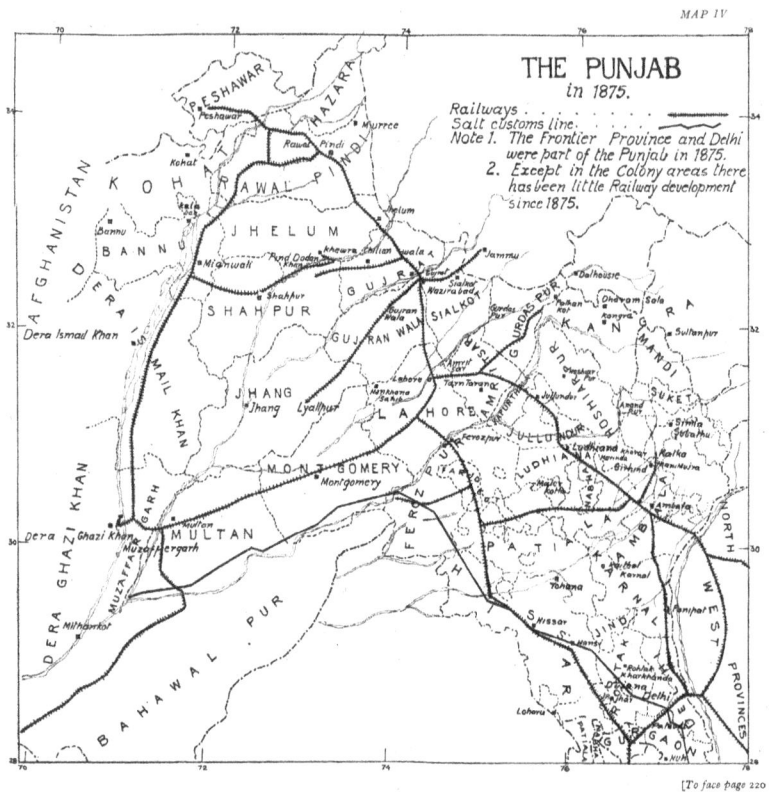

Figure 3.3 The Punjab in 1875

Source: H.K. Trevaskis, *Land of the Five Rivers* (Oxford: Oxford University Press, 1928), opp. 220.

increasingly subject to the vagaries of not only local climatic factors but also those of regional and international grain markets. In the case of the 1908 epidemic, the dramatic rise in Punjab prices to 'scarcity' levels in 1908 was triggered by drought the preceding year, but also by the export of large quantities of grain out of the province to the neighbouring United Provinces in response to overt famine there. Though ultimately railway transport held the potential of helping mitigate the effects of local harvest failure, it did so at a cost.

Thus, while soaring foodgrain prices *signalled* episodic subsistence crises in the historical records, they do not always provide a quantitative measure of *local* distress, a limitation Christophers stressed:

[W]hilst prices give us some idea of the degree of general scarcity, they fail to point out to us areas especially affected by failure of crops and other adverse conditions, the reason being that there is a very remarkable averaging process in regard to ruling prices so that however severely one area is affected by shortage of crops the prices after a brief discrepancy tend to level up if the other areas are unaffected.[42]

Levels of subsistence

How foodgrain price volatility translated into actual food consumption can be estimated only against a background of normal consumption levels. How close to the wire were the poorer classes in the Punjab? Little reliable data on rural wage rates exist for the earlier decades of the colonial period. But the frequently quoted normative rate of two annas a day for 'occasional wage' labourers itself gives some indication of consumption levels.[43] At the lowest grain prices recorded for the 1868–1908 period (four rupees per 100 seers), a two-anna wage would have bought 2.9 kilograms of wheat – slightly more for the millet grains and gram. Spent entirely on foodgrains, this would provide bare minimum calories for a household of two adults and three children, assuming 2,600 calories per adult member. In other words, under good conditions – low prices and regular employment – daily wages allowed nothing for non-grain foods, non-food expenses, or savings for unemployment periods, illness, or price increases. This does not take into account the possibility of additional family earnings, but the lower wages of women and children at best are likely to have only filled in the gaps for irregular adult male earnings.[44] Harvest labour, paid in kind, was the one period of the year when limited savings were possible, estimated at six kilograms of grain per day.[45] Hence the implications of harvest failure for earnings and subsistence precarity, and the added consequences of associated soaring foodgrain prices. A 1937 income survey found between one-third and one-half of the village households in the Madras presidency were 'underfed' in caloric terms. Among poor tenant households, annual income averaged Rs 50–80, food intake (July–August) averaging 1,664 calories a day, the investigators describing the households 'without exaggeration' to be 'half-starved.'[46]

In the face of recurring famines in the 1860s and 1870s across the subcontinent, a confidential GOI enquiry into the 'economic conditions of the lower classes of the population' was undertaken that asked provincial officials to assess whether the 'frequently repeated (assertion) that the greater proportion of the population of India suffer from a daily insufficiency of food is wholly untrue or partially true.'[47] Given the leading nature of the question, provincial officials generally answered in the negative.[48] But the actual content of the local reports was never made public. Leaked excerpts, however, suggested that daily grain consumption amongst agricultural labourers in the Northwest Provinces ranged from 13 to 22 ounces per day, and in Bihar, roughly 40 per cent of the population – agricultural labourers, tenants, and petty land-holders – subsisted with 'one meal a day instead of two.'[49]

In the case of Punjab, a summary of district officials' testimony appears appended to the 1898 Punjab Famine Commission Report,[50] and again, the official summary was generally sanguine. Several local officials however drew 'a very dismal picture of the state of the people in Shahpur and Gurdaspur. . . . Of the Muhammadan population 4 per cent live at starvation point, and 20 per cent do not get sufficient food.'[51] The Deputy Commissioner of Gurgaon district cautiously offered that '[i]n fair seasons there is not actual want of food, but the standard of living is perilously low, directly prices rise or failing health abridges labour, difficulties begin.[52] It is a grave fact,' he continued,

> that at certain periods of the year there is a considerable portion of the population which eke out their grain food with what they call 'ság' (mainly either grain- or mustard leaf), and . . . wild fruits. . . . [W]e cannot deny there is [an] unsatisfactory mass of low diet in the country even in normal conditions.[53]

British administrators routinely referred to the Punjab as the 'land of the peasant proprietor,' and indeed, estimates for the 1860s suggest that up to three-quarters of the land was cultivated by independent peasants ('owner cultivators').[54] But by the turn of the century, it appears that slightly less than half the area was cultivated directly by peasant owners, and over 40 per cent by tenants-at-will with few or no occupancy rights. To some extent, this reflects more complete registration in later Census surveys. Part of the increase, however, appears to have been real, occurring during the final decades of the 19th century.[55] Over this same period, the terms of tenancy worsened as colonial tenancy laws shifted the balance of economic power further in favour of landlords by making it easier to evict tenants.[56]

The first detailed enquiry into land ownership in the province in the 1920s found that 56 per cent of the agricultural population (owners and tenants) cultivated less than five acres of land, and of these almost half cultivated less than one acre,[57] an amount unlikely sufficient to meet basic subsistence needs even with highly intensive cultivation. 'What was retained by the petty tenant,' Bhattacharya suggests, after paying half or more of the produce as rent, might amount to 'less than the total wage of a regular labourer.'[58] For a substantial part of the agricultural population, then, basic survival was precarious and at least in part dependent on wage labour earnings. This dependency was absolute for the landless, a group which in 1881 was estimated to constitute 11 per cent of the agricultural population.[59] In addition, many traditional village artisans lived at subsistence levels in normal times.[60] Among the weaver communities, livelihood since the mid-19th century had been especially undermined by imports of textiles from Britain.

These various data, despite their limitations, together suggest that a substantial proportion of Punjabi households lived at bare subsistence levels and thus must have been quickly affected by drought-induced unemployment and high foodgrain prices. Traditionally, most wages for labourers and servants in Punjab were paid in kind rather than in cash, and thus were not entirely dependent on the market prices. But this was changing rapidly by the turn of the century.[61] Yet even in the absence of a cash economy, foodgrain prices probably reflected hunger closely. Since harvest wages of agricultural labourers were in many cases a set proportion of the produce, their earnings declined in proportion to the crop failure. Traditional master-servant obligations might provide some kind of buffer, but it is unlikely handouts made up for deficient work and earnings.[62] Moreover, during periods of drought and famine, wages declined not just in real terms but also in nominal levels:[63] in 1877 Sirsa district, wages fell to one anna a day.[64] Neeladri Bhattacharya suggests that this collapse in wage rates in bad years was the basis of the large-scale employment of famine labour at 'starvation wages,' citing 1899 famine relief wages in Hissar district as one-quarter non-famine Public Works Department rates in real terms.[65] Such reductions were probably common historically, but the increasing marketability of grain after 1860 further weakened the position of village labourers.[66]

Even in good years, at least some purchases were unavoidable for the poorer households during agriculturally slack portions of the year, often amounting to loans from wealthier landowners and local moneylenders. For the very poor, of course, who possessed nothing in the way of collateral, except their children, borrowing in times of harvest failure was hardly an option. Loans to those so likely to succumb in times of drought were clearly an extremely 'bad risk,' and if given at all, were available only at exorbitant interest rates of as much as 200 per cent.[67] As a respondent to the 1880 Famine Commission pointed out, the field labourer 'has no resources, and having no security to offer is generally unable to borrow, and thus is seldom in debt. But a famine at once throws them on public or private charity.'[68]

Trends in wage levels

This period also saw a distinctly new phenomenon in price behaviour as well. Compounding subsistence vulnerability still further, grain prices in the final years of the 19th century increasingly failed to return to pre-famine levels (Figure 3.4a). The gradual rise was unmatched by corresponding increases in wage levels until well into the 20th century. Employing data from the *Prices and Wages* series, Bhattacharya found a substantial decline in real wage rates in Punjab from the late 1880s, recovering only after 1910 (Figure 3.4b), a pattern seen also in the Madras Presidency.[69] In commenting on the rise of prices in Punjab, the Sialkot Settlement officer in 1895 questioned the assumption that increases brought general prosperity, suggesting the majority of cultivators in the district were not benefitted by the higher prices. 'They require every grain they can produce for the support of themselves, their families and their cattle. . . . [t]hose who profit being the middle men and petty traders.'[70]

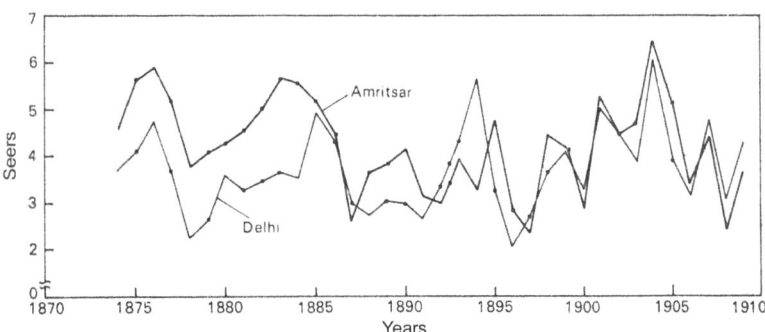

Figure 3.4a Daily wages of agricultural labourers in *seers* of bajra, Punjab, 1874–1909

Source: N. Bhattacharya, 'Agricultural Labour and Production: Central and South-east Punjab, 1870–1940,' in K.N. Raj et al., *Essays on the Commercialization of Indian Agriculture* (Delhi: Oxford University Press, 1985), p. 143. Reprinted with permission of N. Bhattacharya.

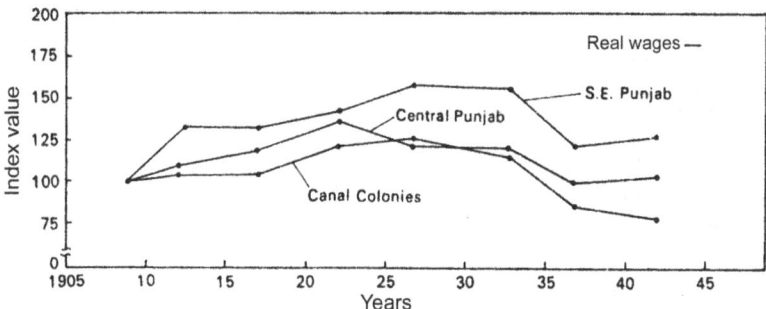

Figure 3.4b Real wages, agricultural labour, Punjab, 1909–1940

Source: N. Bhattacharya, 'Agricultural Labour and Production,' p. 144. Reprinted with permission of the author.

For those households with no reserves, the relationship between foodgrain prices and calorie intake was that much more stark – a doubling of price meaning, in effect, a halving of purchasing power.[71] While the relationship between foodgrain prices and acute hunger became more complex across the period of major malaria epidemics between 1868 and 1908, for many poorer households, access to food became even more insecure in the context of the general rise both in level and volatility of foodgrain prices induced by market conditions outside the region. Despite limitations as an actual measure of acute hunger prevalence in a given epidemic year, market foodgrain prices nonetheless constitute an important marker, precisely because such a substantial portion of the population was so close to the line of caloric insufficiency even in years of low prices.

Christophers's choice of wheat as the foodgrain with which to track 'scarcity' reflects the fact that it was the only grain for which data was available for all 24 plains districts. Wheat was not, however, the main staple foodgrain in much of the province. Primarily a winter crop, wheat was grown increasingly as an export crop with expansion of canal irrigation along with sugarcane and to a limited extent cotton. By the turn of the 20th century, wheat represented 41 per cent of the cropped area in the western districts, compared with one-fifth in the eastern half of the Province. Non-wheat foodgrain crops such as gram (a variety of chickpea known as Bengal gram), bajra (pearl millet), and jowar (sorghum) made up the primary staple food crops, the acreage of each varying greatly among districts (Table 3.2).[72] Even in the major wheat-growing western districts, the staple foodgrains consumed in poorer households were millets and gram.

Table 3.2 Per cent acreage, wheat, gram, bajra, jowar, 1903–1904, Punjab

	Wheat	*Gram*	*Bajra*	*Jowar*
Province-level	41	15	12	8
% irrigated	52	21	11	20
Region/district				
Southeast – Hissar	5	21	41	16
Central – Jullundur	47	19	0.1	1.5
Northern – Sialkot	49	5.2	3.8	8.4
Southwest – Multan	63	4.6	6.6	10.7

Source: *Season and Crop Report*, Punjab, 1903–1904.

Unlike wheat, the 'country' grains grown mainly in non-irrigated tracts were generally cheaper, but correspondingly were also more subject to the vicissitudes of the monsoon. In this sense, non-wheat crop prices could be expected to reflect acute hunger more closely than wheat; hence their inclusion in the district-level regression analysis. For most of the 1868–1908 period, price levels of the millet grains and gram, though slightly lower in normal times than for wheat, followed closely those for wheat in times of drought and poor harvests.[73]

In the present study, regression analysis is conducted separately for each of three main non-wheat food crops, bajra, jowar, and gram, in addition to wheat, in each case including those districts where price data are available. As in the case of rainfall, no continuous price series exists for the entire 1868–1940 period, even for the principal export crop, wheat. However, the provincial Sanitary Commissioner reports include district-level foodgrain price data for the years 1868 to 1898 for each of the four main foodgrains, which may well have been the source of Christophers's wheat price data. For the years 1899 to 1908, district-level figures for the four foodgrains have been calculated as the mean of January, March, May, July, September, November from data available in the *Punjab Gazette*. For the years 1909–1940 regression analysis, wheat price alone is employed, based on district data available in the Punjab annual *Season and Crops* reports.[74]

Foodgrain prices generally were reported in seers per rupee (one seer = 0.93 kg). These rates have been converted to rupees per hundred seers to obtain a series in which numerical trends correspond to a rise or fall in actual prices.

Notes

1 S.R. Christophers, 'Malaria in the Punjab,' *Sci. Mem. Off. Med. Sanit. Dept.*, 46 (Calcutta: Superintendent Government Printing Office, 1911) [hereafter, MP].

2 Separate districts until 1885, Sirsa and Hissar data are combined as Hissar district for the initial 1868–1885 analysis period. Population expansion in the western canal colonies prompted creation of two new districts: Lyall-pur in 1905 and Sheikhupura in 1920, divided off from Jhang and Gujran-wala districts, respectively. All data for these new districts are combined under the original district name.

3 For the purposes of this study, post-1940 data sources include *Annual Punjab Health Report for the Year, 1947*, Simla (1951); Director-General of Health Services, [GOI] *Report for the Quadrennium, 1949–1952*; __, *Health Statistics of India, 1951–1953, 1954–1955*; Director of Health Services, *Report on the Public Health Administration, Punjab for the Year 1956 (1957–1960); India Census, 1951*, Vol. VIII, Part 1-A; *Census of India, 1961*. Punjab. District Census Handbooks.

4 B. Parthasarathy, N.A. Sontakke, A.A. Monot, D.R. Kothawale, 'Droughts/Floods in the Summer Monsoon Season Over Different Mete-orological Subdivisions of India for the Period 1871–1984,' *Journal of Climatology*, 7, 1987, 57–70; R. Chambers, R. Longhurst, A. Pacey, eds., *Seasonal Dimensions to Rural Poverty* (London: Frances Pinter, Institute of Development Studies, 1981), 13–17.

5 Chambers, Longhurst and Pacey, *Seasonal Dimensions*, 17; Parthasarathy, 'Droughts/Floods,' 66.

6 *Report of the Indian Irrigation Commission*, 1901–1903 (London: HMSO, 1903), 4.

7 *Report of the Indian Irrigation Commission*, 4; T. Kessinger, *Vilyatpur 1848–1969, Social and Economic Change in a North Indian Village* (Berkeley: University of California Press, 1974), 11–13; H. Bannerji, *Agrarian Society of the Punjab* (New Delhi: Manohar, 1982), 20.

8 N. Bhattacharya, 'Pastoralists in a Colonial Economy,' in D. Arnold, Ramachandra Guha, eds., *Nature, Culture, Imperialism: Essays on the Environmental History of South Asia* (New Delhi: Oxford University Press, 1995), 58–63, at 61.

9 Bhattacharya, 'Pastoralists,' 61, 65.

10 S.R. Christophers, 'Malaria in the Punjab,' *Sci. Mem. Off. Med. Sanit. Dept.*, 46 (Calcutta: Superintendent Government Printing Office, 1911), 2–3 [hereafter, MP].

11 P.W. Paustian, *Canal Irrigation in the Punjab* (New York: Columbia University Press, 1930), 29.

12 See ch. 9.

13 C.A. Gill, 'The Role of Meteorology in Malaria,' *IJMR*, 8, 4, 1921, 633–693, at 640; C.A. Gill, *The Genesis of Epidemics and Natural History of Disease* (London: Bailliere, Tindall & Cox, 1928), 150–151, Charts X and XI.; E.P. Hicks, S. Abdul Majid, 'A Study of the Epidemiology of Malaria in a Punjab District,' *RMSI*, 7, 1, 1937, 1–43, at 27. M. Yacob and S. Swaroop found all three months' rain significantly predicted autumn fever death rate, August rainfall showing the highest correlation; 'Malaria and Rainfall in the Punjab,' *JMII*, 6, 3, June 1946, 273–284.

14 W.E. Baker, T.E. Dempster, H. Yule, *Report of a Committee Assembled to Report on the Causes of the Unhealthiness Which Has Existed at Kurnaul*, (1847); in 'Collected Memoranda on the Subject of Malaria,' *RMSI*, 1, 2, Mar. 1930, 1–68.

15 MP, 54, 62, 106. In subsequent studies, autumn malaria transmission was found associated with a second 'wave' of splenic enlargement involving progressively greater size of spleen and considered to be 'the result of *falciparum* relapses,' what in modern terms are referred to as recrudescence; G. Covell, J.D. Baily, 'The Study of a Regional Epidemic of Malaria in Northern Sind,' *RMSI*, 2, Dec. 1932, 279–322, at 297.

16 The presence of parasites typically fluctuates during acute infection, declining as specific immunity develops. Thus, a parasite rate of over 50 percent in a population is generally viewed as indicating near-universal levels of infection; Hicks and Majid, 'A Study of the Epidemiology of Malaria,' 31.

17 *Report on the Season and Crops of the Punjab* (Lahore: Civil and Military Gazette Press) [hereafter *Season and Crops Report*].

18 MP, 19, 111, Appendix.

19 M. Yacob, S. Swaroop, 'Investigation of Long-Term Periodicity in the Incidence of Epidemic Malaria in the Punjab,' *JMII*, 6, 1, June 1946, 39–51.

20 See ch. 6, note 72, for discussion of estimating non-malarial autumn fever mortality.

21 Ibid., 41.

22 I. Mills, 'The 1918–1919 Influenza Pandemic – the Indian Experience,' *IESHR*, 23, 1, 1–40.

23 In his 1882 treatise on fever, Sir Joseph Fayrer, President of the Medical Board at the India Office, described malarial fever '[i]n the robust and plethoric young Englishman . . . [as] followed by a well-marked remission. . . . In less robust individuals . . . the patient passes into a low tremulous typhoid state, the fever assum[ing] a continued form . . . whilst in the sthenic forms cerebral symptoms . . . may appear'; *On the Climate and Fevers of India*, Croonian Lecture (London: J&A Churchill, 1882), 96–97. See also W.R. Cornish, *Report of the Sanitary Commissioner for Madras for 1877* (Madras: Government Central Branch Press), 1878, 142, xxix [hereafter *MSCR*].

24 *PSCR* 1888, 11; *PSCR* 1876, 56. In 1893, the Hoshiarpur Civil Surgeon noted that '[t]he largest number of deaths from diarrhoea and dysentery were in the months of August, September and October, that is at the same time when malarial fevers were most rife, showing a distinct connection with the malarial poison'; *PSCR* 1893, 15. See also, Fayrer, *Fevers of India*, 64, 62, 24.

25 *The Punjab Famine of 1899–1900*, Vol. 1 (Lahore: Punjab Revenue Department, 1901), 14–15.

26 *PSCR* 1922, Appendix F, xiii.

27 *PSCR* 1908, 13. On epidemic malaria presenting with gastrointestinal symptoms, see also R. Briercliffe, *The Ceylon Malaria Epidemic, 1934–1935* (Colombo: Ceylon Government Press, 1935), 51. Hamlin also discusses the historical diagnostic quandary and its larger implications in asking 'What is cholera really?'; *More Than Hot: A Short History of Fever* (Baltimore: Johns Hopkins University Press, 2014).

28 See ch. 4 at pp. 147–48 for further discussion.

29 MP, 107 [italics in original].

30 Recent European and Asian demographic history research also confirms strong association between short-term prices surges (price 'shocks') and mortality

among populations no longer subject to frank famine; T. Bengtsson, M. Dribe, 'New Evidence on the Standard of Living in Sweden During the Eighteenth and Nineteenth Centuries: Long-Term Development of the Demographic Response to Short-Term Economic Stress,' in R. Allen, T. Bengsston, M. Dribe, eds., *Living Standards in the Past: New Perspectives on Well-Being in Asia and Europe* (Oxford: Oxford University Press, 2005), 341–371, at 350.

31 A. Sen, *Poverty and Famines: An Essay on Entitlement and Deprivation* (Oxford: Oxford University Press, 1981).

32 A.M. Guntupalli, J. Baten, 'Inequality of Heights in North, West, and East India 1915–1944,' *Explorations in Economic History*, 43, 2006, 578–608.

33 H.D. Craik, *Final Report of the 4th Regular Settlement of the Amritsar District, 1910–1914* (Lahore: Punjab, Revenue Department, 1914), 1.

34 See also, R. Gopinath, 'Aspects of Demographic Change and the Malabar Economy, 1871–1921,' *EPW*, Jan. 1987, PE-30–36; R. Lardinois, 'Famine, Epidemics and Mortality in South India: A Reappraisal of the Demographic Crisis of 1876–1878,' *EPW*, 20, Mar. 16, 1985, 454–465.

35 H.K. Trevaskis, *The Punjab of Today*, Vol. 2 (Lahore: Civil and Military Gazette Press, 1931–1932), 44.

36 *MSCR* 1878, 7–8.

37 While river transport was less expensive relative to overland carriage, it was slower, particularly upstream, and highly seasonal, depending on post-monsoon river flows; T. Raychaudhuri, 'Inland Trade,' in T. Raychaudhuri, I. Habib, eds., *Cambridge Economic History of India*, Vol. I (Cambridge: Cambridge University Press, 1982), 325–359 [hereafter *CEHI*].

38 J.E. O'Conor, *Prices and Wages in India* (Calcutta: Department Finance and Commerce, GOI Press, 1886), 7, 11, 19.

39 One graphic account of 18th-century price behaviour describes 'violent fluctuations of prices in great central markets, such as Delhi. . . . 'while, in places remote from any metalled road, their movement upwards was limited only by the price of a man's life, after a series of bad harvests; and by the value of the grain as fuel, after a series of good harvests'; A. Marshall, *Industry and Trade* (London: Palgrave Macmillan, 1919), App. I, as quoted by H.K. Trevaskis, in 'Wheat Forecasts in the Punjab,' *Agricultural Journal of India*, 29, 3, 1924, 235.

40 In 1863, the coefficient of variation of district wheat prices in British India was .47; by 1890, .18; J. Hurd, 'Railways and the Expansion of Markets in India, 1861–1921,' *Explorations in Economic History*, 12, 1975, 263–288.

41 For the 1878–1920 period, Nico den Tuinder found only a weak inverse relationship between rainfall and bajra prices in Kheda district, Gujrat; 'Population and Society in Kheda District (India), 1819–1921: A Study of the Economic Context of Demographic Developments,' Doctoral dissertation, University of Amsterdam, 1992, 132.

42 Simla Conf., 39, 40.

43 A 'labouring man consumes two pounds of grain daily when he can afford his full allowance,' a two-anna wage allowing, at then-prevailing grain prices, an additional few vegetables, oil and salt; J.B. Peile, 'Notes of the Economic Condition of the Agricultural Population of India,' in *Famine*

Commission Report (London: HMSO, 1880), Appendix I, Miscell. Papers, 162–166, at 163.

44 Neeladri Bhattacharya suggests that even under normal conditions, the earnings of village servants and artisans were insufficient to provide minimum household consumption needs and that wives and children routinely participated in field work and gathering of grass and firewood for sale; 'Agricultural Labour and Production: Central and South-East Punjab, 1870–1940,' in K.N. Raj, et al., eds., *Essays on the Commercialization of Indian Agriculture* (New Delhi: Oxford University Press, 1985), 105–152 at 113.

45 Peile, 'Notes of the Economic Condition,' 166.

46 W.R. Aykroyd, B.G. Krishnan, 'Diets Surveys in South Indian Villages,' *IJMR*, 24, 3, Jan. 1937, 667–688.

47 Confidential Circular, 44 F. – 8.1, dated Aug. 17, 1887; Resolution of the Government of India, 96-F/6–59 dated Oct. 19, 1888. See ch. 5, note 41.

48 'Précis of the Reports received on the enquiry made into the conditions of the lower classes of the population, Appx. A, G.G. in C. to S. of S., 30 Oct. (Famine No. 3) 1888, enclo. Appx II, *Summary of the Principal Measures of the Viceroyalty of Lord Dufferin, Department Of Revenue & Agriculture*, Vol. II (Simla 1888), I.O.R. (9) 3021/2'; cited in P. Bandyopadhyay, *Indian Famine and Agrarian Problems: A Study of the Administration of Lord George Hamilton, Secretary of State for India, 1895–1903* (Calcutta: Star Publishers, 1987), 95–127.

49 W. Digby, *'Prosperous' British India: A Revelation from Official Records* (London: T. Fisher Unwin, 1901), 308–309, 472, 511. B.M. Bhatia gives an account of William Digby's effort to access the content of these reports and summarises his findings; *Famines in India* (New Delhi: Asia Publishing House, 1963), 356–357, 147–149.

50 Government of Punjab, *Report on the Famine in the Punjab in 1896–1897* (Lahore: Civil and Military Gazette Press, 1898), Appendix II, 'Normal condition of the poorer classes,' xxxvii–xlii, 263 S., dated Simla, June 23, 1888.

51 Ibid., xl.

52 Ibid., xxxviii.

53 Digby, 'Prosperous India,' 465.

54 N. Hamid, 'Dispossession and Differentiation of the Peasantry in the Punjab During Colonial Rule,' *Journal of Peasant Studies*, 10, 1, 1982, 65; based on data in B.H. Baden-Powell, *Land Systems of British India*, Vol. 3 (Oxford: Clarendon Press, 1972).

55 N. Bhattacharya, 'The Logic of Tenancy Cultivation: Central and South-East Punjab, 1870–1935,' *IESHR*, 20, 2, Apr.–June 1983, 121–170.

56 Bhattacharya describes how in the late 19th century, tenants were increasingly required to pay some or all of the revenue demand in addition to handing over half the produce as rent; also, that by the 1880s, landlords were claiming part or all of the straw, previously collected by tenants, as its commercial (transportable) value increased; ibid.

57 H. Calvert, *The Size and Distribution of Cultivators' Holdings in the Punjab* (Lahore: Board of Economic Inquiry, 1928) [hereafter BEI].

58 Bhattacharya, 'Agricultural Labour and Production,' 121–123.

59 S.J. Patel, *Agricultural Labourers in Modern India and Pakistan* (Bombay: Current Book House, 1952). Bhattacharya cautions that the Census data fail to reflect seasonal dependence on wage labour of small peasants and artisans as well as the shift over time from permanent to casual labour; 'Agricultural Labour and Production,' 129–136. The 1911 census counted 9.8 per cent of the population as belonging to the depressed castes of the Chamars and Chahras; K.K. Ghose, *Agricultural Labourers in India: A Study in the History of their Growth and Economic Condition* (Calcutta: Indian Publications, 1969), 157.

60 Kessinger estimated 25 per cent of adult males in late 1800s Vilyatpur village belonged to landless labourer or servant/artisan households; *Vilyatpur*, 156.

61 K.K. Ghosh, *Agricultural Labourers in India*, 157, citing *Moral and Material Progress Report* (Calcutta: Central Bureau of Information, GOI Press, 1911–1912), 394; Kessinger, *Vilyatpur*, 156, 217.

62 For discussion of the limits to traditional village risk-sharing amongst classes in times of shortage, see W.I. Torry, 'Mortality and Harm: Hindu Peasant Adjustments to Famines,' *Social Science Information*, 25, 1, 1986, 125–160; __, 'Drought and the Government-Village Emergency Food Distribution System in India,' *Human Organization*, 45, 1, 1986, 11–23.

63 M. Mukherjee, *The National Income of India: Trends and Structure* (Calcutta: Statistical Publishing Society, 1969), cited in A. Heston, 'National Income,' in D. Kumar, ed., *Cambridge Economic History of India*, Vol. 2, 445.

64 Punjab Revenue Department, *Settlement Report: Sirsa, 1879–1883*, Lahore, 1891, 184; Bhattacharya, 'Agricultural Labour and Production,' 146. For similar observations in the Madras Presidency, see D. Kumar, *Land and Caste in South India: Agricultural Labour in the Madras Presidency during the 19th Century* (Cambridge: Cambridge University Press, 1965), 146, 160.

65 Bhattacharya, 'Agricultural Labour and Production,' 146–148.

66 Punjab Revenue Department, *Karnal Settlement Report, 1872–1880* (Allahabad: Pioneer Press, 1883).

67 For thorough discussion of usury and merchant-money-lending in Punjab, see N. Bhattacharya, 'Lenders and Debtors: Punjab Countryside, 1880–1940,' *IESHR*, 1, 2, 1985, 305–342.

68 Peile, 'Notes of the Economic Condition,' 165. '[E]very village population,' C.A. Bentley observed, 'can be divided into three classes: (a) lenders, (b) borrowers and (c) persons too poor either to lend or to borrow: *Report of the Royal Commission on Agriculture in India* (London: HMSO, 1928), Vol. IV, Evidence: Bengal, 240.

69 N. Bhattacharya, 'Agricultural Labour and Production': 105–162, Figs. II (b), III; H. Banerjee, *Agrarian Society of the Punjab (1849–1901)* (New Delhi: Manohar, 1982), 191; Kumar, *Land and Caste*, 162–167; O'Conor, *Prices and Wages in India*, 44.

70 *Sialkot Settlement Report*, 1886–1895; cited in B. Narain, *Eighty Years of Punjab Prices* (Lahore: Board of Economic Inquiry, 1926), 13, 49.

71 *MSCR 1877*, 10. In post-Independence India, a family is considered to be living under the poverty line if, by spending 75 per cent of total family

income on the least expensive source of calories (650 gms of foodgrains), they are unable to meet minimum caloric requirements set at 2,250 kilocalories per consumption unit; V.M. Dandekar, N. Rath, *Poverty in India* (Pune: Indian School of Political Economy, 1971). The definition assumes that all medical and education needs are provided by the State, and excludes any animal foodstuffs (milk, eggs, meat) as well as lentils and vegetables. Poverty is thus a measure directly based on caloric undernourishment (hunger). 48 per cent of the population was considered officially to be below the poverty line in the 1970s.

72 Ajit K. Dasgupta, 'Agricultural Growth Rates in the Punjab, 1906–1942,' *IESHR*, 18, July–Dec. 1981, 341.

73 W.H. Myles, *Sixty Years of Panjab Prices, 1861–1920* (Lahore: BEI, 1925), 22; *PLRA* 1899–1900, 2.

74 *Season and Crops Report of the Punjab* (Lahore: Superintendent, Government Printing Office, 1901–1945).

4 Testing the rain-price epidemic malaria model

This chapter summarises the findings of the quantitative analysis of Punjab malaria epidemicity, beginning with descriptive aspects relating to the three variables employed: levels and trends in annual monsoon (July–Sept.) rainfall, foodgrain prices, and autumn Oct.–Dec. fever death rate (Oct.–Dec. FDR) across Punjab for the 1868–1940 period (Table 4.1). This is followed by results from the regression analysis that explores the relationship between rain and price and annual fever (malaria) mortality, and the changing nature of these relationships after 1908.

Descriptive analysis

Sanitary officials and malaria researchers of the colonial period saw the phenomenon of Punjab 'fulminant' malaria in terms of two characteristics: heightened malaria mortality in affected tracts and broad geographic influence, hence the term 'regional' epidemics (Figures 2.8 and 2.9). Thus, epidemic severity in a given year was gauged applying a province-wide tally of autumn fever mortality. We begin by first exploring province-level patterns of the three variables, a perspective that corresponds to Christophers's original analysis. This allows for testing of his general conclusions, and for identification of the major epidemics in the province across the 41-year period, 1868–1908. Aggregate-level analysis, however, inevitably obscures important regional differences in the interplay of the factors triggering fulminant conditions, and thus is followed by analysis of epidemic behaviour at district level.

Province-level

Oct.–Dec. fever death rate

When mean Oct.–Dec. fever death rate for the 23 plains districts[1] is graphed for 1868–1940, marked fluctuations are evident across much of the earlier period (Figure 4.1). Superimposed on this 'saw-tooth'

Table 4.1 Mean Oct.–Dec. fever death rate (per 1,000), crude death rate (per 1,000), July–Sept. rain (inches), wheat price (Rs/100 seers), 1868–1940*, 24 plains districts**, Punjab

Year	Oct.–Dec. FDR (per 1,000)	July–Sept. rain (in)	Wheat price (Rs/100 seers)	CDR (per 1,000)	Year	Oct.–Dec. FDR (per 1,000)	July–Sept. rain (in)	Wheat price (Rs/100 seers)	CDR (per 1,000)
1868	2.5	8.0	6.1	16.0	1905	4.8	9.7	6.7	47.9
1869	8.6	15.5	8.3	26.5	1906	8.2	16.5	5.9	36.9
1870	6.7	11.5	7.3	24.8	1907	6.3	9.9	9.5	62.9
1871	3.6	8.4	4.8	21.5	1908	20.2	23.7	9.0	51.6
1872	6.6	19.0	4.9	25.8	1909	6.4	16.8	6.8	31.1
1873	4.8	17.2	4.6	21.4	1910	4.8	14.9	6.3	33.6
1874	4.0	12.6	4.5	18.9	1911	3.2	6.8	7.4	34.1
1875	7.3	25.2	4.1	26.9	1912	4.1	12.3	7.7	26.6
1876	11.6	15.7	4.0	30.2	1913	5.7	11.7	8.0	30.2
1877	3.7	6.2	4.3	20.6	1914	5.3	19.6	8.8	32.2
1878	14.4	17.7	6.4	37.8	1915	3.9	7.8	8.2	35.8
1879	11.2	10.5	7.5	38.8	1916	7.0	18.4	8.8	30.5
1880	5.7	11.6	6.8	27.1	1917	14.4	26.9	9.6	38.7
1881	9.0	16.2	5.7	30.7	1918		6.1	13.9	81.0
1882	7.7	17.4	4.6	27.2	1919	6.1	14.9	12.2	28.3
1883	4.3	11.3	4.5	25.4	1920	4.6	8.6	16.2	29.8
1884	13.6	16.6	4.3	37.5	1921	5.6	14.0	14.1	28.5
1885	6.9	11.6	4.2	28.3	1922	4.9	14.1	9.5	22.4
1886	5.6	13.2	5.2	27.8	1923	8.6	14.9	9.1	31.3
1887	10.5	17.9	6.8	36.0	1924	7.5	17.0	12.8	44.3
1888	7.5	15.4	6.3	31.0	1925	5.9	14.3	12.0	30.5
1889	9.0	13.1	5.1	32.1	1926	8.0	16.7	12.2	37.5
1890	17.0	16.4	5.4	49.8	1927	4.4	10.6	10.7	27.6
1891	6.5	11.4	6.2	29.4	1928	4.0	10.1	10.9	24.6

Year					Year				
1892	17.0	21.8	7.0	50.2	1929	7.6	14.1	7.7	28.7
1893	6.6	18.4	5.8	29.0	1930	6.0	13.1	3.8	29.9
1894	9.8	16.1	4.1	38.3	1931	5.6	13.9	5.2	25.8
1895	5.9	10.3	4.7	29.4	1932	4.7	14.4	6.9	24.5
1896	4.3	8.2	7.8	30.8	1933	8.4	25.0	5.2	28.4
1897	9.8	12.9	8.5	31.3	1934	5.6	12.3	5.4	27.9
1898	6.3	11.7	6.4	31.6	1935	4.5	13.7	5.7	25.0
1899	5.0	4.4	6.3	29.8	1936	4.2	14.0	7.5	24.1
1900	18.6	20.5	8.3	50.9	1937	4.1	9.6	5.6	23.6
1901	11.1	11.8	6.6	36.7	1938	4.1	7.5	5.9	26.7
1902	7.0	12.1	6.2	45.1	1939	4.4	7.1	6.7	25.7
1903	9.9	15.7	6.1	50.2	1940	6.3	12.1	7.3	28.2
1904	5.1	8.8	5.7	50.6					

Source: 1. Annual Oct.-Dec. fever death data, Annual crude death rate: *Annual Report of the Sanitary Commissioner, Punjab (PSCR)*; after 1921, *Report on the Public Health Administration of the Punjab*. 2. July–Sept. rain: PSCR (1868–1899); *Report of the Land Revenue Administration of the Punjab* (1900); *Report on the Season and Crops of the Punjab* (1901–1940). 3. Wheat price: PSCR (1868–1898); *Punjab Gazette* (1899–1908); *Report on the Season and Crops of the Punjab* (1909–1940).

* 1918 is omitted from the analysis, autumn influenza deaths confounding malaria mortality estimates. See ch. 3, pp. 102–03.
** Mean figures for the years 1868–1911 include 24 districts; for 1912–1940, 23 districts (without Delhi).

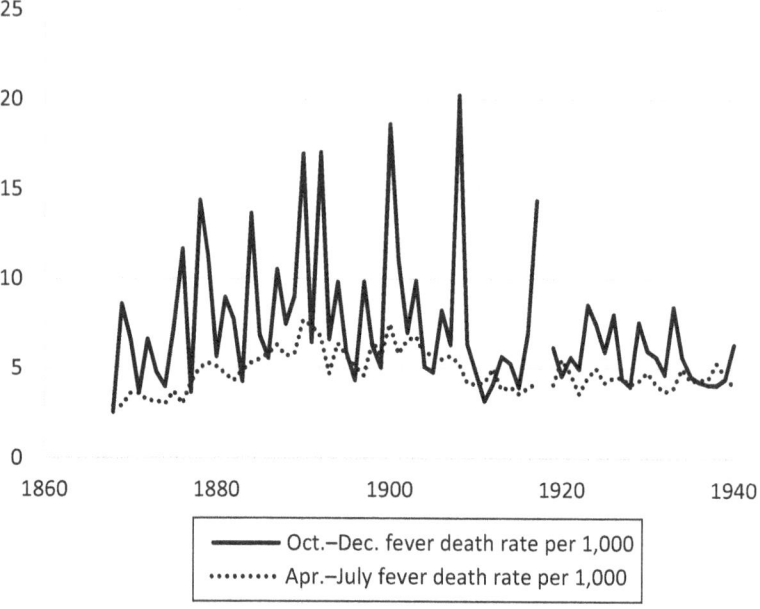

Figure 4.1 Mean annual Oct.–Dec. fever death rate, Apr.–July fever death
rate, 1868–1940, 23 plains districts, Punjab

Note: 1918 omitted.

Source: *PSCR*, 1868–1908; *PPHA*, 1922–1940.

pattern are two trends: first, a gradual increase in mortality levels
across the earliest years, and second, pronounced decline in autumn
fever mortality across the final decades. The initial rise in autumn
mortality is likely attributable in large part to improvements in vital
registration coverage. Levels of reporting were low in the initial years:
one-quarter of all villages in some western districts still were not providing any mortality returns a decade after initiation of vital registration. From the later 1870s, however, coverage and completeness
of vital registration reporting was improving, and by the end of the
century, death returns in some districts had reached an estimated completeness rate as high as 97 per cent.[2]

That the rise in autumn fever death rate evident across the 1870s
is related to improved registration is suggested also by trends in other
demographic indices. A similar increase, for example, can be seen in
the April–July fever death rate (Figure 4.1), and in overall (crude) death
rates (Figure 4.2) through the late 1860s and 1870s. Change in vital

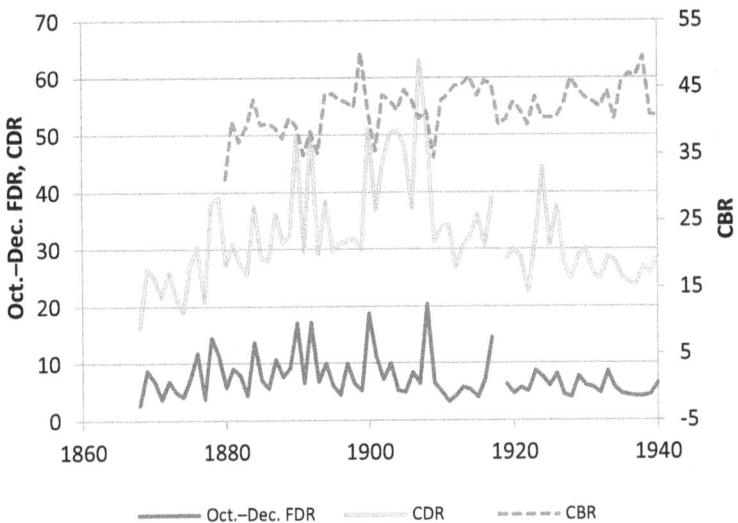

Figure 4.2 Mean annual Oct.–Dec. fever death rate, crude death rate, crude birth rate, 1868–1940, 23 plains districts, Punjab

Source: See Figure 4.1.

registration coverage, however, is an unlikely explanation for post-1908 decline in autumn fever death rates. Attenuation of autumn epidemic intensity is evident after World War I. Year-to-year fluctuation in Oct.–Dec. fever death rate in the decades 1920–1940 is approximately one-third the level prevailing up to 1908. Crude birth rate figures however remain essentially unchanged through to 1940 (Figure 4.2).

Monthly (seasonal) fever mortality, pre- and post-1920

Marked diminution in autumnal fever deaths after 1908 is evident also when seasonal patterns of mean fever mortality are compared across the two periods: the October rise in fever deaths, which is such a prominent demographic feature in the 1868–1908 period, is still evident post-1908 but is no longer the predominant season of recorded fever deaths (Figures 4.3a and b).

Epidemic trend

In an effort to take into account changes in vital registration completeness and other residual effects, a detrended series was created for

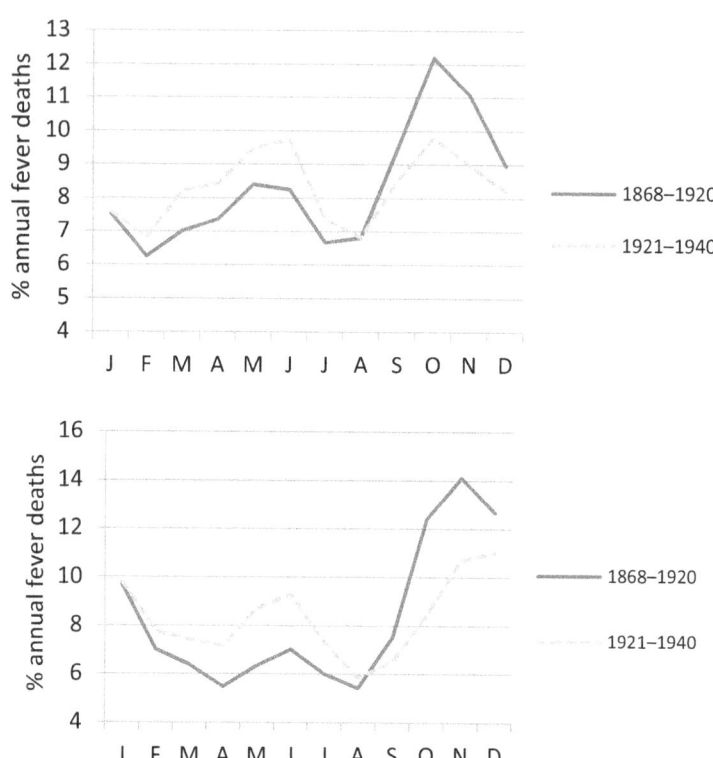

Figure 4.3a Per cent distribution of fever deaths, by month, 1868–1920, 1921–1940, Hissar district, Punjab

Source: See Figure 4.1.

Figure 4.3b Per cent distribution of fever deaths, by month, 1868–1920, 1921–1940, Shahpur district, Punjab

Source: See Figure 4.1.

Oct.–Dec. fever death rate for the 1868–1940 data set, using the Loess procedure (local polynomial regression fitting). To adjust for skewness in mortality data, a log transformation was applied. Annual epidemic malaria mortality is calculated as deviation from this autumn fever trend line.[3] In the detrended data series for the pre-1909 period, relatively low mortality levels related to under-registration are evident in the first several years of the series, but are less prominent than in the raw data series. On the other hand, the post-1917 decline in autumn fever mortality remains pronounced (Figure 4.4).

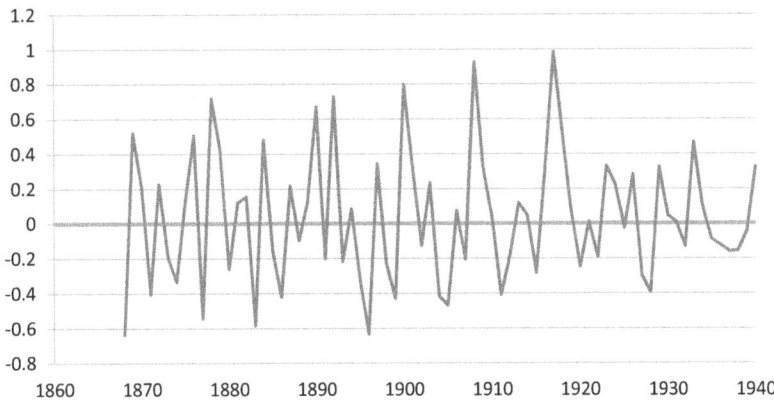

Figure 4.4 Mean annual Oct.–Dec. fever death rate (detrended), 1868–1940, 23 plains districts, Punjab

Source: See Figure 4.1.

In both the raw and detrended data sets, eight of the 41 years between 1868 and 1908 stand out as prominent mortality peaks, with a ninth year (1879) obscured visually, adjacent to the peak in 1878.[4] These nine years correspond closely to narrative accounts of severe epidemics as documented in the annual provincial administrative records.[5] One further major epidemic, that of 1917 in the later 1909–1940 period, is of comparable severity to those of the pre-1909 period. The year was marked by both record-high monsoon rainfall and grain prices, triggered not primarily by harvest failure but by World War I hyper-inflation.[6]

Rain (July-Sept.) and Oct.–Dec. fever death rate

A close relationship between monsoon (July-Sept.) rainfall (24-district mean) and annual Oct.–Dec. fever death rate is readily evident (Figure 4.5). Most epidemic years are associated with above normal rainfall; conversely, years of below average rains are generally free of fever epidemics. This relationship, however, was not exact. Between 1868 and 1940, there were five years when mean monsoon rainfall for the 24 districts exceeded 20 inches (Table 4.1). Only three were major epidemic years, those preceded by severe drought (1892, 1900, 1908). The remaining two heavy rainfall years (1875 and 1933) were not associated with fulminant malarial conditions. In both cases,

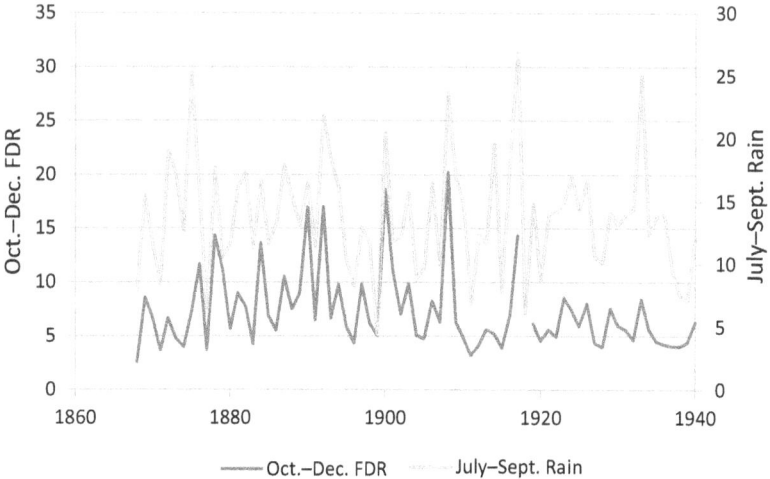

Figure 4.5 Mean annual Oct.–Dec. fever death rate, July–Sept. rain, 1868–
1940, 23 plains districts, Punjab

Source: See Table 4.1.

heavy monsoon rains were not preceded by conditions of harvest failure. Conversely, a single epidemic year, that of 1879, was associated
with below normal July-Sept. rainfall: 10.5 inches, compared with an
1868–1908 mean of 13.7 inches.

After 1908, the close relationship between July-Sept. rainfall and
autumn fever death rate appears to continue, though the actual level of
mortality in years of excess July-Sept. rainfall is much lower.

Wheat price and Oct.–Dec. fever death rate

Mean annual wheat price for the 24 districts also shows marked fluctuation, with seven prominent surges across the 1868–1908 period
(Figure 3.2). In many cases, duration of the price rise can be seen to
extend across a period of three years. Within this pattern, a general
trend of rising prices is evident from the 1890s, price levels often failing to return to previous low levels after episodic peaks. The final
three decades of the study period, 1910–1940, were marked by yet
more pronounced trends: wheat prices soared during the four years
of World War I, remained high through the 1920s, then declined pre-
cipitously in 1930 with the global economic depression. Within this

pattern, short-term fluctuations continued, although price surges now tended to be limited to two, or even single, years.

An association between prices (wheat) and autumn fever mortality is evident for the 1868–1908 period, if less consistent than for rainfall (Figure 4.6). Six of the seven major surges in foodgrain prices in the 1868–1908 period was associated with a major epidemic, generally occurring in the peak year of the price surge. On the other hand, three epidemics of the 41-year period occurred when wheat prices were low (1876, 1884, and 1890). After 1920, an association between wheat price and autumn fever mortality is less apparent.

Annual malaria mortality and general (crude) death rate

A close relationship is evident between annual autumn (Oct.–Dec.) fever death rate and total annual mortality (crude death rate), until the turn of the 20th century (Figure 4.2). Mortality levels were notably affected by the 1897 outbreak of plague in the wheat-exporting provinces of British India, an epidemic that was most severe in Punjab and continued through to the late 1920s. As an epidemiologically exceptional disease – one not normally contributing to general levels of mortality – plague mortality thus tends to obscure the general pattern of

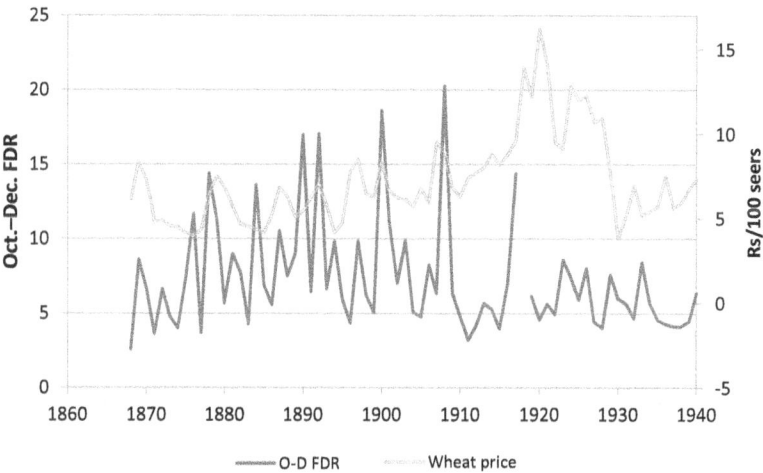

Figure 4.6 Mean annual Oct.–Dec. fever death rate (per 1,000), wheat price, 1868–1940, 23 plains districts, Punjab

Source: See Table 4.1.

death rates over the early decades of the 20th century. Plague deaths, however were generally considered identifiable, typically occurring in the early spring months of the year,[7] and from 1901 were recorded under a separate heading in the annual sanitary reports. Subtracting the registered plague deaths from total annual mortality, the relationship of crude death rate and Oct.–Dec. fever death rate appears considerably closer (Figure 4.7). Fitting a regression line for the two measures gives an R-square of .80.[8]

District-level

July-Sept. rain

Mean July–September (third-quarter) rainfall for the 1868–1908 period varies from over 20 inches in the eastern and northeastern (submontane) districts to less than five inches in the southwest (Figure 4.8). July-Sept. rainfall in the plains shows little decline over the 77-year period, 1868–1944: mean July–September rain for the 23 plains

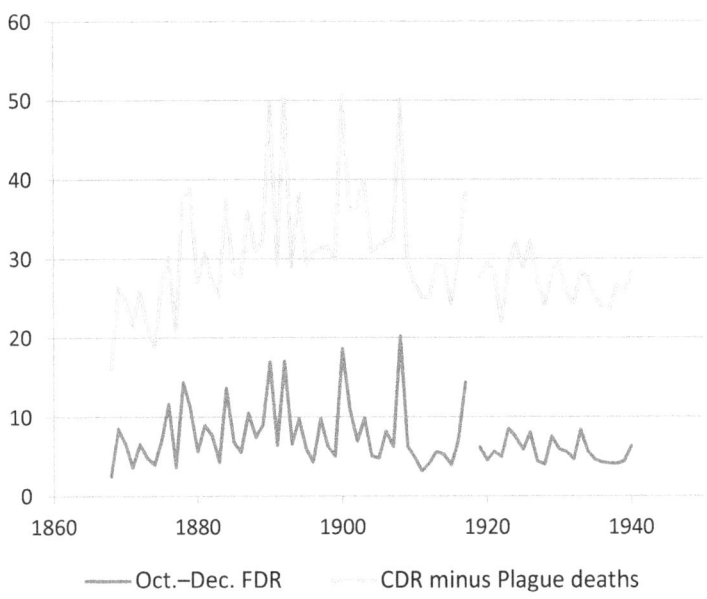

Figure 4.7 Mean annual Oct.–Dec. fever death rate, crude death rate (plague deaths, 1918, omitted), 1868–1940, 23 plains districts, Punjab

Source: See Table 4.1.

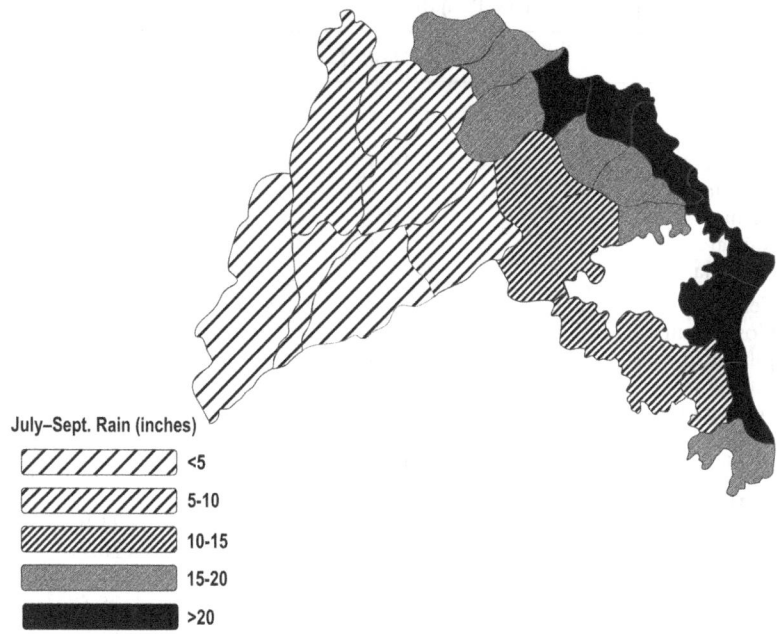

Figure 4.8 Mean July-Sept. rain (inches), by district, 1868–1908, 24 plains
districts, Punjab

Source: See Table 4.1.

district (omitting Delhi for which data are not available after 1911)
is 13.8 inches for the 1868–1908 period, and 13.7 inches between
1909 and 1944 (Table 4.2). A slight decline is evident for some eastern
districts in the post-1908 period, but also a comparable increase for
several districts in the western half of the province. A regression line
was fitted to the 73 years' 23-district mean July-Sept. rainfall data,
showing there to be no significant decline.[9]

Wheat price

In contrast to third-quarter rain, mean district wheat price levels for the
1868–1908 period show only slight geographic variation (Table 4.3),
suggesting a high degree of market integration already by the final
third of the 19th century.

Table 4.2 Mean July–Sept. rain (inches), 1868–1908, 24 districts; 1909–1944, 23 plains districts, Punjab

	1868–1908	*1909–1944*
Southeast:		
Hissar	10.7	10.5
Rohtak	14.3	13.6
Gurgaon	18.7	17.7
Delhi	20.2	
Karnal	20.5	20.2
Amballa	21.8	20.8
Central:		
Hoshiarpur	23.8	22.6
Jullundur	18.3	17.4
Ludhiana	18.3	17.3
Ferozepur	11.9	10.4
Lahore	12.2	12.6
Amritsar	16.5	14.3
North:		
Gurdaspur	23.1	21.9
Sialkot	21.7	20.7
Gujrat	15.7	17.1
Gujranwala	15.2	15.5
Jhelum	16.0	17.6
Southwest:		
Shahpur	8.0	8.9
Jhang	6.2	6.1
Montgomery	6.7	6.7
Multan	4.1	4.2
Dhera Ismail Khan	4.6	6.4
Muzaffargarh	3.4	4.3
Dhera Ghazi Khan	3.2	3.6

Source: See Table 4.1.

Table 4.3 Mean annual wheat price (Rs/100 seers), 1868–1908, 24 plains districts, Punjab

	Rs/100 seers	*Regional mean*
Southeast:		6.3
Hissar	6.3	
Rohtak	6.5	
Gurgaon	6.6	
Delhi	6.4	
Karnal	6.0	
Amballa	5.8	

	Rs/100 seers	Regional mean
Central:		5.8
Hoshiarpur	5.7	
Jullundur	5.6	
Ludhiana	5.5	
Ferozepur	6.0	
Lahore	6.0	
Amritsar	5.8	
North:		5.8
Gurdaspur	5.5	
Sialkot	6.0	
Gujrat	5.8	
Gujranwala	6.0	
Jhelum	5.8	
West/Southwest:		6.2
Shahpur	5.9	
Jhang	6.2	
Montgomery	6.1	
Multan	6.6	
Dhera Ismail Khan	6.2	
Muzaffargarh	6.3	
Dhera Ghazi Khan	6.4	

Source: See Table 4.1.

Autumn fever death rate

Mean district-level autumn fever death rates are similar across much of the province for the 41-year period, 1868–1908 (Table 4.4). Somewhat lower mean levels, however, are seen in the western region of the province. When mean Oct.–Dec. fever death rates are calculated omitting the first decade of greatest vital registration under-reporting, some regional east-west difference in levels remains (Figure 4.9). In several districts (Dhera Ghazi Khan and Dhera Ismail Khan), the lower figures appear to be due in part at least to greater levels of under-registration, birth rate figures also appearing low.[10] Western districts such as Shahpur, Jhang, and Montgomery, however, have crude birth rate levels similar to those in the eastern half of the province, suggesting that the lower mortality figures may reflect actual lower autumn fever (malaria) and general mortality levels compared with eastern Punjab.

General mortality levels, as measured by crude death rate, are somewhat higher in the eastern half of the province as well (Figure 4.10).

Table 4.4 Mean Oct.–Dec. fever death rate (per 1,000), 1868–1908, 1880–
1908, 24 plains districts, Punjab

District	1868–1908	1880–1908	Regional mean, 1880–1908
Southeast:			9.4
Hissar	7.1	8.3	
Rohtak	8.3	8.6	
Gurgaon	9.0	9.4	
Delhi	9.3	10.0	
Karnal	9.3	10.6	
Amballa	8.4	9.5	
Central:			9.0
Hoshiarpur	8.6	8.4	
Jullundur	8.8	7.6	
Ludhiana	8.7	9.4	
Ferozepur	8.9	10.3	
Lahore	8.5	8.8	
Amritsar	9.3	9.7	
North:			9.1
Gurdaspur	9.4	9.7	
Sialkot	9.2	10.0	
Gujrat	7.1	8.1	
Gujranwala	8.5	9.3	
Jhelum	7.8	8.4	
Southwest:			7.9
Shahpur	6.9	7.6	
Jhang	6.7	7.0	
Montgomery	6.4	6.7	
Multan	7.6	8.4	
Dhera Ismail Khan	7.5	8.2	
Muzaffargarh	9.3	10.3	
Dhera Ghazi Khan	6.1	7.2	

Source: See Table 4.1.

Trends in Oct.–Dec. fever death rate, 1868–1940

Province-level

Change point

The close relationship between autumn malaria mortality and crude
death rate suggests timing of epidemic malaria decline is an important
aspect of the region's demographic history. At province-level, decline in
Oct.–Dec. fever death rate fluctuation from trend is evident from 1919
on: year-to-year fluctuation continues after 1919, but at a notably

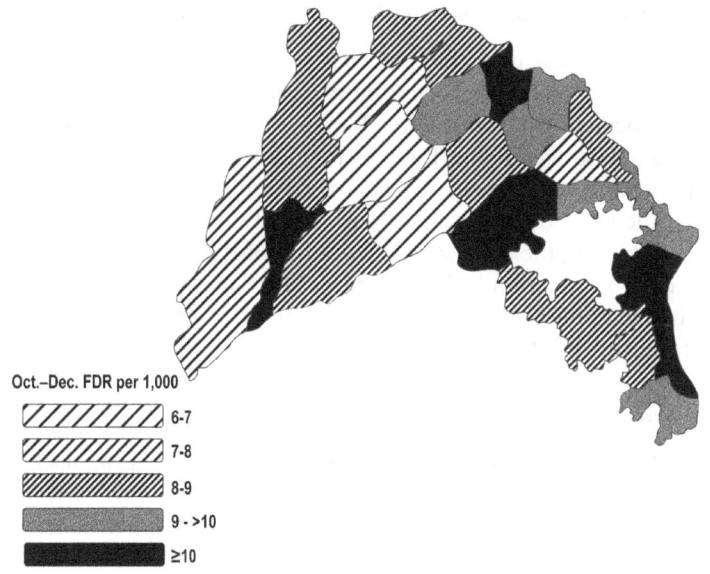

Oct.–Dec. FDR per 1,000

⧄	6-7
⧄	7-8
⧄	8-9
▦	9 - >10
■	≥10

Figure 4.9 Mean Oct.–Dec. fever death rate, 1880–1908, 24 plains district, Punjab

Source: See Table 4.1.

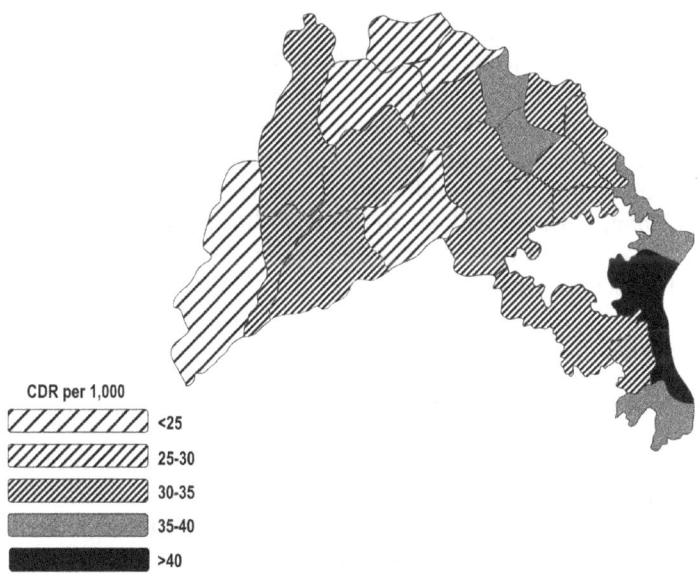

CDR per 1,000

⧄	<25
⧄	25-30
⧄	30-35
▦	35-40
■	>40

Figure 4.10 Mean crude death rate, 1880–1908, 24 plains districts, Punjab

Source: See Table 4.1.

lower level. Assessing a possible earlier change point for malaria mortality in the province is confounded, however, by the exceptional events associated with World War I. Hyper-inflation pushed foodgrain prices to record levels, and the war period culminated in famine and the influenza pandemic in 1918. To investigate change points, we applied the Pruned Exact Linear Time (PELT) method, an exact algorithm for finding the optimal segmentation of the data with respect to the likelihood function.[11] Applying the PELT method identifies 1917 as a change point in both the raw and detrended province-level Oct.– Dec. fever death rate series.

District-level

Exploration of epidemic trends at district-level allows for a clearer assessment of decline in the various regions of the province. A detrended series for annual fever death rate (Oct.–Dec.) was created for each of the plains districts, as was done for the aggregate province-level data set. Marked fluctuation from trend is evident across the 1868–1908 period for all districts (Figures 4.11a–d). Decline in fluctuations in autumn fever mortality is evident in most districts from the early decades of the 20th century, in some central and eastern regions of the province amounting to an almost flattening of the autumn fever death rate curve after 1908 (Hoshiarpur, Amballa, Jullundur, Ludhiana, Lahore). Elsewhere, attenuation is more evident after 1917. As noted earlier, a major epidemic occurred in 1917, associated with record-high monsoon rainfall extending into the western half of the province, war-time inflation, and record grain prices. In contrast to trends in much of the eastern half of the province, substantial year-to-year fluctuation continued in the southwestern districts (Muzaffargarh, Dhera Ghazi Khan, Dhera Ismail Khan) in the 1930s, associated again with westward extension of heavy monsoon rainfall and severe flooding in several epidemic years (1929, 1933).

Quantifying district-level malaria epidemicity

Calculation of decadal coefficients of variability for autumn fever mortality, by district, offers another method of assessing change point in epidemic mortality patterns for different regions of the province. Here the coefficient is computed as the standard deviation of mean Oct.– Dec. fever death rate fluctuation from trend for each decade divided by the decadal mean, omitting 1918.[12]

Marked fluctuation in autumn fever mortality for the four-decade period, 1871–1910, is seen throughout much of the eastern two-thirds

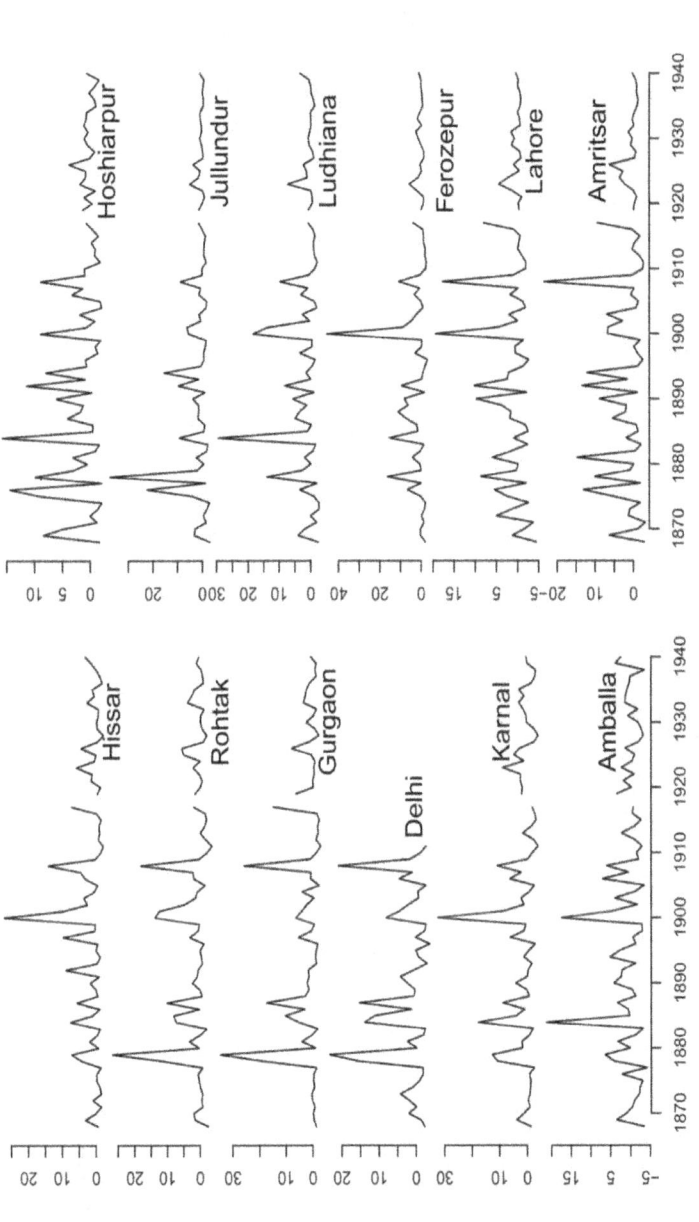

Figure 4.11a–d Annual Oct.–Dec. fever death rate, fluctuation from trend, by district, Southeast/Central/Northern/Southwest Punjab, 1868–1940

Source: See Table 4.1.

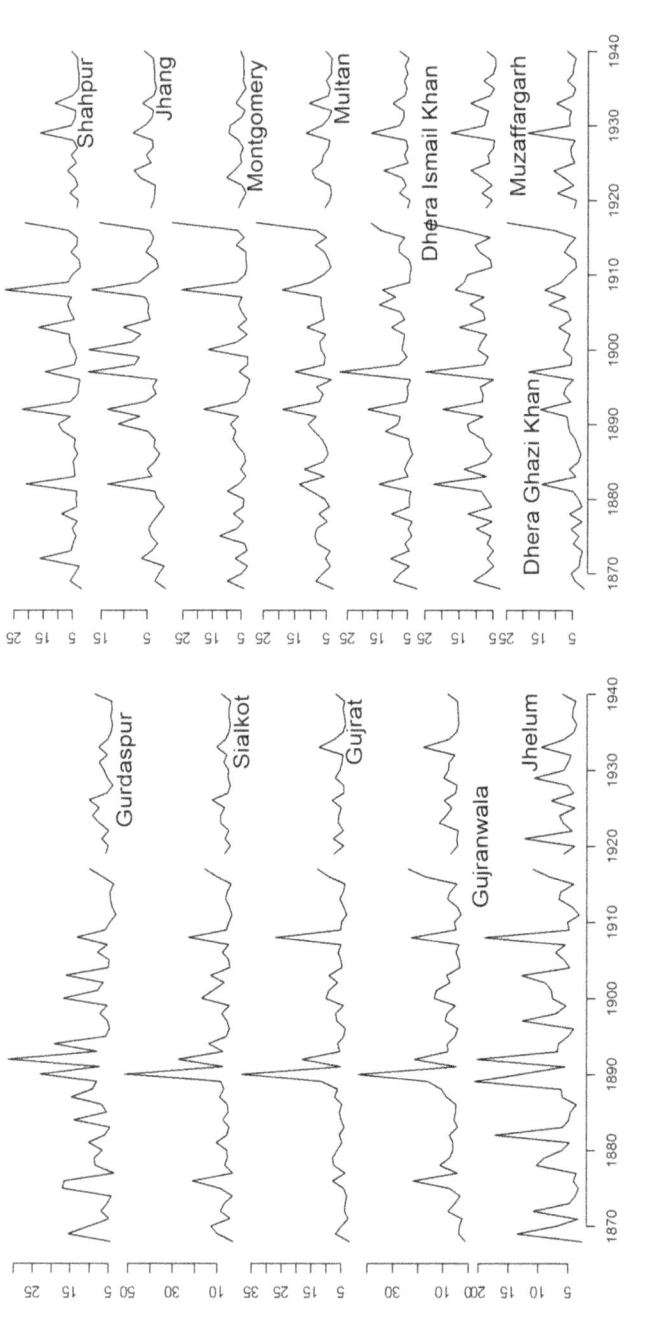

Figure 4.11a–d Continued

of the province (southeastern, central, and northern regions) (Table 4.5). In general, the southwestern districts show considerably lower year-to-year variability in autumn fever mortality, the spatial pattern of such differences appearing to correspond to a mean third-quarter rainfall level of less than 10 inches (Figure 4.8). A pattern of overall decline in fluctuations from trend is apparent after 1920. In many of the eastern and central regions of the province, marked decline is evident from 1910; in the western districts, from 1920. By the 1930s, most districts show lower coefficients of autumn fever death rate variability compared with the pre-1910 period. Two exceptions are Multan and

Table 4.5 Decadal coefficient of variation, Oct.–Dec. fever death rate, 1871–1940, 24 plains districts, Punjab

District	1871–1880	1881–1890	1891–1900	1901–1910	1911–1920	1921–1930	1931–1940
Southeast:							
Hissar	0.71	0.49	0.94	0.54	0.54	0.39	0.30
Rohtak	1.07	0.50	0.58	0.69	0.38	0.41	0.27
Gurgaon	1.33	0.54	0.35	0.48	0.89	0.44	0.28
Delhi	0.86	0.58	0.45	0.62			
Karnal	0.85	0.60	0.57	0.45	0.37	0.48	0.33
Amballa	0.59	0.71	0.39	0.47	0.34	0.41	0.34
Central:							
Hoshiarpur	0.68	0.58	0.56	0.43	0.18	0.21	0.17
Jullundur	1.07	0.44	0.69	0.52	0.24	0.33	0.13
Ludhiana	0.71	0.84	0.69	0.67	0.22	0.44	0.28
Ferozepur	0.94	0.49	1.11	0.52	0.45	0.39	0.20
Lahore	0.46	0.44	0.75	0.50	0.92	0.42	0.46
Amritsar	0.63	0.55	0.65	0.56	0.76	0.36	0.26
North:							
Gurdaspur	0.60	0.56	0.80	0.52	1.10	0.36	0.21
Sialkot	0.74	1.28	0.75	0.51	0.53	0.35	0.23
Gujrat	0.43	1.15	0.63	0.85	0.57	0.34	0.18
Gujranwala	0.73	1.07	0.60	0.78	0.42	0.31	0.33
Jhelum	0.51	0.70	0.61	0.56	0.63	0.40	0.37
West/Southwest:							
Shahpur	0.71	0.80	0.93	0.84	0.56	0.26	0.51
Jhang	0.45	0.71	0.67	0.53	0.80	0.37	0.62
Montgomery	0.52	0.35	0.85	0.94	0.42	0.43	0.35
Multan	0.32	0.39	0.56	0.50	1.04	0.64	0.58
Dhera Ismail Khan	0.48	0.59	0.82	0.44	0.60	0.50	0.25
Muzaffargarh	0.36	0.49	0.60	0.32	0.66	0.48	0.34
Dhera Ghazi Khan	0.43	0.62	0.55	0.34	0.88	0.58	0.30

Note: 1918 omitted.

Source: See Table 4.1.

Table 4.6 Rank order, mean decadal coefficients of variation, Oct.–Dec. fever death rate (per 1,000), by district, 1871–1910, mean July–Sept. rain (inches), 1868–1908, 24 plains districts, Punjab

District	Region	Coeff. of variation	July–Sept. rain (in)
Shahpur	NW	0.83	8.0
Gujrat	NC	0.81	15.7
Montgomery	SW	0.80	6.7
Gujranwala	NC	0.79	15.2
Rohtak	SE	0.70	14.3
Ludhiana	CE	0.70	18.3
Sialkot	NC	0.66	21.7
Ferozepur	CE	0.64	11.9
Delhi	SE	0.62	20.2
Hissar	SE	0.61	10.7
Jullundur	CE	0.60	18.3
Amritsar	C	0.58	16.5
Jhelum	NW	0.58	16.0
Gurgaon	SE	0.57	18.7
Gurdaspur	NC	0.57	23.1
Jhang	W	0.56	6.2
Karnal	SE	0.54	20.5
Lahore	CE	0.52	12.2
Dhera Ismail Khan	SW	0.51	4.6
Amballa	CE	0.50	21.8
Hoshiarpur	CE	0.49	23.8
Multan	SW	0.47	4.1
Dhera Ghazi Khan	SW	0.41	3.2
Muzaffargarh	SW	0.38	3.4

Source: See Table 4.1.

Jhang districts, where the coefficient for 1931–1940 is similar to that of 1881–1890, likely reflecting record flooding in 1933. Nonetheless, the absolute level of Oct.–Dec. fever death rate for the later decade in both cases is one-half that for the 1880s (4.7 cf 8.3 per mille, and 3.9 cf 7.0).

Ranking mean decadal coefficients of variation for the initial four-decade period 1871–1910 (Table 4.6) suggests greatest variability in autumn fever mortality in the northern region of the province, and least in the southwestern with lowest rainfall. However, regional location is not a consistent predictor of variability.

Regression analysis

Province-level

The close relationship of autumn fever mortality to monsoon rainfall and prevailing wheat price observed graphically for the 1868–1908 period is borne out in aggregate regression analysis. Mean Oct.–Dec. fever death rate (detrended) for the 24 plains districts was regressed on mean July–Sept. rainfall and mean wheat price.[13] Both July-Sept. rainfall and wheat price are highly significant predictors of autumn fever mortality, together explaining 59 per cent of year-to-year variation (Table 4.7).

District-level

Repeating the regression analysis at district-level allows identification of important regional differences in the relationship between epidemic malaria, monsoon rainfall, and economic stress, differences obscured in the aggregate analysis. The 1868–1908 interval initially was chosen for quantitative analysis in order to replicate and test Christophers's statistical results. This periodisation has been retained for the district-level regression analysis as well in light of the different epidemic dynamic evident for most districts after 1908.

1868–1908

For each district, a detrended annual series was created for annual Oct.–Dec. fever death rate and for each of the four foodgrain price series, using the Loess procedure. Death rate deviation from trend was regressed on district-level July–Sept. rain and annual district-level foodgrain price. In each case, a log form of the mortality data was used because it gives residuals closer to normal distribution (Table 4.8).

Third-quarter rainfall is seen to be a highly significant ($p < 0.01$) predictor of Oct.–Dec. fever death rate for all 24 plains districts. Rain coefficients are highest in the western districts, a finding consistent with Christophers's observation that epidemicity in this region was limited to those years where the 20-inch rain isohyet extended further west than normal. Wheat price, on the other hand,

Table 4.7 Mean Oct.–Dec. fever death rate (per 1,000), regressed on July–Sept. rain (inches), wheat price (Rs/100 seers), 24 plains districts, Punjab, 1868–1908

	Estimate	*Std. error*	*t-value*	*p-value*
(Intercept)	–1.37	0.22	–6.29	<0.001
Rain	0.06	0.01	6.55	<0.001
Wheat Price	0.09	0.03	2.87	0.007

Source: See Table 4.1.

Table 4.8 District Oct.–Dec. fever death rate (per 1,000), regressed on district July–Sept. rain (inches) and wheat price (Rs/100 seers),* 24 plains districts, Punjab, 1868–1908

District	Rain			Wheat			R-sq.
	Coeff.	Std. error	p-value	Coeff.	Std. error	p-value	
Southeast:							
Hissar	0.032	0.012	0.008	0.134	0.042	0.003***	0.39
Rohtak	0.023	0.010	0.030	0.123	0.049	0.017**	0.23
Gurgaon	0.031	0.010	0.004	0.109	0.050	0.039**	0.31
Delhi	0.036	0.007	<0.001	0.063	0.038	0.109*	0.47
Karnal	0.022	0.009	0.020	0.085	0.047	0.077*	0.21
Amballa	0.025	0.008	0.004	0.046	0.046	0.052**	0.24
Central:							
Hoshiarpur	0.026	0.007	0.001	0.065	0.043	0.138	0.33
Jullundur	0.036	0.008	<0.001	0.031	0.048	0.527	0.33
Ludhiana	0.025	0.009	0.002	0.098	0.048	0.048**	0.26
Ferozepur	0.028	0.013	0.037	0.083	0.052	0.117	0.19
Lahore	0.052	0.009	<0.001	0.091	0.038	0.020**	0.51
Amritsar	0.038	0.006	<0.001	0.071	0.040	0.085*	0.51
North:							
Gurdaspur	0.034	0.006	<0.001	0.083	0.039	0.039**	0.52
Sialkot	0.048	0.007	<0.001	0.096	0.044	0.037**	0.56
Gujrat	0.050	0.009	<0.001	0.095	0.038	0.017**	0.54
Gujranwala	0.043	0.012	0.001	0.099	0.062	0.118	0.28
Jhelum	0.026	0.012	0.039	0.083	0.048	0.09*	0.21
West/Southwest:							
Shahpur	0.092	0.018	<0.001	0.053	0.046	0.264	0.41
Jhang	0.067	0.015	<0.001	−0.085	0.054	0.122	0.35
Montgomery	0.043	0.017	0.013	0.103	0.058	0.085*	0.33
Multan	0.086	0.015	<0.000	0.062	0.036	0.090*	0.47
Dhera Ismail Khan	0.085	0.019	<0.001	0.056	0.035	0.120	0.39
Muzaffargarh	0.120	0.019	<0.001	0.081	0.032	0.016**	0.58
Dhera Ghazi Khan	0.086	0.023	0.001	0.072	0.045	0.116	0.28

* p-value < 0.1*; < 0.05**, < 0.01***
Source: See Table 4.1.

is a significant predictor ($p < 0.05$) of malaria mortality in only 10 districts of the 24; 15 districts at $p < 0.1$. Unlike for rainfall, major regional differences are apparent in the wheat price-malaria mortality relationship. Wheat price most strongly predicts malaria mortality in the southeastern region of the province: in two districts (Hissar and Rohtak) the significance of wheat price is marginally higher than that for rainfall. But wheat price is also a significant predictor in the central region districts of Lahore and Ludhiana, in three contiguous submontane districts in the north (Gurdaspur, Sialkot, Gujrat), Jhelum in the northwest, and a single southwestern district, Muzaffargarh. In a single district, Jhang, the price coefficient is negative, a western district where irrigation coverage at 92.8 per cent was at the highest level in the province, most based on large government canals. Together, rainfall and wheat price explain from one-fifth and to over one-half of year-to-year variation in district Oct.–Dec. fever death rate for the 1868–1908 period.

The regression analysis was repeated using price data for each of the three additional foodgrains, gram (black gram, *urad dal*),[14] bajra (pearl millet), and jowar (sorghum), consumed locally as staple grains. These crops were grown generally on unirrigated land and often made up only a small portion of all crops sown. Nevertheless, because they were more subject to the vicissitudes of the monsoon, in some districts, their price levels likely reflect local economic stress triggered by poor rains more closely than the major irrigated cash crop, wheat.

Of the 17 districts for which data are available, 12 districts show gram price to be a significant predictor of autumn fever mortality variable at the $p < 0.1$ level, eight at $p < 0.05$; for jowar, nine (and six) districts, respectively, and bajra, eight (and five), reflecting perhaps the more localised cropping patterns of these latter foodgrains (Table 4.9). Price significance, once again, is most common in the southeastern districts, but as with wheat, price significance of the non-wheat foodgrains is apparent across all regions of the province. In 13 of the 24 districts, one or more of the four foodgrains is a significant predictor of Oct.–Dec. fever death rate at the $p < 0.05$ level; in an additional five districts, at the $p < 0.1$ level. In the remaining six districts (Jullundur, Ferozepur, Gujranwala, Shahpur, Jhang, and Dhera Ghazi Khan), none of the four foodgrains significantly predict malaria mortality, at $p < 0.1$.

1909–1940

District-level regression analysis of autumn fever mortality, third-quarter rain, and foodgrain price levels was carried out for the subsequent 31-year period, 1909–1940 (1918 omitted), in this case for wheat price alone. As for the earlier period, a detrended series was used for both fever death rate and price.

Table 4.9 Summary of price significance levels: District Oct.–Dec. fever death rate (per 1,000) regressed on July–Sept. rain (inches), price (wheat, gram, bajra, jowar) (Rs/seer), 24 plains districts, Punjab, 1868–1908*

District	p-value				
	Wheat	Gram	Bajra	Jowar	$p < 0.1$ value for one or more foodgrains
Southeast:					
Hissar	0.003	<0.001	0.014	0.001	$p < 0.01$
Rohtak	0.017	0.016	0.045	0.031	$p < 0.05$
Gurgaon	0.038	n.a.	n.a.	n.a.	$p < 0.05$
Delhi	0.101	0.082	0.173	0.096	$p < 0.1$
Karnal	0.077	0.001	0.782	0.006	$p < 0.01$
Amballa	0.052	0.010	0.060	0.062	$p < 0.01$
Central:					
Hoshiarpur	0.138	0.102	0.279	0.933	$p < 0.1$
Jullundur	0.527	0.558	0.991	0.586	
Ludhiana	0.048	0.013	0.050	0.037	$p < 0.05$
Ferozepur	0.117	0.215	0.613	0.262	
Lahore	0.090	0.005	0.012	0.008	$p < 0.01$
Amritsar	0.122	0.064	0.090	0.180	$p < 0.1$
North:					
Gurdaspur	0.039	n.a.	n.a.	n.a.	$p < 0.05$
Sialkot	0.037	0.088	0.108	0.239	$p < 0.05$
Gujrat	0.017	n.a.	n.a.	n.a.	$p < 0.05$
Gujranwala	0.118	n.a.	n.a.	n.a.	
Jhelum	0.091	0.011	0.080	0.041	$p < 0.01$
West/Southwest:					
Shahpur	0.264	0.252	0.278	0.194	
Jhang	0.122	0.932	0.391	0.291	
Montgomery	0.085	0.113	0.106	0.084	$p < 0.1$
Multan	0.090	0.154	0.269	0.345	$p < 0.1$
Dhera Ismail Khan	0.120	0.040	0.047	0.246	$p < 0.05$
Muzaffargarh	0.016	n.a.	n.a.	n.a.	$p < 0.05$
Dhera Ghazi Khan	0.116	n.a.	n.a.	n.a.	

* $p < 0.05$ in bold
Source: See Chart 4.1.

Monsoon rainfall remains a strong predictor of malaria mortality (Table 4.10). By contrast, in none of the 23 districts is wheat price a significant predictor of autumn fever mortality; indeed, in 13 districts, the price coefficient is negative. This change in the relationship between wheat price and malaria mortality (Oct.–Dec. fever death rate) after 1908 is apparent as well from Figure 4.6, certainly after 1917.

Table 4.10 District Oct.–Dec. fever death rate (per 1,000), regressed on district July–Sept. rain (inches) and wheat price (Rs/100 seers), 23 plains districts, Punjab, 1909–1940

District	Rain			Wheat			R-sq.
	Coeff.	Std. error	p-value	Coeff.	Std. error	p-value	
Southeast:							
Hissar	0.043	0.007	<0.001	0.001	0.013	0.938	0.57
Rohtak	0.016	0.007	0.032	0.010	0.019	0.601	0.16
Gurgaon	0.029	0.011	0.011	0.007	0.025	0.781	0.21
Delhi							
Karnal	0.019	0.008	0.030	0.006	0.025	0.820	0.16
Amballa	0.014	0.009	0.138	0.025	0.024	0.314	0.10
Central:							
Hoshiarpur	0.007	0.003	0.049	−0.005	0.011	0.664	0.13
Jullundur	0.016	0.005	0.003	−0.001	0.012	0.968	0.27
Ludhiana	0.022	0.005	<0.001	−0.002	0.015	0.900	0.37
Ferozepur	0.025	0.011	0.025	−0.031	0.019	0.116	0.19
Lahore	0.021	0.007	0.009	−0.007	0.018	0.717	0.23
Amritsar	0.025	0.008	0.002	0.010	0.016	0.551	0.20
North:							
Gurdaspur	0.020	0.005	0.001	−0.009	0.017	0.615	0.35
Sialkot	0.031	0.007	<0.001	−0.002	0.018	0.926	0.44
Gujrat	0.043	0.006	<0.001	0.011	0.013	0.421	0.69
Gujranwala	0.050	0.012	<0.001	−0.012	0.025	0.646	0.39
Jhelum	0.030	0.007	<0.001	0.003	0.015	0.833	0.44
West/Southwest:							
Shahpur	0.065	0.014	<0.001	−0.017	0.023	0.456	0.45
Jhang	0.056	0.014	<0.001	0.000	0.017	0.991	0.38
Montgomery	0.069	0.014	<0.000	−0.003	0.020	0.856	0.48
Multan	0.071	0.017	<0.001	−0.012	0.022	0.059	0.39
Dhera Ismail Khan	0.059	0.016	0.001	−0.017	0.019	0.398	0.33
Muzaffargarh	0.068	0.011	<0.001	−0.028	0.017	0.123	0.57
Dhera Ghazi Khan	0.097	0.016	<0.001	0.014	0.014	0.330	0.58

Source: See Table 4.1.

Crude death rate and price

For comparative purposes, district-level analysis of crude death rate and wheat price for the 1868–1908 period was also explored, employing detrended annual crude death rate, with plague deaths again subtracted (Table 4.11).

Fewer of the 24 districts show wheat price to be a significant predictor of crude death rate fluctuations compared with Oct.–Dec. fever death rate: seven at $p < 0.05$, and four additional districts at $p < 0.1$ Again,

Table 4.11 Annual crude death rate (per 1,000) regressed on wheat price (Rs/100 seers), 24 plains districts Punjab, 1868–1908

District	Coeff.	Std. error	p-value*	R-sq
Southeast:				
Hissar	0.090	0.026	**0.001**	0.240
Rohtak	0.076	0.028	**0.009**	0.170
Gurgaon	0.065	0.031	**0.049**	0.120
Delhi	0.038	0.022	0.092	0.070
Karnal	0.044	0.024	0.077	0.080
Amballa	0.009	0.024	0.719	0.000
Central:				
Hoshiarpur	0.022	0.022	0.312	0.030
Jullundur	–0.001	0.026	0.983	0.000
Ludhiana	0.046	0.025	0.080	0.080
Ferozepur	0.062	0.024	**0.014**	0.150
Lahore	0.050	0.024	**0.047**	0.100
Amritsar	0.041	0.027	0.140	0.060
North:				
Gurdaspur	0.036	0.025	0.157	0.050
Sialkot	0.029	0.031	0.348	0.020
Gujrat	0.052	0.031	0.100	0.070
Gujranwala	0.022	0.036	0.550	0.010
Jhelum	0.073	0.027	**0.010**	0.160
West/Southwest:				
Shahpur	0.050	0.024	**0.041**	0.100
Jhang	0.023	0.029	0.437	0.020
Montgomery	0.067	0.035	0.066	0.080
Multan	0.016	0.024	0.514	0.010
Dhera Ismail Khan	0.021	0.033	0.526	0.010
Muzaffargarh	0.045	0.038	0.242	0.040
Dhera Ghazi Khan	0.032	0.040	0.426	0.020

* $p < 0.05$ in bold
Source: Table 4.1.

the higher R-square and price significance levels are found in the southeastern districts (Hissar, Rohtak, Gurgaon, Delhi, Karnal). But price is a significant predictor as well in other regions (Ludhiana, Gurdaspur, Sialkot). As with fever death rate, in one district, the price coefficient is negative, in this case, Jullundur, also an irrigation-'secure' district.

Interpretation

Quantitative analysis of autumn (Oct.–Dec.) fever mortality as an estimate of epidemic malaria mortality for the 1868–1908 period suggests that Christophers was correct in concluding that the malaria epidemic of 1908 was not an exceptional event, but part of a more general phenomenon characterising this region and period. At least as far back as the 1860s, severe malaria epidemics were a recurring feature of the region's health and demographic history, and a primary contributor to the high, and highly variable, death rate in the region (Figures 4.11a–d).[15] One of the more remarkable findings evident from the district-level analysis is the broad geographic prevalence of such 'fulminant' malaria epidemics. Despite marked differences in rainfall and other ecological features, mean autumn fever death rates are similar across much of the province for the pre-1909 period of recurring epidemics (Table 4.4, Figure 4.9), a pattern reflected also in high decadal coefficients of variation for Oct.–Dec. fever death rate through the four decades 1871–1910 (Table 4.5).

A somewhat different dynamic, however, is seen in the near-rainless southwest where year-to-year fluctuation in fever mortality in a number of districts is less pronounced (Figure 4.11d). These geographic differences also correspond to Christophers's view regarding the lower epidemic vulnerability of the western districts, likely related to low rainfall and thus lower flood risk as well as greater harvest security through high levels of crop irrigation.[16]

At the same time, the district-level quantitative results also support Christophers's 1911 conclusion that greater malaria endemicity and presumed higher levels of acquired immunity did not appear to offer protection from epidemicity. Of the four districts considered by sanitary officials as notoriously affected by waterlogging and high malaria endemicity, two (Gujranwala, Gujrat) fall within the highest district rankings for mean coefficient of variation for the 1871–1910 period (Table 4.6) and the remaining two, Gurgaon and Gurdaspur, in the mid-range of variability. Mean 1868–1908 Oct.–Dec. fever death rate is also well above average province levels (8.1 per mille) for Gujranwala, Gujrat, and Gurgaon districts (Table 4.4).[17]

One relatively minor discrepancy between the present study's findings and Christophers's relates to his assessment of greater 'epidemic potential' in the northern plains districts compared with the southeast.[18] As we have seen, mean autumn fever death rates (Oct.–Dec.) for the 1868–1908 period were similar across both regions (Table 4.4), with autumnal fever mortality fluctuations as frequent and large in the southeast of the province as in the northern districts. It seems likely Christophers's view of greater northern epidemicity derives from his use of the Epidemic Figure measure to assess regional epidemicity differentials and its inherent limitations, as outlined in chapter 3. As a ratio of autumn fever mortality divided by a comparable early summer mortality, the measure introduces an under-estimation bias in famine-prone districts where death rates leading up to the monsoon period tended to be higher than in districts with greater access to well irrigation, an exaggerated example of this bias evident in the 1900 famine year (Table 4.12).

With respect to etiological factors underlying epidemic patterns in the 1868–1908 period, regression analysis supports Christophers's 1911 broad conclusions: a strong role for rainfall in predicting malaria mortality throughout the Punjab plains, but as well an independent

Table 4.12 Crude death rate, Oct.–Dec. fever death rate, Apr.–July fever death rate (× .75), epidemic figure*, 1900, 24 plains districts, Punjab

District	CDR	Epidemic figure*	Oct.–Dec. FDR	Apr.–July FDR (× .75)
Southeast:				
Hissar	96.4	2.2	32.4	14.7
Rohtak	68.0	1.5	19.6	12.9
Gurgaon	49.7	2.0	13.1	6.6
Delhi	53.9	2.4	16.1	6.6
Karnal	92.9	2.8	40.1	8.4
Amballa	50.7	4.7	24.9	3.1
Central:				
Hoshiarpur	40.8	4.6	15.0	3.3
Jullundur	37.6	3.2	10.6	3.3
Ludhiana	60.4	4.9	24.1	5.0
Ferozepur	86.8	7.5	51.4	5.1
Lahore	59.4	5.4	25.4	4.7
Amritsar	46.0	2.8	13.2	4.7
North:				
Gurdaspur	46.0	4.9	16.7	3.4
Sialkot	44.4	4.3	16.7	3.9
Gujrat	33.8	2.4	9.9	4.1
Gujranwala	44.8	2.0	13.5	6.6
Jhelum	33.7	1.5	7.6	5.0
West/Southwest:				
Shahpur	28.9	1.1	4.5	4.2
Jhang	59.1	2.2	17.6	8.1
Montgomery	38.6	7.0	16.4	2.4
Multan	28.6	1.6	6.8	4.3
Dhera Ismail Khan	31.0	1.3	6.9	5.3
Muzaffargarh	27.4	2.1	9.6	4.6
Dhera Ghazi Khan	27.3	1.7	7.8	4.5

* Oct.–Dec. fever death rate divided by the Apr.–July death rate (× .75)
Source: Table 4.1.

role for foodgrain prices in most districts over and above that of rainfall. The highly significant role for third-quarter rain across the province is not an unexpected finding, given the direct and immediate role of monsoon rainfall in malaria transmission in the Punjab plains.[19] Nor is it surprising that the enabling role of rainfall would continue through the final four post-1908 decades of colonial rule, though the *amount* of fever mortality it was predicting was much lower. But the strong significance of rainfall in predicting autumn fever mortality in districts with such a wide range of normal rainfall levels also suggests that the role of third-quarter rain was related less to absolute amounts than to *relative* increase above normal levels, amounts that potentially overwhelmed local surface drainage capacity.[20]

The relationship of prices to malaria mortality, in contrast to that of rain, is less consistent: in six of the 24 plains districts, price fails to predict 1868–1908 autumn fever mortality for any of the four foodgrains. The spatial pattern of this opposite relationship between foodgrain price and malaria mortality, however, is not random, but corresponds closely to variation in agricultural economies across the province. Grain prices are significant predictors of autumn fever mortality in districts where cultivation depended to a large extent on direct rainfall – as was the case in much of the rest of the Indian subcontinent. Here, market prices were a marker of crop failure *and* agricultural paralysis (drought-triggered unemployment), in addition to the costliness of staple foodgrains. Conversely, all six districts where foodgrain price does not predict autumn fever mortality were located in the north-central and southwestern regions, tracts with a higher proportion (>40 per cent) of crops under irrigation (Figure 4.12).

This spatial pattern to price significance in predicting autumn fever mortality closely parallels the 1903 Irrigation Commission's categorisation of Punjab districts as agriculturally 'secure' or 'insecure.'[21] The designation was based upon the proportion of cropped area protected by irrigation: 'secure' districts were those north-central districts where well-/canal-irrigation predominated (Hoshiarpur, Jullundur, Amritsar, Gujranwala), and in the southwest, inundation-/canal-irrigation (Shahpur, Multan, Montgomery, Jhang, Dera Ghazi Khan) (Table 3.1). The remainder of the Punjab plains districts the Commission designated as harvest 'insecure.'

In the 'secure' districts, the more powerful trigger of harvest failure and agricultural paralysis was *excess* rainfall and associated flooding, the economic consequences of which were well understood within the administration. In his 1892 district Settlement report, W.E. Purser observed that Jullundur district 'has not suffered severely from famine

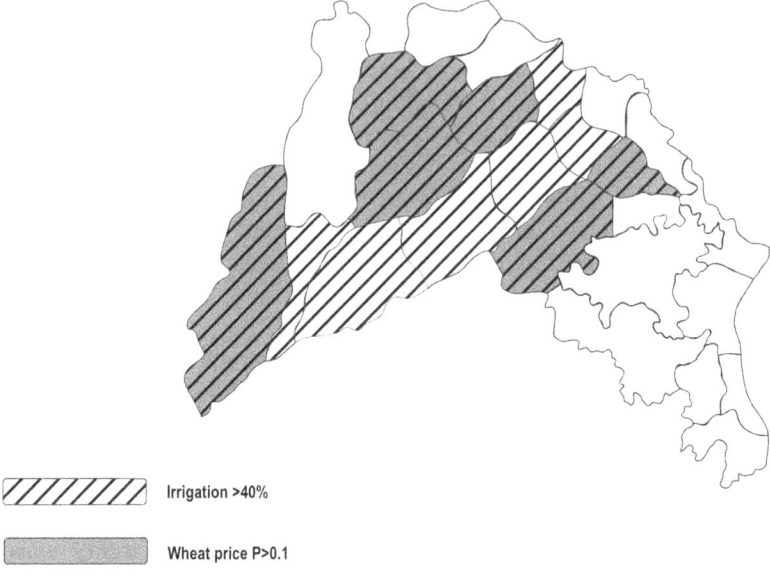

Irrigation >40%

Wheat price P>0.1

Figure 4.12 Per cent irrigated area, 1904; wheat price (*p* > 0.1), 1868–1908, 24 plains districts, Punjab

Source: See Tables 3.2, 4.1, 4.10, 4.11.

in living memory of man, and is not likely ever to suffer much. . . . [The] greater part of the soil requires little rain to yield some return.'[22] In neighbouring Amritsar district, officials similarly observed that

> failure of the summer rains may mean a shortage of fodder and pulse crops, but in the greater part of the district an excess monsoon, such as occurred in 1908 and 1909, causes more extensive loss and suffering . . . [t]he evil effects of [which] . . . may last for years.[23]

Yet the heavy rains that caused such damage also spelled favourable harvest conditions elsewhere in the region and thus were associated with low or falling market grain prices in general across the province, including in the highly irrigated districts.

The near-rainless southwest region of Punjab province also was relatively insulated from harvest failure. As in the north-central region, economic paralysis and severe malaria epidemics were associated with exceptional floods rather than drought. But here severe flooding was less frequent by virtue of generally much lower rainfall levels, destructive flooding occurring mainly in years when the 10-inch monsoon isohyet extended markedly westward. This quite different profile to agricultural prosperity and malaria epidemicity appears to be reflected both in the region's lower mean Oct.–Dec. fever death rates and smaller decadal coefficients of variation. (Tables 4.4, 4.5).

A partial exception in this regard is Muzaffargarh, the single southwest district where price is a significant predictor of autumn fever mortality. This may reflect the district's distinctive geography as a narrow tract bounded by two major river systems of the region, a district particularly subject to destructive flooding despite minimal direct rainfall: a tract where the added economic stress of famine-level prices may have been felt more acutely than elsewhere in the southwest. At 9.3 per 1,000, mean Oct.–Dec. fever death rate for the 1868–1908 period in Muzaffargarh is the third highest of the 24 districts, and year-to-year fluctuation in autumn fever death rate is as pronounced as in many of the eastern districts.[24]

In sum, while district-level regression results confirm the importance of price behaviour in predicting malaria epidemicity in much of the province across the first half of the colonial period, they also underscore limitations to foodgrain prices as a *measure* of acute hunger – failing, for example, to capture economic hardship in those districts where harvests were more seriously affected by flooding than drought. This pattern of price non-significance – rain as the sole predictor of malaria lethality – is consistent with a much more complex meaning to rainfall in the epidemic model, one that is economic as well as entomological. Moreover, this dual dimension to the effect of monsoon rainfall on malaria epidemicity was not limited to harvest-secure districts. While 'excess rain' was particularly detrimental in the highly irrigated and waterlogged tracts of the province, above normal rains could trigger destructive flooding in virtually any of the plains districts.[25]

The district-level regression results highlight, in other words, major limitations to the rain-price model itself for understanding malaria epidemicity in the province: with respect to both independent variables (rain and price), there exist additional, or paradoxical, relationships with the condition each was intended to measure (malaria transmission and acute hunger, respectively).

The question, then, as to *how much* epidemic mortality in the earlier 1868–1908 period was hunger – rather than malaria transmission – mediated is one that cannot be resolved through statistical methods alone. Distinguishing economic from entomological factors in epidemic causation must rest upon additional methods.

Two avenues are pursued in this study: first, more detailed exploration of individual major epidemics in the pre-1920 period, in particular, those which appear as outliers to the rain-price model, a subject explored in the chapter that follows, and second, that of placing the experience of 1868–1908 fulminant malaria in the context of post-1908 epidemic decline, exploring what factors change after 1908 and which do not, questions addressed in detail in Parts II and III of the study.

With respect to the question of post-1908 epidemic decline, quantitative analysis of the 1909–1940 period offers a useful starting point. Decline in autumn fever mortality in the early decades of the 20th century is evident for all regions of Punjab. Coefficients of variability after 1910 are one-half to one-quarter the levels experienced in the pre-1910 period (Table 4.5). As remarkable perhaps as the size of this decline is its geographic extent, a decline evident across regions with very different ecological and rural agricultural economies. It seems unlikely the minimal changes in monsoon rainfall noted earlier could have altered entomological conditions or flooding incidence substantially; especially in the context of the very much greater differences in normal rainfall levels across the province.[26] Indeed, as will be traced in subsequent chapters, post-monsoon malaria transmission continued unabated in the province through to the early 1950s.

As for scarcity, a fundamental shift in the relationship between market foodgrain prices and autumn fever mortality is apparent in the final decades of the colonial period, with no districts showing a statistically significant relationship between the two after 1908. It is unlikely that the link between staple foodgrain prices, acute hunger, and malaria mortality ceased altogether after 1908. Marked foodgrain price fluctuations continued, but such swings were influenced more by global forces than by local harvest and employment conditions, hence 'diluting' further the value of the major market price data as indicators of acute destitution.[27] Increased variability in price behaviour after 1910 has been noted by some observers.[28] Change in price behaviour is suggested in the present study as well, with price fluctuations generally limited to two- or even single-year episodes post-1908 compared with the more prolonged three-year surges evident in the earlier decades of the colonial period (Figure 4.6).

It is worth noting at this point that Punjab province was not alone in the decline in epidemic mortality in the early decades of the 20th century. In its timing, the attenuation of malaria mortality in Punjab is similar to that seen in other parts of the subcontinent after 1920 for other epidemic diseases. Ortega has analysed trends in yearly fluctuations in epidemic mortality across the colonial period in selected

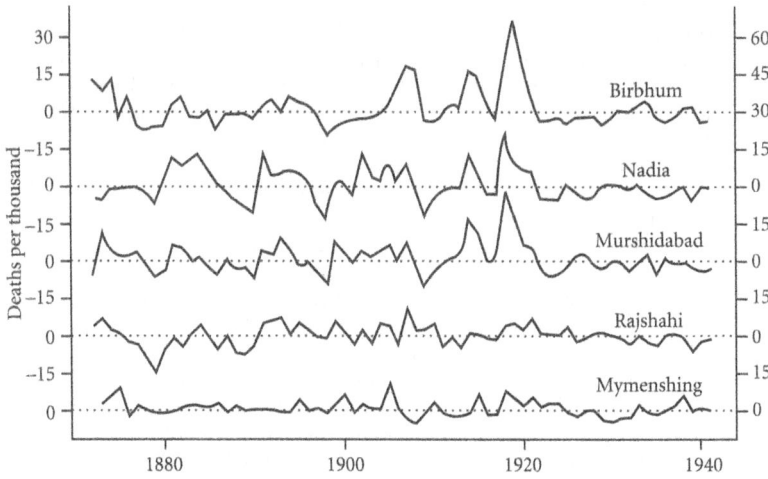

Figure 4.13 Annual crude death rate (fluctuations from trend), selected Bengal districts, 1872–1941

Source: J.A. Ortega Osona, 'The Attenuation of Mortality Fluctuations in British Punjab and Bengal, 1870–1947,' in T. Liu et al., eds., *Asian Population History* (2001), 319, Figure 15.1. Reprinted with permission of Oxford University Press.

districts of Bengal and Punjab. He found that while the magnitude of fluctuations from trend is smaller in Bengal through the first half of the colonial period, a notable decline also is evident after 1920 (Figure 4.13).[29] As Ortega concludes, attenuation in mortality fluctuations (crises) appears to have been a central aspect of the broader phenomenon of demographic transition in South Asia more generally.

Before turning to investigate the range of factors, in the case of Punjab malaria, that contributed to epidemic decline, we turn to examine the statistically 'anomalous' epidemic years, outliers to the rain-price model, for the additional insights they offer beyond those elucidated in the regression analysis.

Notes

1 The district-level regression analysis of the 1868–1908 period includes Christophers's original 24 districts, whereas analysis of trends to 1940 includes only 23 districts, Delhi district no longer within the jurisdiction of Punjab province after 1911.

2 T. Dyson, M. Das Gupta, 'Demographic Trends in Ludhiana District, Punjab, 1881–1981: An Exploration of Vital Registration Data in Colonial

India,' in T. Liu, et al., eds., *Asian Population History* (Oxford: Oxford University Press, 2001), 79–104.

3 Using R version 3.1.0 and standard bandwidth of .67. For discussion of limitations of trend lines as 'normal' mortality levels, see J.A. Ortega Osona, 'The Attenuation of Mortality Fluctuations in British Punjab and Bengal, 1870–1947,' in Liu, et al., eds., *Asian Population History*, 306–349.

4 In the raw data graph (Figure 4.1) the 1869 epidemic is less prominent due to markedly incomplete reporting in this initial period of vital registration.

5 Two additional epidemic years are prominent in the sanitary records, 1887 and 1897, with Oct.–Dec. FDR registered at or above 10 per mille, a 25 per cent increase over the 41-year mean of 8.1 per mille. The 1887 epidemic was anomalous in not being preceded by harvest failure; in the case of 1897, famine conditions were limited to the southeast corner of the province, limiting the province-level figure.

6 One additional year of marked autumn 'fever' mortality occurred in 1918, associated with the influenza pandemic, deaths recorded under the 'fever' vital registration category. Coinciding in Punjab with both severe drought (undeclared famine) and war-time hyper-inflation, Oct.–Dec. FDR reached the extraordinary level of 54.8 deaths per mille. Because autumn malarial deaths cannot be distinguished from influenza mortality, the year 1918 is excluded from the analysis.

7 Christophers, 'Malaria in the Punjab,' *Sci. Mem. Off. Med. San. Dep.*, 46 (Calcutta: Superintendent, Government Printing Office, 1911), 6–7 [hereafter MP].

8 The regression equation is $\mu_y = -7.09 + 0.49x$, where μ_y is FDR and x is CDR for a given year.

9 Mean third-quarter rain trend line (23 plains districts) for the 1868–1943 period is $y = 14.33–30.0154x$ (P = .69).

10 Mean 24-district crude birth rate for 1885–1908 is 41.7 per 1,000; for Dhera Ghazi Khan, 31.0, and Dhera Ismail Khan, 35.9 per 1,000.

11 R. Killick, P. Fearnhead, I.A. Eckley, 'Optimal Detection of Changepoints with a Linear Computational Cost,' *Journal of the American Statistical Association*, 107, 500, 2012, 1590–1598.

12 For discussion of methods of quantifying vital registration data variability, see Ortega, 'Attenuation of Mortality,' 315–317. He identifies 1922 as the crude death rate change point for Hoshiarpur, Jullundur, and Ludhiana districts. See as well, C. Guilmoto, 'Towards a New Demographic Equilibrium: The Inception of Demographic Transition in South India,' *Indian Economic and Social History Review*, 28, 3, 1992, 247–289, at 265.

13 A detrended wheat price series was created, again using the Loess procedure.

14 *Vigna mungo* (L.) (syn *Phaseolus mungo*).

15 Christophers, MP, 7. A partial exception is the contributing role of plague mortality for two and a half decades from the turn of the century.

16 Christophers, MP, 71. It is possible that lower deaths rates in the major canal colonisation districts of Shahpur, Jhang, and Montgomery (Figure 4.9, 4.10) partly reflect differences in age profile of the population, migration into the region with canal development resulting in proportionately greater numbers of young adults, an age group with lowest relative malaria mortality risk.

17 Only Gurdaspur shows mean Oct.–Dec. FDR below the 24-district mean, at 6.4 per mille. An off-shoot from colonial discussions on the role of acquired immunity in Punjab malaria epidemicity was interest in epidemic periodicity. Here, we can note that the detrended time-series of 1868–1940 FDR suggests intervals of six to nine years between major epidemics. Applying the White Noise test to the 72-year series suggests an eight-year cycle but a result that is not statistically significant. The Kolomogorov-Smirnov test statistic for Oct.–Dec. FDR is 0.152; for third-quarter rain, 0.145. If a periodic cycle exists, it cannot be detected due to "noise" in the data.

18 MP, 72.

19 The power of 'excess' rainfall in predicting major epidemics at the provincial level lay in part in its association with westward extension of the 10-inch isohyet, which meant a greater portion of the province with favourable entomological conditions but also affected economically by flood conditions, together increasing the aggregate (provincial) mortality tally in a given year.

20 Certainly, in the normally near-rainless southwest, severe flooding was associated with the main post-1908 epidemics of 1929 and 1933.

21 Canal-irrigated area quadrupled in the final decades of the 19th century, from 943,043 acres in the early 1880s to 4,123,548 acres by the turn of the century, mainly in the dry western districts. The 1903 Irrigation Commission would describe agriculture in the 'rainless' districts of Muzaffargarh, DI Khan, DG Kahn, Multan, Montgomery, Shahpur, Jhang as dependent on 'snow-fed rivers' and 'not liable to failure even in seasons of intense drought. The districts in this tract cannot, therefore, be considered as liable to famine, though they are often affected by unfavourable conditions in the river supply'; *Report of the Indian Irrigation Commission* (London: HMSO, 1903), 2, 6.

22 W.E. Purser, *Final Report of the Revised Settlement of the Jullundur District in the Punjab* (Lahore: Punjab Revenue Department, 1892), 64.

23 H.D. Craik, *Final Report of the 4th Regular Settlement of the Amritsar District, 1910–1914* (Lahore: Punjab, Revenue Department, 1914), 1.

24 Control of famine after 1920 likely had a greater impact on malaria epidemicity in the more harvest 'insecure' eastern portion of the province compared with the southwest, where major epidemics were limited to years of exceptional westward extension of the 20-inch monsoon isohyet. The most severe southwest epidemic, in 1917 (Figure 4.11d), saw record monsoon rainfall in Muzaffargarh, Multan, and Shahpur districts, set against a background of war-time famine-level foodgrain prices. Two further post-1908 western epidemics were associated with record rainfall in southwestern districts (1929), and near-record levels across the province (1933).

25 '[I]n the eastern half of the Punjab it is doubtful,' Christophers observed, 'whether any large tract however situated can be considered free from the possibility of flooding should an unusually heavy monsoon rain happen to fall there'; MP, 3.

26 Yacob and Swaroop found no significant decline in July–Aug. rain in Punjab for the period 1914–1943, but a 10-inch decline in total annual rainfall between 1867 and 1943; 'Malaria and Rainfall in the Punjab,' *Journal of the Malaria Institute of India*, 6, 3, June 1946, 273–284 at 278. It is difficult to see how a decline of this magnitude, if real, would not have been

noted by officials. A possible explanation is inadvertent inclusion on the part of the investigators of rain data from the new canal districts (Lyallpur in 1905 and Sheikapura in 1920) carved out of the large low-rain western districts in annual rain calculations, thus weighting mean levels downward; also, possible inclusion of Delhi district data up to 1911, a district with rainfall above the 24-district mean. In later years, Punjab officials analysed rainfall data for possible trends. McKenzie et al. found no trend for any individual month for the period 1903–1938; E. McKenzie Taylor, M.L. Mehta, 'Some Irrigation Problems in the Punjab,' *Indian Journal of Agricultural Science*, 11, 1941, 137–169. Blyn later found a decline in rainfall at Simla of 0.18 per cent per year for the period 1891–1946, suggesting a 10 per cent decline over the 54-year period, but no significant trend for Lahore district in the plains; G. Blyn, *Agricultural Trends in India, 1891–1947* (Philadelphia: University of Pennsylvania Press, 1966), 182. More recently, Parthasarathy reports no apparent decline in frequency of 'flood years' across the colonial period, as measured by June–Sept. rainfall >25 per cent above normal; B. Parthasarathy, N.A. Sontakke, A.A. Monot, D.R. Kothawale, 'Droughts/Floods in the Summer Monsoon Season Over Different Meteorological Subdivisions of India for the Period 1871–1984,' *Journal of Climatology*, 7, 1987, 57–70, 54; as cited in Menno J. Bouma, H. van der Kaay, 'The El Niño Southern Oscillation and the Historical Malaria Epidemics on the Indian Subcontinent and Sri Lanka: An Early Warning System for Future Epidemics?' *Tropical Medicine and International Health*, 1, 1, Feb. 1996, 86–96, at 91.

27 Price behaviour in the final decades of the colonial period was powerfully affected by external influences with war-time inflation and the post-1929 global economic depression; A.K. Ghosh, *Prices and Economic Fluctuations in India 1861–1947* (New Delhi: S. Chand, 1979). Thus, the value of price data as an indirect gauge of rural employment, livelihood, and earnings ('exchange entitlements') for a good portion of this period is limited.

28 Ashoka Mody notes increased variability of foodgrain prices between 1922–1933 in some Punjab districts (e.g., Ludhiana, though not Muzaffargarh); 'Population Growth and Commercialisation of Agriculture: India, 1890–1940,' *Indian Economic and Social History Review*, Dec. 1982, 237–266, at 249.

29 Ortega, 'Attenuation of Mortality.' For discussion of similar timing in epidemic mortality decline in the Madras Presidency, see Guilmoto, 'Towards a New Demographic Equilibrium.'

5 'Outlier' malaria epidemics

Among the nine major epidemics identified in the 1868–1908 period, we have seen that five conform to the 'excess' rain-'scarcity' model: three occurring during years of officially declared famine in 1869, 1878, and 1900, and another two, 1892 and 1908, in years of soaring foodgrain prices, though famine was not formally declared. Four epidemics, of the nine, however, stand out as exceptions to the general scarcity-rainfall pattern. Two, in 1876 and 1884, occurred in years when foodgrain prices were low and rainfall only marginally above average. A third, in 1879, was the only epidemic in the 41-year period to occur in a year of relative drought: monsoon rainfall 10.5 inches compared with a 24-district mean of 13.9 inches. And a fourth outlier, that of 1890, was a year where both grain prices and third-quarter rain were only moderately elevated: prevailing economic distress only partially reflected in aggregate rainfall or market price levels. To what extent do the 'anomalous' epidemics undermine the hypothesis linking epidemic occurrence to acute hunger? In what ways do they offer additional insights into epidemic aetiology?

1876 and 1884: exceptions to the 'scarcity'-epidemic model

Among price-'anomalous' epidemics, that of 1876 is perhaps the most striking. Foodgrain prices were at the lowest level of the entire 1868–1908 period, and monsoon rainfall at 15.7 inches was only marginally above normal (Table 4.1). Yet autumn fever mortality was severe, as attested by numerous accounts of intense malarial fever in both the revenue administration and sanitary reports.[1] Analysis of variance in the study data set confirms that 1876 was highly unusual in the rain-price regression model, standing out as a marked outlier in scatter plots of residual values, an epidemic Christophers also saw as anomalous:

> though the rainfall in 1875 was extraordinarily heavy the epidemic conditions were slight, whereas in the same area less heavy rain the next year caused a severe epidemic. It would be interesting to trace out the actual facts were one able to do so, as, for example, whether floods in 1875 did not damage crops to such an extent as to bring about local scarcity. Whichever way one looks at the matter, the year 1876 is quite unique.[2]

'[A]ctual facts,' as Christophers anticipated, do shed light upon pre-existing economic hardship. The preceding year, 1875, had been one of record monsoon rainfall levels for the 1868–1908 period, with 'disastrous flooding' and widespread crop damage. In the northern districts of Gurdaspur, Amritsar, and Sialkot, the summer crops 'almost totally failed' due to the rains, and in others, 'low-lying tracts remained submerged so long that they could not even be sown for the spring crop of 1876.' In some areas, whole villages were swept away by flood waters, 'lands [became] heavily mortgaged, crops lost and cattle destroyed.'[3] Yet the Oct.–Dec. fever death rate in 1875 was only moderately elevated, with economic conditions leading up to the heavy third-quarter rains having been favourable. Despite the 1875 *kharif* crop losses, harvest prospects for the province as a whole in 1876 were good by virtue of the previous year's rains, and prices remained low. Following the 1876 summer rains, however, autumn fever deaths soared in the irrigation-'secure' north-central districts and contiguous submontane region, the recorded mortality highest in Jullundur district (Table 5.1).[4]

The 'actual facts' surrounding the 1876 epidemic, moreover, also included fiscal and administrative aspects. In the aftermath of the 1875 flooding, the provincial administration refused most applications for suspension of land revenue (tax) collections, arguing

> there is every reason to hope that the people are so well off as to be able to meet the calamities of one disastrous season without requiring the direct interposition of Government by remission or suspension of revenue. . . . It is possible that the people who suffered were not pressed beyond their power, and were able to pay their revenue, though their crops failed.[5]

Token remissions were granted for only two of the eastern districts: in Jullundur district on 930 acres and in Gurgaon for 13,000 acres.

Table 5.1 Oct.–Dec. fever death rate (per 1,000), 1876; % normal July–Sept. rain, 1875, 1876, 24 plains districts, Punjab

District	Oct.–Dec. FDR (per 1,000), 1876	% normal July–Sept. rain	
		1876	1875
Southeast:			
Hissar	3.6	127	186
Rohtak	5.4	84	203
Gurgaon	4.1	122	230
Delhi	4.2	59	197
Karnal	4.3	70	101
Amballa	8.3	99	138
Central:			
Hoshiarpur	20.3	106	158
Jullundur	29.0	103	274
Ludhiana	9.6	44	174
Ferozepur	11.1	88	245
Lahore	12.5	144	221
Amritsar	19.2	167	239
North:			
Gurdaspur	16.5	127	219
Sialkot	20.9	201	208
Gujrat	7.7	174	148
Gujranwala	21.9	154	258
Jhelum	4.1	68	145
West/Southwest:			
Shahpur	5.1	86	77
Jhang	4.6	77	154
Montgomery	6.6	109	13
Multan	8.1	107	66
Dhera Ismail Khan	4.7	84	125
Muzaffargarh	9.9	187	129
Dhera Ghazi Khan	5.4	212	159

Source: See Table 4.1.

Others that had also suffered heavy losses, such as Delhi, Amritsar, Hoshiarpur, Gurdaspur, and Sialkot, were granted none, district officials blaming local Indian revenue agents who were said to dislike the extra paperwork involved.[6] Nor were relief measures sanctioned in 1875 for flood-affected districts. Thus, when seasonal malaria transmission again peaked in the autumn months of 1876, it was visited upon a peasant population that had suffered many months of cumulative economic paralysis in addition to crop losses. Those areas hard hit by floods the year before, such as Jullundur, Hoshiarpur, Amritsar,

Gurdaspur, and Sialkot districts, experienced the most intense fever mortality.

Thus, though atypical in the rain-price statistical model, the 1876 epidemic is hardly anomalous with respect to the acute hunger thesis of malaria mortality, and thus it highlights a major limitation to foodgrain prices as a measure of destitution. But it demonstrates as well the contingent nature of heavy rainfall as epidemic trigger. Autumnal fever mortality in 1875, though elevated, does not appear to have been exceptionally high despite record rains and flooding, conditions seemingly conducive for malaria transmission. Good economic conditions going into a heavy rainfall season provided some physiological buffer, it appears, to the disrupting impact of floods and malaria transmission. When flooding was preceded, on the other hand, by severe harvest losses, as in 1908 triggered by drought, it was associated with severe mortality.

This element of contingency becomes apparent also for Jullundur district in 1878. Third-quarter rainfall at 35 inches was well above normal, but considerably lower than in 1875 (49 inches). Yet with grain prices at famine level, the 1878 autumn fever death rate rose to 43.8 per mille, compared with 10.7 per mille three years earlier (Table 5.2).[7]

A second price-'anomalous' epidemic was that of 1884. As in 1876, foodgrain prices were low and monsoon rainfall at 16.7 inches was only moderately above normal (24-district mean: 13.9 inches). Autumn fever mortality, however, was the sixth highest of the 41-year period. Unlike 1876, agricultural conditions leading up to the 1884 epidemic had been dominated by severe drought in the eastern third of

Table 5.2 July–Sept. rain (inches), Oct.–Dec. fever death rate (per 1,000), Jullundur district, Punjab, selected years

	July–Sept. rain (in)*	Oct.–Dec. FDR (per 1,000)
1875	49.0	10.7
1876	18.4	29.0
1878**	35.0	43.8
1892**	25.0	15.4
1933	31.6	5.4

Source: See Table 4.1.

*1868–1940 Mean July–Sept. rain = 17.7 inches.

**'scarcity'/famine-level prices

the province, in some districts (Karnal and Amballa) by two preceding years of failed harvests.[8] In its 'narrative' overview of recent famines, the 1898 Famine Commission Report would later refer to 1884 as a year of 'famine.' Little relief, however, had been instituted. A proposal for agricultural loans was refused by the provincial Government, the 1898 Commission concurring with officials at the time that 'it would be a great mistake . . . to encourage the people to run largely into debt for this purpose. . . . [Hence] the people must be left to themselves in this matter.' Nor was tax relief granted, except in the single district of Hissar.[9]

The 1882–1883 drought conditions afflicting eastern Punjab, however, were localised. Harvests elsewhere in the province, and generally in the subcontinent, had been good. Thus, agricultural distress in the Delhi Division was not reflected in province-level grain prices, and only marginally in market prices in the afflicted southeast.

In the event, much of the excess rainfall in the summer months of 1884 fell in this eastern region. Amballa district received 41 inches, one rural station, Jagadri, receiving 71 inches of rain.[10] Karnal district to the immediate south also was hit by 'very heavy' late September rains when the crops were nearly ripe. 'A terrible epidemic of fever was the result,' the provincial sanitary commissioner reported, which 'prostrated quite one-fourth of the population and greatly delayed harvesting . . . [A]round Karnal [town] the water lay for miles like a lake.'[11] Economic hardship in much of the eastern region of the province, in other words, was dual: extended drought followed by severe flooding. It was in the high rainfall districts that autumn fever mortality was especially severe (Table 5.3).[12]

Table 5.3 Oct.–Dec. fever death rate (per 1,000), % normal July–Sept. rain, by district, Punjab, 1882–1884

	1884		% normal July–Sept. rain		
	Oct.–Dec. FDR	July–Sept. rain	1884	1883	1882
Hissar	12.1	10.1	95	80	110
Rohtak	12.6	14.1	101	66	76
Gurgaon	10.9	21.4	117	73	67
Delhi	21.0	34.7	172	53	105
Karnal	24.1	32.6	161	58	77
Amballa	28.3	41.2	193	56	71

Source: See Table 4.1.

Christophers himself would single out the 1884 epidemic as atypical. '[T]hough the prices given suggest prosperity, I find the year recorded as one in which the very districts concerned (Umballa) underwent great hardship owing to failure of crops.' It was on this basis, it appears, that he chose to omit 1884 from his correlation calculations.[13] It may, in fact, have been the 1884 epidemic he had in mind when pointing out, at the 1909 Simla malaria conference, the limitations of price data due to the 'very remarkable averaging process in regard to ruling prices' at the major district markets if crop failure was limited in geographic extent.[14]

In addition, then, to their 'outlier' status, the 1876 and 1884 epidemics are notable for highlighting the continuing reluctance of the colonial administration to respond to famine conditions limited in their extent to only portions of a province, or indeed even to acknowledge their human cost. '[T]hat this [1884] scarcity,' the 1898 Famine Commission sanguinely remarked,

> arising as it did from a very extensive failure of two successive harvests . . . should have been tided over at such small expense to the State and resulted in so little distress, speaks well of the staying power and resources of the agriculturalists of the south-eastern Punjab.[15]

That 'staying power,' however, did not extend to the 120,000 whose fever deaths were recorded in excess of the 35,000 mean in the autumn months of the year.

1879: an exception to the diluvial epidemic model

Beyond rigid taxation and 'stringent' famine relief policies there was a further economic dimension to colonial governance influencing epidemic patterns across this period: the entry of South Asian foodgrains onto international grain markets. The impact, in Punjab, is dramatically seen in a third outlier epidemic, that of 1879. The 1879 epidemic represented the final phase of three years of hardship in northwest India in the late 1870s. Severe drought in 1875–1876 across southern India had triggered widespread famine there in 1876–1877, with pressure on foodgrain prices felt across the subcontinent. Punjab province itself experienced drought and severe failure of the *kharif* harvest one year later in 1877, mean third-quarter rainfall falling to 6.2 inches. Return of good summer rains (17.7 inches) in 1878 brought epidemic malaria mortality, in classic fashion, in the autumn months of the year.

Yet despite improved harvest conditions, foodgrain prices across the province failed to return to normal.[16] Famine-level prices continued to prevail throughout the region for a third year, and the summer monsoon rains of 1879 brought a second year of fulminant malaria conditions in train (Table 5.4).

The 1879 malaria epidemic was exceptional in a number of ways. It is notable epidemiologically as an outlier to the rain-price model, the year being one of relative drought (10.5 inches), the single instance of soaring autumn fever mortality in the province following a monsoon season of below normal rains. But it is notable also

Table 5.4 Oct.–Dec. fever death rate (per 1,000), July–Sept. rain (inches), 24 plains districts, Punjab, 1879

District	Oct.–Dec. FDR, 1879	July–Sept. 1879 rain	
		inches	% of normal
Southeast:			
Hissar	11.3	9.4	88
Rohtak	31.7	15.9	114
Gurgaon	39.6	20.4	111
Delhi	29.9	26.7	132
Karnal	18.3	18.2	90
Amballa	12.8	12.6	59
Central:			
Hoshiarpur	9.0	9.8	42
Jullundur	8.6	14.2	79
Ludhiana	8.9	7.2	40
Ferozepur	4.7	8.1	72
Lahore	7.3	10.8	87
Amritsar	7.2	10.2	66
North:			
Gurdaspur	8.6	11.8	52
Sialkot	5.2	16.6	78
Gujrat	7.6	14.5	89
Gujranwala	7.3	10.0	65
Jhelum	8.9	18.5	111
West/Southwest:			
Shahpur	3.5	7.6	90
Jhang	1.3	1.9	37
Montgomery	4.3	2.6	39
Multan	4.0	1.7	41
Dhera Ismail Khan	4.3	3.1	56
Muzaffargarh	5.4	0.0	0
Dhera Ghazi Khan	2.1	0.9	26

Source: See Table 4.1.

economically, in highlighting – in the bright glare of vital registration accounts – market price dynamics very different from the 'classic' pattern: grain prices remaining at famine level after the return of normal rains in 1878.

Despite being a year of relative drought, narrative descriptions of the autumn fever mortality in 1879 leave little doubt as to the malarial character of the epidemic, or to its intensity. Sanitary officials described 'the universal prevalence of fever of a severe and fatal character all over the Punjab,'[17] the autumn fever death rate in 1879 ranking eighth in severity of the nine major epidemics. Soaring fever mortality shows the typical monthly autumnal rise occurring simultaneously across the eastern half of the Punjab plains.

Autumn fever mortality in 1879 was highest in the southeast, the Oct.–Dec. FDR in several districts rising to between 30 and 40 deaths per 1,000, from a non-epidemic mean of 6.3, one person in thirty in the population succumbing. And only in this region did monsoon rainfall in 1879 approach near-normal levels (Table 5.4). Elsewhere in the province, where third-quarter rainfall was in marked deficit, there was little autumnal rise in fever mortality, although very high general (crude) death rates prevailed across much of the province throughout the year. The one exception was the irrigated southwest.

In this respect, the epidemic of 1879 in Punjab appears to be an example of the 'enabling' role of monsoon rains on malaria transmission, and conversely the limiting impact of drought. Still, the question remains why fever mortality in the southeast was so severe when rainfall even there reached barely average levels. At 20.4 inches, third-quarter rainfall in Gurgaon district was only marginally above the district mean of 18.1 inches. In Karnal district, also quite severely affected by fever mortality in the autumn months of 1879, rainfall was slightly below normal levels. Accounts of flooding appear nowhere in the narrative administrative reports. Entomological conditions, in other words, do not appear to have been exceptional in any of the epidemic-affected tracts.

On the other hand, numerous accounts of debility and medical symptomatology of severe starvation are described in district Land Revenue officials reports. 'The people look ill – out of heart, and badly nourished,' one official observed, with 'dropsical swelling' and 'large ulcers on the legs so bad, as to be fatal.'[18] Others noted relative protection from the epidemic among canal-irrigated villages, which

> had not suffered from failure of their crops . . . and had escaped the scarcity and semi-starvation which in the high lands had

lowered the health of the people and rendered them, from their weakened and debilitated condition, unable to resist the effects of a fever which climatic occurrences have rendered unusually prevalent and severe.[19]

The *Gurgaon District Gazetteer* later would recount that

[S]carcity caused by the failure of harvests [in 1877] hardly deepened into actual famine, although there were some deaths from starvation, and a large portion of *the population was greatly weakened by want; but it was followed in 1878 and 1879 by a dreadful epidemic of fever.*[20]

From the epidemiological standpoint, the 1879 epidemic suggests that 'excess' rainfall was not required for autumn malaria to take on intense form *if* economic stress were severe enough. Quite possibly it was this epidemic Christophers had in mind when he observed at the 1912 Madras malaria conference that, 'the mortality [caused] by the epidemic is very much increased *even if the epidemic is not strong* by a condition of stress among the people in the previous year.'[21] Here he appears to be using the word 'epidemic' in the limited microbiological sense of malaria transmission, contrasting this with malaria lethality.

But the 1879 epidemic was unusual in another way as well: it is one of the few instances of two consecutive severe epidemics in the same rural region. Districts, and indeed specific villages, severely affected in 1879 had experienced high fever mortality the previous year as well.[22] This suggests that, where scarcity conditions continued to prevail, any protective effect of acquired immunity from a previous year's epidemic was readily overwhelmed.

Beyond epidemiological considerations, from the standpoint of political economy, the malaria epidemic of 1879 confirmed the grave implications of the change in behaviour of market prices on public health. Railway construction over the preceding decade had brought about rapid integration of South Asian foodgrains into international markets (Figure 3.1).[23] In 1873, the government had repealed the export duty on wheat, actively encouraging the export of foodgrains from India.[24] Now, a single poor harvest was sufficient to trigger soaring prices, where in the past only consecutive years of harvest failure did so. The effects were starkly evident in the severe southern India famine in 1876–1877, and in the north, a year later.

In fact, though July–September monsoon rainfall was in marked deficit in 1877 across Punjab, rainfall earlier in the year had been well above normal and the *rabi* (winter) harvest had been good. These were hardly typical famine conditions. Yet by 1878, foodgrain prices in the province had soared to near-record levels, setting the stage for the severe epidemic in the autumn of that year. Within the administration, confusion prevailed as to what to term the entire three-year period of famine-level prices. Still working with local crop failure as the basis for assessing agricultural 'stress,' Punjab district officials did not officially declare famine in 1878 because crop losses the previous year were insufficient under existing guidelines to qualify. Nor was famine declared in 1879 because harvests had been good the year before. And once again, the Land revenue was collected with equal thoroughness, with several district officials noting, 'with great oppression.'[25]

Notwithstanding official reluctance to formally term 1878–1879 a famine in northwest India, similar conditions in the western districts of the neighbouring Northwestern Provinces and Oudh (United Provinces) had prompted authorities to undertake a 'famine census' to determine the class profile of famine mortality. The results would be submitted in a confidential memorandum which reported that approximately 80 per cent of famine deaths came from the labouring classes, with many of the remaining deaths among cultivators with marginal holdings of less than three acres.[26]

This sequence of late 1870s famines, first in southern India in 1876–1877, then in the northwest in 1878–1879, would prompt a prominent commission of inquiry. The resulting Famine Commission Report of 1880 led to formulation of the first comprehensive famine relief legislation, the provisional Indian Famine Code in 1883. However, as we will consider in Part III of the study, the broader economic forces underlying the lethality of malaria in 1878 and 1879 in Punjab would fail to be addressed under the new Famine Code, and fulminant malaria epidemics continued (Figure 1.2).

1890: further limitations to the rain-price model

The decade or so following release of the 1880 Famine Commission Report was a period of generally favourable rains across much of the subcontinent. Yet autumn fever mortality in Punjab province in 1890 would approach that seen in 1908, despite only moderately elevated levels of monsoon rainfall (16.4 inches) and foodgrain prices (Rs 5.4 per 100 seers).

Monsoon rainfall in 1890 was heaviest in the northern submontane districts of Sialkot, Gujrat, and Gujranwala, and it was here where autumn fever mortality would be most intense. However, mortality rates were already very high well in advance of the malaria season. In Sialkot district, for example, mortality over the first nine (pre-malaria) months of the year averaged 51 per mille. Autumn fever mortality would push that rate even further, to 101.2 per mille, over 10 per cent of the population dying over the course of the year. General mortality levels were high, in fact, across the entire province in 1890, virtually double those levels prevailing only several years earlier. Indeed, at 50 deaths per 1,000 population, the provincial crude death rate was comparable to that during the 'great' famines at the turn of the century.

Surprisingly little information appears in the sanitary or administrative reports to explain the high level of mortality leading up to the autumn 1890 epidemic. Nor does it appear to have been due to sudden improvement in vital registration reporting: crude birth rates are unchanged, for example, through this period. In terms of agricultural conditions, one has to go back five years in the administrative records to identify a single year of poor rains. Yet grain prices had been extremely high throughout the later years. In the absence of references to other epidemic diseases in the early months of 1890, it is difficult not to conclude these death rates reflected general underlying economic stress induced by scarcity-level grain prices.[27] Indeed, three years earlier, there had been another epidemic, 'anomalous' for prices being at famine-level in the absence of major harvest failure. In order to better understand the 1890 epidemic, it is useful to look back at the 1887 epidemic, about which much more contemporary commentary exists.

Christophers did not include the 1887 epidemic in his list of 'fulminant' epidemics, although the Oct.–Dec. fever death rate was just marginally lower at 10.5 per mille than that of 1879 (11.2 per mille). Again, monsoon rainfall in 1887 at 17.9 inches was only moderately above the mean of 13.6 inches. Foodgrain prices, however, were at famine level, despite good harvests the year before. And as in 1890, death rates were already high well before the autumn fever season, in some districts mortality for the year reaching 62 deaths per 1,000. Rising grain prices initially had been triggered two years earlier by poor monsoon rains in 1885 in the north-central region of the province. Good harvests returned in 1886; however, prices did not recover. Instead, they continued to climb, reaching famine level in 1887.

That there was severe economic stress across the province leading up to the autumn 1887 epidemic is clear from administrative reports. But it appears to have been precipitated not by harvest failure but by soaring exports of foodgrains leading to depletion of local stocks. In the early 1880s, exports of wheat from Karachi, the main port exporting Punjab grain, had amounted to less than 10,000 tons. With increasing rail construction linking district grain markets, international exports had risen to 350,000 tons by 1885–1886,[28] a point at which India was supplying 23 per cent of Britain's imports of wheat (Table 5.5).[29] The effect on local grain prices at this time was felt especially in the southeast of Punjab province where rail lines had recently linked local markets to the burgeoning international export grain trade. Despite indifferent harvests in the south-east in 1886, exports continued through 1887, triggering 'grave apprehensions' on the part of district-level officials over 'the large depletion of food stock reserves, the great demand for exportation coupled with speculative time-dealings in wheat, and the increased use of facilities of transit of the last year.'[30] Not only were wheat prices now affected by demand in neighbouring markets, remarked the Karnal Deputy Commissioner,

> but produce even is tapped by buyers and brokers from distant centres including Bombay and Kurráchi themselves. . . . The Punjab Steam Navigation Company, under the patronage of the Western Jumna Canal Authorities, have maintained a flotilla of barges by which a marked stimulus has been given to exportation . . . and the Grand Trunk Road . . . has assumed a new phase as a Railway feeder precisely corresponding to the extension of Railway traffic itself. . . . It cannot, I think, any longer be said . . . that there is not sufficient outflow for the produce of abundant years to countervail the pressure of seasons of local scarcity.[31]

Table 5.5 Annual wheat outturn and exports (tons), Punjab, 1885–1886 to 1896–1897

	Wheat outturn (tons)	*Wheat exports (tons)*
1885–1886	n.a.	526,345
1886–1887	1,361,915	153,916
1887–1888	1,668,507	45,796
1888–1889	2,054,074	217,279
1889–1890	1,603,176	367,066
1890–1891	2,071,239	316,173
1891–1892	1,392,146	535,473
1892–1893	2,235,611	170,012
1893–1894	2,560,341	289,902
1894–1895	2,395,353	457,524
1895–1896	1,715,873	354,318
1896–1897	1,676,606	102,994

Source: *Report of the Land Revenue Administration of the Punjab*, 1885–1886, 1897–1898, xi; Moral & Material Progress. Condition of India, 1891–1892, p. 440.

More alarming still, in the two years leading up to the 1887 epidemic, export demand had extended beyond wheat, the primary cash crop, to include staple 'millets which form so large a proportion of the actual food of the local population.'[32] With equal alarm, the Deputy commissioner of Hissar district noted that '[t]he harvests during the year were good, but if the price of any grain fell, it was immediately exported.'

> There is now little grain of any kind in store; and dealers do not now buy in quantity to keep for years, but only to keep for a month or two until they can make a fair profit. It is understood that with the facilities for transport given by the Railway, fortunes cannot now be made by storing grain for a famine.[33]

Thus, despite the good *kharif* harvest in 1887, prices even for the coarser foodgrains remained high. 'By March nearly the whole available stores of the district had been bought up,' the Deputy Commissioner of Amballa district reported, adding,

> it is impossible to watch the tendency to sell off standing stocks, without some misgiving as to the result in future years. . . . [T]here can be little doubt that the poorer classes are being exposed to the risk of much distress from the sensitiveness of a market which is in danger of being entirely dependent on the supply grown from year to year.[34]

In his sweeping study of the late 19th-century famines in South Asia, China, and Brazil, Davis has described the global imperial context for these profound shifts in foodgrain supply and commerce. By the mid-1870s, he observes, 'The grain trade under the leadership of great cartels like Bunge and Dreyfus for the first time achieved authentically global scope and integration.'

> [T]he Liverpool Corn Trade Association and the Chicago Board of Trade (Wheat Exchange), with their new-fangled invention of 'futures' trading became the twin poles of a single world market in subsistence. . . . The new, globally integrated grain trade, moreover, ensured that climate shocks and corresponding harvest shortfalls were translated into price shocks that crossed continents with the speed of a telegraph. . . . The Punjab had become an important shock absorber for Britain and to a lesser extent, continental Europe in face of poor harvests and higher prices in the

US wheat belt. The coincidence of drought in North America and South Asia was particularly dangerous for poor Punjabis.[35]

Local sanitary officials were well aware of the effects of these altered market conditions, but it would be some years before the British Raj would acknowledge and seek to address their effects.

As familiar patterns of local market behaviour collapsed, speculation and anxiety by the late 1880s had become 'rife.' 'The tendency,' observed the Karnal deputy commissioner in his 1887 report, 'is . . . to enhance what I may call relative internal prices, that is to say, the absolute cost to local consumers of certain staples.'[36] Here, the delicate inference was that price levels in rural villages – 'internal' markets where information on trade conditions and potential access to external supplies could not reach – may have been much higher still.

Perhaps the clearest expression of concern over the 'immense demand for export' came from the Gurgaon district deputy Commissioner, J.R. Maconachie. 'I am not going beyond the subject,' he wrote in his annual report for 1887, 'when I note the grave apprehensions that existed [during the year],'

> Depletion of stocks is a thing which under the present circumstances of supply and demand in the India wheat trade seems likely to occur not seldom, and anything which renders such a dangerous condition more pronounced or more frequent is to be deprecated. To discourage such speculations may be difficult, but the subject is worth considering in connection with the question of refunds* which are now so liberally given on exports of grain from our trade centres.[37]

In his appended footnote, marked by an asterisk, Maconachie went on to cautiously suggest that

> [i]f refunds were allowed only when grain was sent out of the town within a certain period (say two months) of purchase, the difference thus made in favor of steady trade, might turn the scale of profit in many transactions.[38]

Though a fleeting reference, the Deputy Commissioner's citing of 'refunds' suggests some form of direct subsidising of the export grain trade. If so, this would have been additional to a 'bounty' also given to exporters in the form of highly subsidised freight rates as well as public cesses (taxes) levied by the provincial government to make up for an annual railway operating deficit of £400,000.[39] *Laissez-faire* in practice in 1880s Punjab was a decidedly one-sided 'free-trade' affair.

More remarkable still, Maconachie's remarks would expressly link mortality patterns to the export trade:

> In the early months of 1888 the stock of grain in hand in Gurgaon was almost *nil*, and had the *rabi* proved poor, there must have been at least inconvenience, as neighbouring districts were in the same case. Such inconvenience . . . would mean distress to numbers of the poorer portion of the working population, and *such distress means greater susceptibility to disease, and consequent greater loss of life.*[40]

Though delicately phrased as possible future hardship, such effects already were taking place, mortality across the district having soared to 62 per mille in 1887, 1 in 16 in the district succumbing.[41]

It is difficult to see the malaria epidemic of 1887, then, as an exception to the scarcity-epidemic mortality pattern, except in this case prevailing economic hardship leading up to the autumn malaria transmission season was market-induced rather than a character of the seasons. General (crude) death rates for the year were high across the province. But autumn death rates were highest in the southeast, a function it appears of both above normal rainfall in this region – in two districts, Rohtak and Karnal, double the normal level – but also soaring local grain prices triggered by sudden intense export pressures on local supplies: the Rohtak district deputy Commissioner ruefully observing that '[t]he excellent rabi harvest would have caused prices of gram, wheat and barley to have fallen off largely, if it had not been that stocks had become completely exhausted by an immense demand for export.'[42]

Such transparency on the part of district-level officers would fade from the administrative reports after 1888. Fulminant malaria, however, did not. The 1887 epidemic would be only a prelude to a series of even more severe epidemics through the subsequent two decades, including that of 1890. And like the 1887 epidemic, those districts most severely affected in 1890 would coincide with further penetration of rail lines in the northwestern districts of Sialkot, Gujrat, and Jhelum.[43] – the epidemic the culmination of a number of years of export-driven hardship compounded in the worst affected districts by severe localised flooding.

The 1892 epidemic

The 1892 epidemic was remembered in the province 'as the great fever,' a spatial map of which Christophers also included in his 1911 report, alongside that for 1908 (Figure 2.9).[44] Despite good rains and harvests in 1890, prices had continued to climb, reaching famine level a year later. The *kharif* harvest was poor in 1891, but favourable winter rains and good harvests returned in early 1892 and monsoon rainfall later in the year, at 21.4 inches, was above normal levels across the province.[45]

Although conditions for malaria transmission in 1892 likely were favourable throughout much of the province, autumn fever mortality was highest in the northern submontane region of the province, a tract corresponding to the heaviest monsoon rainfall in absolute terms.[46] But even here, Christophers noted, 'Sialkot which was severely affected is far to the west of the centre of precipitation,' adding that 'rainfall was not so excessive as would be imagined from the extent of epidemic malaria.' He concluded, 'We can see clearly that there are other factors determining the exact distribution and intensity of epidemics.'[47] The 'other factors' Christophers had in mind likely encompassed flooding. But they undoubtedly also included three preceding years of famine-level prices. Death rates in 1892, in fact, were extremely high long before the onset of the autumn malaria season across the province.

What instead preoccupied district officials in their accounts of the year, rather than flooding, were price levels and grain stores.[48] Harvests in 1890 and the early *rabi* harvest in 1891 had been good. But due to badly timed rains the *kharif* harvest in the autumn of 1891 was poor: in the northern district of Sialkot, crops had failed in two consecutive sowings.[49] In 1891–1892, the provincial wheat harvest fell to 1.39 million tons from an average of just under 2 million tons. Despite the shortfall, however, rail exports of wheat continued to climb, reaching 535,000 tons.[50] In neighbouring Shahpur district, the stress of high prices on the poor prompted official relief works organised 'not as Famine Relief, but at the usual rates for such work.'[51] In their 1892 reports the Deputy Commissioners of Ludhiana and Jullundur districts warned that

[p]rices were generally high throughout the year, but the reason was not the scarcity of produce but heavy exports to Europe by the European firms of Ralli Brothers, McKinch and Co. and others. Prices having risen . . . [and] show no sign of falling. Even the

abundant rain we have had this year seems to have had no effect upon them, and though cultivators and traders largely benefit by them, the labourers and artizans appear to suffer considerably.

. . . [T]he high prices prevailing in consequence . . . have benefited the agricultural classes, but have been severely felt by the poorer classes 1891 and by those receiving a fixed income in money.[52]

As these district-level warnings were being recorded, the vital consequences already were being played out in epidemic form, as in the case of 1887. The provincial Sanitary Commissioner, A. Stephens, in his annual report for 1892, concluded that the 'scarcity of food . . . reducing as it did the physical powers of the poorer classes, was doubtless a predisposing cause of the excessively severe outbreak of fever.'[53] Thus, even though the 1892 epidemic conformed to the usual rain-price model on the surface, in fact it was a partial outlier to the extent that the economic hardship was not driven primarily by drought, but was a function of export-driven price levels.

Interestingly, the revised Settlement report for Jullundur district, published in 1892, would refer to indebtedness in the district, attributing 'the cause . . . [among] agriculturalists to be the purchase of food in the various bad seasons with which so much of the province has been afflicted during the last 25 years.' The report noted 'much sickness of late years in Jullundur' and attributed this to waterlogging in particular tracts, and

want of proper sanitary precautions facilitated by the work of cholera. But elsewhere, as for instance at Kuleta in the Phillour tahsil, no special reason for the excessive mortality is apparent. It may be hoped that the deterioration of the health of the district is only temporary, as there is nothing in the situation, soil or climate, which should be adverse to the human situation.[54]

But if the Settlement officer was reluctant to cite the impact of grain exports and famine prices, the 'Native' Press definitely was not. Protest against the export trade filled their pages across this period,[55] writers 'constantly reproach[ing] the Government for not finding a remedy.'[56] By this point, however, the provincial administration had been read the riot act. In his review of the 1891–1892 Land Revenue report, the Punjab Lieutenant-Governor maintained the official line, making it clear to district officers that criticisms of foodgrain exports were 'one-sided' and would no longer be tolerated. '[T]he vast majority of the agricultural population,' he insisted, 'usually derive a large profit from [high prices].'

> In short, the case is simply one of those, unfortunately too common in this world, in which one man's gain is another man's loss, . . . (and) any attempt by the Government to adjust matters . . . would, except under the most extraordinary circumstances, be altogether unacceptable.[57]

If a 'great depletion of stocks in India . . . [led to] absolute famine,' he conceded, the government might be compelled to

> check exportation. . . . But it is clear that nothing short of such an extraordinary concurrence of untoward circumstances would warrant the interference of the Government, and it is well that this should be plainly understood by all concerned.[58]

One year later, however, he would express surprise at the severity of the 1892 autumn epidemic and the markedly greater lethality observed amongst the poor.

> The most remarkable feature of the [epidemic] . . . is not that fever prevails so extensively among the natives of the Province, but that it should prove so often fatal to them. Europeans and Eurasians suffer very severely from fever in the Punjab, but they very rarely die of it. The difference is, it is impossible to doubt, due to a great measure to the fact that a European or Eurasian getting fever has the advantage of being properly treated, fed and nursed. . . . Something is no doubt also due in a year of high prices like that under report to the poorest classes of the population being compelled to live in a lower way than usual, and being thus less able to resist the approach of illness.[59]

Grain exports would decline in 1893 (Table 5.5), and prices quickly fell. So, too, did fever and overall death rates. Price volatility, however, would take even more exaggerated form in the later years of the decade as large exports resumed and recurring severe drought returned to the subcontinent. In April 1897, the provincial administration expressed further 'surprise,' this time

> that a reduction in area of crops [in 1896] by only one-fifth . . . should be attended by a rise in prices equal to or in some cases

exceeding one hundred percent . . . a somewhat remarkable circumstance which deserves a more detailed study.[60]

As these remarks were being recorded, the province was plunging headlong into frank famine, to be followed in 1900 by an even more severe 'great' famine, both associated with classic 'fulminant' malaria epidemics upon return of the rains.

In the period after 1908, one further 'outlier' epidemic can be identified, in 1917. The year was marked by record levels of both monsoon rainfall and grain prices. But as in 1887 and 1890, economic stress had not been triggered by preceding harvest failure, but rather by three years of war-triggered hyper-inflation. Fever mortality rose throughout the province in the autumns months of the year but was highest in the southwestern region, where above normal rains, flooding, and *kharif* crop destruction were greatest (Figure 4.11d).[61] For all seven southwestern districts, the 1911–1920 decadal Oct.–Dec. fever death rate coefficient of variation is the highest of the entire 73-year period (Table 4.5). Given the extreme shortage of administrative personnel, with many colonial officials drafted for military service elsewhere in the empire, flood relief efforts are likely to have been minimal.

What conclusions, then, can be drawn from the epidemics that do not conform to the scarcity-excess rainfall model? In each of the three instances of fulminant malaria when grain prices were low, severe economic hardship can be identified from the administrative records in the period leading up to the autumn epidemic. Rather than undermining the hunger-malaria mortality hypothesis, price-'anomalous' epidemics thus lend additional support to the hunger-'fulminancy' thesis of malaria mortality in the province.

As for the role of rainfall, the epidemic of 1879, a year of below average monsoon rains, offers a somewhat more nuanced understanding of the relationship of rainfall to epidemic malaria mortality. The geographic pattern of autumn fever mortality evident across the province in 1879 strongly suggests the entomologically enabling effect of a minimum level of summer rain for epidemic malaria mortality conditions to arise: though death rates were high throughout the year in all districts, fever mortality rose markedly in the autumn months only where the summer rains were not in marked deficit. Yet even in the worst affected epidemic districts rainfall was only marginally above normal levels, in Rohtak and Gurgaon districts, two inches in 'excess.' This suggests that in the eastern half of the province where fulminant epidemics were more common, the entomological conditions conducive to effective malaria transmission within a district could be achieved with *average* ('normal') rainfall levels. No doubt the likelihood of rapid multiplication of malaria transmission was more assured in years of higher rainfall. But widespread transmission does not appear to have depended on excessive rainfall. This, in turn, adds weight to the view that the role of flooding was as much, or perhaps more, economic than entomologic in nature.

Interestingly, Christophers also was quite aware of exceptions to the 'excess' rain formula, pointing out that 'there have been fever years with by no means excessive rainfall.'[62] Moreover, while flooding was a potent amplifier of epidemic lethality, even here such amplification was largely contingent on pre-existing economic hardship: the 1875 epidemic suggests favourable entomological conditions were a necessary but not sufficient condition for fulminant malaria. But then so, too, does the post-1920 experience of marked decline in epidemic mortality. That economic stress was the common feature underlying the most lethal epidemics of this period is supported as well by a consistent pattern of differential malaria impact on the very poor, the least food secure, a subject explored in more detail in the chapter that follows.[63]

A second pattern that emerges from analysis of local (district-level) conditions in outlier epidemics is that the economic hardship underlying many of the major epidemics of this period stemmed not from 'classic' (harvest-induced) famine but rather reflected economic shifts wrought by the international commercialisation of South Asian agriculture. The 1879 epidemic can be seen to signal a fundamental break from the historical relationship between price behaviour and local harvest failure: 'scarcity'-level grain prices no longer dependably falling with the return of good local harvests. Broader forces were now at play determining local prices and undermining traditional methods of local grain storage. Severity of subsequent epidemics, in 1887, 1890, and 1892 – and as we will see ahead in relation to the two 'great' famines at the end of the 19th century – were, to a considerable extent, cumulative expressions of these broader shifts, bringing into sharp relief the largely unmitigated human cost of the new agroeconomic order. Though the price effects of commercialisation were province wide and continent wide, a greater impact was often seen locally, in tracts most recently connected by rail and suddenly exposed to uncharted pressures on village supplies, and additionally 'picked out' by above normal rains – extreme effects not necessarily reflected in aggregate price and rain averages.

As we will consider in the second part of the study, the decline in epidemic malaria mortality in the years after 1908 brings further light to bear on the role of acute hunger in fulminant malaria. But before turning to the post-1908 period, one further example, the 1881 Amritsar epidemic, merits inclusion in this survey of 'outlier' epidemics for the insights it offers into a different epidemiological form of economic stress underlying 'fulminant' malaria: endemic destitution.

Endemic starvation and 'exalted' malaria: Amritsar, 1881

The year 1881 was not included in Christophers's list of nine epidemics of fulminant intensity, although it was an epidemic he drew attention to both in his 1911 report and earlier at Simla. The 1881 epidemic was anomalous not in terms of rain or even price, but rather in affecting primarily an urban population. Though limited geographically to Amritsar city and its peri-urban area,[64] epidemic mortality was sufficiently high in the district to push up the autumn fever death rate for the province as a whole (Table 4.1). The Amritsar epidemic prompted an inquiry, conducted by the province's deputy Sanitary Commissioner. Surgeon-Major J. Bennett's findings, appended to the 1881 provincial Sanitary Commission report, provide one of the few detailed accounts of conditions during the course of a severe epidemic.[65]

As a major grain trade and rail centre for the province, Amritsar was a key administrative centre and held the largest urban population in the province. It was also a city where malaria was a major concern because of long-standing drainage problems and waterlogging associated with high levels of irrigation nearby. Monsoon rainfall in 1881 across the district was extremely heavy, recorded at 53.8 inches compared to a normal 15.3 inches. Amritsar city itself received 38 inches in July and August, triggering widespread flooding and bringing economic activity and livelihood to a standstill.[66] Leading up to the floods, economic stress had also been prevalent. Foodgrain prices for the preceding three years had been extremely high, triggered by the famines of 1876–1877 and 1877–1878.

Throughout the district, autumn fever death rates soared in the autumn months of 1881, climbing much higher still in Amritsar town itself. In October–November, 6,810 fever deaths were recorded, compared with an average of 500 deaths in non-epidemic years.[67] At the peak of the epidemic, 13 medical officers were treating over 10,000 civilian cases daily. Initial increase in fever deaths in the city itself was evident in the final days of August, mortality soaring in September, and further doubling in October.[68] 'Two forms of the disease were met with,' Bennett observed, 'common intermittent fever, and the ever dangerous remittent form to which so many of the city people succumbed.'

> In the vast majority of cases examined by me the fever was undoubtedly intermittent, . . . the ordinary autumnal fever of this country. . . . [But] [i]n many cases [of the remittent form], especially amongst the poorer people, the body was much emanated [emaciated] from the combined effects of fever and insufficient and inappropriate diet. In almost all, the signs of inanition as well as of malarial cachexia were more or less marked . . . and not unfrequently dropsical swellings of the lower limbs.[69]

Few data on differential mortality rates within the urban population apparently were recorded. A recurring observation, however, was that despite 'universal' infection where 'not a single native or European in the city or civil station appears to have escaped attack,' mortality was 'greatest amongst the poorer classes of Hindus and Muhammadans.' Amongst the poor, officials observed, fever mortality was 'disproportionately' greatest among Muslim households. This was explained 'by the fact that a large proportion of the Muslim population is made up of poor, ill-fed and badly clad Kashmiris, on whom the disease fell heaviest, and committed its greatest ravages.'[70] As in 1908 nearly two decades later, it was in the Kashmiri wards where the highest mortality rates were registered.[71]

Attributing the epidemic to 'massive flooding in and around the city,' the Deputy Sanitary Commissioner acknowledged that it was 'not improbable that there may have been other agencies at work.'

> [T]he vast majority of this class, owing to their inability to earn money to buy food, were found in the most impoverished conditions, and suffering as much from the effects of chronic starvation as from fever. . . . Although the poor classes in all parts of the city, no doubt, suffered much from deficiency of food, no where did I see the results of poverty and chronic starvation so plainly manifest as amongst the Kashmiri Shawl-weavers. . . . In that part of the city . . . almost the whole of the population appeared to be suffering more or less, from the depressing effect of malaria cachexia and chronic starvation.[72]

Destitution was not a new phenomenon to the Kashmiri shawl weaver community, having emigrated as famine refugees in the 1830s. However, by 1880, the shawl weaving industry was in rapid decline, a result of intense competition from cheaper British textile imports, a decline deepened further in the 1870s by the sudden loss of its European markets due to the Franco-Prussian war. '[T]he position of the weavers went from bad to worse [as] the shawl industry became a sweated industry,' Gadgil describes, so that 'by 1895 the industry was already a mere tradition – a memory of the past.'[73] Christophers similarly concluded that 'the severity of the [1881] outbreak was associated with economic conditions affecting the large bodies of Kashmiri workers who about this time were adversely affected by the decay of the shawl trade in Amritsar.'[74]

Added to industrial decline, three years' cumulative famine-level prices meant that for many, foodgrain stores and physiological reserves had been exhausted long before. Though prices in 1881 had begun to moderate, they were still well above normal levels. Moreover, at this point, staple foodgrains would have been unprocurable by the destitute, irrespective of market price. Severe flooding in and around the town brought livelihood to a standstill for many of the poor, economic paralysis further intensified by universal malaria infection and debility.

Mortality amongst young children was 'appallingly high,' Bennett observed, noting 'wasting of the tissues' and a 'peculiarly marked susceptibility' to the disease.

> The worst forms of [starvation] were seen . . . particularly amongst infants at the breast, many of whom, their mothers having lost health and strength from frequent or prolonged attacks of fever, were seen to be literally dying of inanition. . . . It would probably be no exaggeration to say that two-thirds of the infantile population have died.[75]

The relationship between malaria mortality and hunger portrayed in Bennett's report is stark, with graphic descriptions of terminal stage starvation leading to 'dropsical swelling,' what today is termed 'marasmic kwashiorkor,' a physical state compounded by malarial-induced anaemia. Autopsy findings showed a 'peculiar form of degeneration (of the intestinal mucous membrane), which has been described as characteristic of chronic starvation . . . having lost, to a great extent, the power of absorbing food.'[76] It is unlikely that acute malaria infection could cause such severe clinical and pathological states of undernourishment in the absence of pre-existing undernourishment. More likely, malaria infection simply tipped the balance nutritionally for many of those already subsisting on inadequate food intake, conditions Christophers would refer to as 'an exaggerated human factor . . . among the labouring and artizan classes in Amritsar City, especially among the Kashmiris, [where] the pinch of poverty is severely felt.'[77] Municipal response to the epidemic took the form of soup kitchens, officials nonetheless acknowledging that 'charity will not reach those most in need of it.'[78]

The 1881 Amritsar malaria epidemic presents an epidemiological profile of hunger quite different from 'classic' famine, or scarcity associated with the regional (rural) epidemics such as that of 1908. Economic downturns in urban industries could bring cycles of destitution, and soaring prevalence of semi-starvation, independent of rural agricultural conditions, and, in turn, a general, rather than episodic, heightened vulnerability to epidemic disease. The distinction between short-term epidemic starvation associated with harvest failure and endemic semi-starvation was one Christophers would explicitly highlight at the October 1909 Simla conference, devoting a separate section to urban 'squalor and poverty.'[79] The two were, of course, related because urban mortality was generally higher than rural in regional epidemics such as 1908. Certainly, the impact of high prices was felt that much more acutely among the urban poor because of their much greater dependence on the market for staple foodgrains. But also, because of specific conditions of work that left many endemically weakened and readily destitute. Here, he pointed out that it was among the small towns that 'the worst effects of the [1908] epidemic were recorded,' 1 in 12 succumbing, even though exposure to malarial infection was unlikely to have been greater than in rural areas.[80]

Christophers's attentiveness to endemic destitution undoubtedly stemmed from an investigation conducted one year earlier into the 'exalted' malaria conditions prevailing in the Duars northeastern tea plantation labour camps. That inquiry had also led to the conclusion that destitution among the labourers was the central factor underlying the intense form and extreme lethality of the disease on the tea estates – conditions specifically related to the indentured labour system – rather than factors of vector transmission.[81]

Indentured labour recruitment was not limited, however, to the hill plantations. It was prevalent in many industrial centres in the Indian plains as well, including in the towns and canal labour camps of Punjab. An 1869 inquiry into a cholera epidemic in Amritsar during the 1868–1869 famine, for example, similarly linked the vulnerability of the Kashmiri weaver community to destitution under indentured labour conditions prevalent in the industry.

> The ravages of the cholera commenced, and were most apparent in the . . . quarter which are chiefly inhabited by Cashmeeries . . .

and the distressing condition of the Cashmeeree shawl-weavers, who by the system of advances which prevails in the trade, are the bond slaves of their wealthy employers, predisposed them for disease. Famine-stricken, ill-clothed, and worse lodged, it is not a matter of surprise that they fell an easy prey.[82]

By including the 1881 Amritsar epidemic in his analysis of epidemic malaria in Punjab, Christophers was explicitly highlighting the larger dimensions of the 'scarcity'-related malaria problem, pointing to the 'malariogenic' effects of endemic destitution *in general* across the subcontinent.

In subsequent chapters, the relationship between labour conditions and 'exalted' malaria will be explored in more detail through accounts such as the Duars inquiry, and as well, the impact of such observations upon formulation of malaria control policies through the remaining decades of the colonial period. But here we return to the biomedical domain to consider a range of possible physical mechanisms linking lethality of malaria and destitution.

Notes

1 Civilian autumn fever mortality, described as 'appalling', was the seventh highest of the 41-year period, at a time when registration was still considerably incomplete; *PSCR* 1876, 56. Fever admission rates amongst 11,888 European troops in the province soared in 1876, though accompanied by only eight deaths; *GOI-SCR* 1875, 1876, Forms XXI–XXII.

2 S.R. Christophers, 'Malaria in the Punjab,' *Sci. Mem. Off. Med. Sanit. Dept.*, 46 (Calcutta: Superintendent Government Printing Office, 1911), 110 [hereafter MP].

3 *Report of the Land Revenue Administration of the Punjab*, 1875–1876, 43–45 [hereafter, *PLRA*].

4 Monsoon rainfall was heavy in several southeastern districts also, but flooding does not appear to have been extreme, possibly because rainfall was only moderate in upstream districts.

5 *PLRA* 1875–1876, 1, 4.

6 Ibid.; Form No. X, A, Statement of Alluvion, Diluvion and Destructive Inundation. A few lower level officials expressed 'regret [at] the rigid pressure of our inelastic [revenue] system,' arguing that they 'could not fairly allow suspension for balance owing to distress and ruin, because it would not have been fair to those who had borrowed the money and "paid up"'; *PLRA* 1875–1876, Extracts from Commissioner's Report, Jullundur Division, 11.

7 Vital registration may have improved over this four-year period, but increased reporting seems unlikely to account for such differences in death rates: crude death rates, and thus overall reporting, were comparable in non-famine years across this period.

8 Harvests in 1883 had been nearly 50 per cent deficit across much of central and southeastern Punjab. Following the 'complete failure' of the summer 1883 *kharif* harvest in Delhi, Karnal, and Amballa districts, 'no crop was expected on non-irrigated' lands for the following 1884 *rabi* harvest; *PLRA* 1883, 2. Sequential failed rains 'had reduced the lowest class of agriculturalists, the labourers and village servants, to a state nearly bordering on destitution'; *PLRA* 1884–1884, 2. By contrast, in Jullundur district, 'the year [1884] was free from seasonal calamities of every sort. There were no floods, no hail, no drought. The health of the people was also exceptionally good, and the autumnal fevers did less harm than usual'; ibid., 32.

9 GOI, *Report of the Indian Famine Commission, 1898*, Simla, Government Central Printing Office [hereafter *FCR* 1898], 'Narrative of Famines which Have Occurred since the Famine Commissioner's Report, 1880,' para. 15. Only locally funded famine relief works were initiated in Hissar district, and tax suspensions granted in Rohtak district; *PLRA* 1884–1885, 2, 5.

10 MP, 110.

11 *PLRA* 1884–1885, 19.

12 *PLRA* 1884–1885, Extracts from Deputy Commissioner rpts [hereafter, Exts.], 35. Interestingly, 1884 autumn fever mortality was greatest in Ludhiana district, considered a relatively drought-secure district that had experienced heavy rains also the preceding year, with 1884 flooding possibly exacerbated from exceptional rains in upstream Amballa district.

13 MP, 110. In an appended table to the 1911 report, data for 1884 is omitted.

14 S.R. Christophers, 'On Malaria in the Punjab,' in *Proceeding of the Imperial Malaria Conference held in Simla, Oct. 1909* (Simla: Government Central Branch Press, 1910), 39 [hereafter, Simla Conf.].

15 *FCR* 1898, para. 15.

16 It is likely military foodgrain demands contributed to continuing scarcity prices. In the Peshawar Division of the province '[d]uring 1878–1879 and 1879–1880 . . . food grains were at famine prices owing to the Afghan War'; *Report on the Famine in the Punjab in 1896–1897* (Lahore: Government Press, 1898), Appendix II, xxxvii–xlii, at xl.

17 In Rohtak district '[t]he fever was described as intermittent . . . killing chiefly by diarrhoea and dysentery, and leaving enlarged spleens which were exceedingly common among the children'; *PSCR* 1879, Appendix C, iv, 107.

18 *PLRA* 1879, Appendix C, iii.

19 *PLRA* 1879, iv.

20 *Gazetteer of the Gurgaon District, 1883–1884* (Lahore: Arya Press, 1884), 131–132.

21 *Paludism*, 4, 1912, 82 [emphasis added]. There is some ambiguity in Christophers's 'excess rain' conclusions. At one point, he suggests 'very heavy precipitation . . . is a necessary condition' for epidemic malaria, elsewhere that 'there have been fever years with by no means excessive rainfall,' possibly with the 1879 epidemic in mind; MP, 107; Simla Conf., 35.

22 In the single village of Chota Thanah, for example, officials would remark upon the '[g]reat mortality last year,' 42 deaths registered in 1878 in a population of 1,216, and another 55 deaths 'upto [*sic*] November this

year,'; *PLRA* 1879, iii. Christophers also notes that the town of Palwal in Gurgaon district was severely affected in the 1878 autumn fever epidemic and again in 1879; MP, 48.

23 H.K. Trevaskis, *Land of the Five Rivers* (Oxford: Oxford University Press, 1928), opp. 220.

24 KN Chaudhuri, 'Foreign Trade and Balance of Payments,' *Cambridge Economic History of India*, Vol. II (Cambridge: Cambridge University Press, 1983), 850 [hereafter *CEHI*].

25 *PLRA* 1878–1879, Exts., 2.

26 Famine Inquiry Commission (India), 'Note on the Results of the Enquiries Made into the Mortality in the North-Western Provinces and Oudh,' Government N.W.P. and Oudh, 596, dated Mar. 17, 1879, in *Report of the Indian Famine Commission. Part 3, Famine Histories* (London: HMSO, 1885), 243–250.

27 Though little reference to grain exports appears in his 1890 report, the Sanitary Commissioner clearly noted 'absolute want' in the province and its relationship to malarial mortality, observing that '[w]ere those suffering from malarial fevers among the general population as carefully treated, fed and nursed as fever patients in Jails and in the Native Army, the mortality from these causes would be very much smaller than it is'; *PSCR* 1890, 9.

28 *PLRA* 1896–1897, xi and accompanying bar-graph.

29 J. Hurd, 'Railways,' *CEHI*, 737–761, at 745; __, 'Railways and Market Expansion in India, 1861–1921,' *Explorations in Economic History*, 12, 3, July 1975, 263–288.

30 *PLRA* 1887–1888, 18; Extracts from Deputy Commissioners' Reports, 10, 9.

31 Ibid., 10. Navtej Singh describes protest in the vernacular press, how the 'enormous demand at a higher price induced the exporters not only to buy up old stocks largely, but also to make "forward" purchases of wheat to be supplied from the new crop at similar prices. . . . purchas[ing] even the standing crops for the purposes of export to Europe'; *Starvation and Colonialism: 1858–1901, A Study of Famines in the Nineteenth Century British Punjab* (New Delhi: National Book Organisation, 1997), 88–89. See also H. Banerji, *Agrarian Society of the Punjab, 1849–1901* (New Delhi: Manohar, 1982).

32 *PLRA* 1887–1888, Exts. 10; *PLRA* 1887–1888, 18.

33 Ibid., Exts, p. 9. Elizabeth Whitcombe observes a similar effect of grain exports in the neighbouring North-West Provinces in this period; *Agrarian Conditions in Northern India, I, The United Provinces Under British Rule, 1860–1900* (Berkeley: University of California Press, 1972).

34 *PLRA* 1887–1888, Exts, 11.

35 M. Davis, *Late Victorian Holocausts: El Niño Famines and the Making of the Third World* (London: Verso, 2001), 120–123.

36 *PLRA* 1887–1888, Exts, 10.

37 Ibid., Exts, 9. Maconachie was becoming clearly uneasy over imperial economic doctrine, having a year earlier 'harden[ed] my heart . . . [against] "paternal kindness"' regarding granting remission of land revenue demand 'by remembering the piteous demoralisation caused by the generosity already shown'; *PLRA* 1886–1887, Exts. 8.

38 Ibid.
39 On this, see A.K. Connell, 'Indian Railways and Indian Wheat,' *Royal Statistical Society*, 48, June 1885, 236–276, at 248–249. Connell describes how the two Punjab rail lines, completed in the late 1870s, were running at a deficit of £400,000 a year because of generous guarantees given to British investors. Government made up this deficit through additional local cesses. This amounted in effect to a 'bounty on all the import and export trade, on wheat going out of, and cotton goods and metals coming into the [province]. . . . The Indus Valley and Sindh Punjab and Delhi Railways are the most signal instances of bounty-supported lines, but to a less extent all the wheat carrying lines are only worked by the help of the State'; ibid., 252–253. See also, Hurd, 'Railways,' 741–743.
40 *PLRA* 1887–1888, Exts., 9.
41 *PSCR* 1887. It is perhaps more than mere coincidence that on the eve of his departure in 1888, the Viceroy, Lord Dufferin, commissioned his confidential Circular enquiring into the 'condition the lower classes of people of India' (Confidential Circular, 44 F. – 8.1, dated Aug. 17, 1887). See ch. 3 at pp. 109–10.
42 *PLRA* 1887–1888, Exts., 9.
43 A branch rail line to Sialkot was opened in 1884; *Administrative Report on the Railways in India for 1887–1888*, Appendix E, p. cxviii.
44 MP, 25.
45 Ibid., 94.
46 Christophers describes an 'enormous' northern epidemic nucleus, but one leaving 'no trace' in the southeast; MP, 25. Epidemic Figure calculations were indeed highest for the northern Gurdaspur and Sialkot districts. Yet autumn fever deaths were high throughout the province, but because fever mortality in the southeast had also been very high throughout the year, there the Epidemic Figure, as a ratio of Apr.–July to Oct.–Dec. fever deaths, were much lower.
47 Simla Conf., 35.
48 *PLRA* 1891–1892, 2. The single district where severe flooding was reported was Shahpur, but while FDR was high (20.2 per mille), autumn fever mortality was considerably higher in the northern districts of Sialkot and Gurdaspur; *PLRA* 1992–1993, 3–5.
49 *PLRA* 1891–1892, 2.
50 *PLRA* 1896–1897, ix, xi.
51 *PLRA* 1891–1892, Exts., 19.
52 *PLRA* 1891–1892, 10, Exts., 19.
53 *PSCR* 1892, 16.
54 W.E. Purser, *Final Report of the Revised Settlement of the Jullundur District in the Punjab* (Lahore: Punjab Revenue Department, 1892), 45, 13.
55 Navtej Singh chronicles an outpouring of criticism in the vernacular press; *Starvation and Colonialism*, 89–90.
56 Proc. of the Lieutenant-Governor of the Punjab in the Home Department (Sanitary) [hereafter PLGP], July 10, 1893, in *PLRA* 1891–1892, 1–2.
57 Ibid.
58 Ibid.
59 PLGP, July 28, 1893, in *PSCR* 1892, 3.

60 PLGP, in the Home Department (Sanitary), Apr. 27, 1897, in *PLRA 1895–1896*, 2. Drought and harvest failure in 1896 was limited to the southeast (Hissar, Rohtak, and Ferozepur districts), which explains the moderate province-level 1897 Oct.–Dec. FDR, though famine was declared in much of the province on the basis of price levels.

61 *Season and Crops of the Punjab*, 1917-18, 1–2; Statement No. I; *PSCR* 1917, 1.

62 Christophers cites 1901 as one example where third-quarter rain was below average levels in the epidemic tracts of Hissar, Rohtak, and Ferozepur, putting to some question, along with 1879, his conclusion elsewhere that 'a deficient [rain]fall is never associated with severe epidemic conditions'; Simla Conf., 35; MP, 107. See also note 22.

63 This is not to suggest that flooding alone did not trigger increased malaria mortality in the ensuing months, simply not the exceptional lethality seen in the major epidemics of the pre-1910 period.

64 MP, 30.

65 *Report on Epidemic, Remittent and Intermittent Fever occurring in the City of Amritsar in the Autumn of 1881*, by Surgeon-Major J. Bennett, Deputy Sanitary Commissioner, Eastern Circle, Punjab; reproduced in *PSCR* 1881, Appendix C.

66 *PSCR* 1881, iii.

67 C.A. Gill, 'The Relationship of Malaria and Rainfall,' *IJMR*, 7, 1920, 618–632, at 631.

68 *PSCR* 1881, i.

69 Ibid., iv.

70 Ibid., iii.

71 Christophers calculated that in the Kashmiri ward of Khazana in 1908, over 9 per cent of the residents died in the three months of Oct.–Dec., compared with 2 or 3 per cent in other wards, some which also were on the periphery of the city and thus potentially more exposed to *Anopheles* breeding sites; MP, 31. These figures are not age-adjusted and so cannot be interpreted as accurate measures of case mortality rates.

72 *PSCR* 1881, iv–v.

73 D.R. Gadgil, *The Industrial Evolution of India in Recent Times, 1860–1939* (Bombay: Oxford University Press, 1971), 34–35.

74 MP, 30–31.

75 *PSCR* 1881, iii–iv.

76 *PSCR* 1881, iv–v.

77 MP, 30.

78 *PSCR* 1881, v.

79 Simla Conf., 38–39.

80 MP, 47–48.

81 S.R Christophers, C.A. Bentley, *Malaria in the Duars: Being the second report to the Advisory Committee appointed by the Government of India to conduct an Enquiry regarding Black-water and other Fevers prevalent in the Duars* (Simla: Government Monotype Press, 1911).

82 F.M. Birch, 'Report Upon an Out-Break of Cholera in Amritsar in A.D. 1869,' *Indian Sanitary Proceedings*, 1870, Range 434, 45, 735–736, as cited in I. Klein, 'Death in India,' *Journal of Asian Studies*, Aug. 1973, 639–659, 648–649.

6 'Intense' malaria
Biological mechanisms

'Many ailments ordinarily trifling, became fatal at such times [of famine]' an official observed in the course of the 1866 Orissa famine.
– *Report of the Sanitary Commissioner for Madras for 1877* (Madras: Govt Press, 1878), Appendix 1, xxviii–xxix.

Analysis of the major malaria epidemics in the province between 1868 and 1908 suggests that, in each case, severe economic hardship preceded heightened fever deaths in epidemic-affected tracts, even where that stress was unreflected in market grain-price levels. Here, we examine the malaria-destitution relationship more closely, considering historical accounts of heightened malaria lethality among the famished as seen in class and gender differentials in fever mortality, and the contribution of 'secondary' hardship: economic paralysis induced by simultaneous malarial morbidity amongst a population. Entomologically mediated explanations for the link between famine and epidemic malaria, such as the 'vector deviation' thesis, also are explored. Finally, we consider the question of Punjab epidemic specificity. To what extent was epidemic malaria intensity in the province a function of the distinctive combination of ecological conditions of the South Asian northwest plains – the region's continental climate, agricultural economy, topography, geology, and soil hydrology? Certainly, in later writing, Punjab was considered entomologically exceptional: a region of highly 'unstable' malaria due to wide fluctuations in yearly transmission and hence in protective acquired immunity levels.

Differential malaria mortality: narrative accounts

Even a cursory survey of the colonial records reveals that highly lethal malaria epidemics were not unique to Punjab, and that malaria's greatest toll lay selectively amongst the famished. Among such accounts, perhaps the most carefully documented – outside the 1911 Punjab study – appears in the annual reports of W.R. Cornish, Sanitary Commissioner for the Madras Presidency during the 1876–1877 South Indian famine. Mortality rates, already high among the lower castes in advance of the monsoon rains, climbed dramatically in the autumn months of 1877. 'The fever,' Cornish concluded, 'is nothing more than the ordinary malarious ague. . . . With the strong and well-to-do it has occasioned very little mortality, but with the weakly and half-starved victims of the famine it has been very fatal. . . . They had no strength or vital force to enable them to rally.'[1]

Cornish interpreted the Madras fever epidemic in 1877 in then-prominent zymotic terms: 'rainfall following on prolonged drought, had set free malarious exhalations from the soil.'[2] But he was also exacting in distinguishing the 'precipitating' role of rainfall from the 'predisposing' conditions of starvation, observing that with the exception of an unusual 'cyclone' in the Madras town area in May of 1877, rainfall across the Presidency had not been exceptional. Among the nine districts worst affected by the famine and high fever death rates, in only two, Tirunelveli and Madurai, had the 1877 rains been considerably above average levels. In Kurnool and Cuddapah, the two districts 'worst' affected by fever and overall death rates, rainfall was slightly below average, and in the remaining five famine districts, in the 'normal' range.[3] There was, he stressed, little relationship between fever death rates and rainfall patterns across the Madras famine region.

Marked class differentials in malaria morbidity were a recurring observation in Punjab as well. As we have seen, Punjab sanitary officials in 1892 observed that '[t]he comparative scarcity of food . . . [amongst] the poorer classes, was doubtless a predisposing cause of the excessively severe outbreak of fever,' adding, 'Europeans and Eurasians suffer very severely from fever in the Punjab, but they very rarely die of it.'[4] A still more stark description appears in an account of the 1868–1869 Rajasthan famine: '[o]n the cessation of the rains a terrible fever struck down the entire population. All the weak and sickly, the old and half-starved children debilitated by famine, were early carried off. The strong and well-to-do only remained. In some cases, half the population died of fever.'[5]

A parallel pattern of class differentials is also evident in accounts of overall famine mortality. Perhaps the most detailed assessment was undertaken in northern India in the wake of the 1877–1878 famine. All three officials deputed to investigate mortality in 224 famine-afflicted villages in the west-central region of the North-western (United) Provinces reported that 80 per cent of deaths had occurred amongst the landless or near landless, a group that made up only one-quarter of the population. '[T]he cultivators proper,' the report noted, 'suffered . . . especially from the loss of cattle but . . . few died of starvation. The landowners were never near the point of famine.'[6] With deaths classified by caste, the inquiry found mortality amongst the labouring castes to be 10 times the rate for Brahmin households. Among weaver (Kori) communities who depended largely on agricultural labour, the death rate was recorded as 80.6 per 1,000.[7] In all cases, mortality was considered under-reported, in part because whole families disappeared leaving no-one to report deaths. The village *chowkidars*, coming from the poorest households and responsible for reporting vital events, were themselves often victims of famine. The previous figures represent total mortality rather than fever deaths. But in light of the general prominence of post-monsoon malaria in the region's famine mortality tolls,[8] such data bear relevance for malaria lethality.

Differential 'fever' death rate data for the army, police, and jail populations were reported in Punjab in 1879, a year of continuing famine in the province (Table 6.1). Malarial fever was common among the many European troops on duty to control looting and rioting at famine relief camps, a group roughly similar in age and exposure to infection to prison populations. Fever death rates were recorded as 6.9 and 7.5 per 1,000, respectively, among the Native and European army troops in 1879, compared with a rate of 47.6 deaths per 1,000 in the provincial jails. The Sanitary Commissioner interpreted the 'high mortality in the Jail population . . . [as] no doubt, due to the depression of spirits under imprisonment, coupled with restricted food and task work, as well as to the defective physique of a considerable proportion of the prisoners.'[9]

Table 6.1 Differential annual fever death rates (per 1,000), by group, Punjab, 1870–1879, 1879

	1870–1879	1879
Jails	14.0	47.6
European Army	4.7	7.5
Native Army	3.5	6.9
Police Force	1.8	2.4
Towns	21.5	52.7
Rural Circles	19.5	36.6

Source: *Ann. Rpt. Sanitary Commissioner*, Punjab, 1880, p. 40.

In this case, differences in access to quinine may account for some of the nearly seven-fold mortality differential. But this is less likely among these groups three decades later. Routine administration of prophylactic quinine to all prisoners was instituted in Punjab jails as early as 1893, but 1907 fever case mortality rates, a non-epidemic year, were still three times higher than among European troops despite 'far more stringent measures of prevention . . . in jails than in regimental lines.' Prisoners, it was generally acknowledged, came from the 'lowest and poorest ranks of society' and were 'greatly inferior to soldiers in physique.'[10]

Age and sex differentials in malaria mortality

The importance of hunger is suggested as well in the age profile of malaria mortality in epidemic years. Mortality rates in the 1908 Punjab epidemic were highest amongst the very young and the aged, based upon burial records for Amritsar city. The largest increase in excess deaths in absolute numbers occurred among infants, with the infant mortality rate rising from 206 to 412 per 1,000, as seen in chapter 2 (Table 2.1). Particularly notable in the Amritsar figures however is mortality among children in the second year of life (13 to 24 months of age), in actual numbers approaching those of infant deaths,[11] and an age group typically the most severely undernourished in impoverished populations, in the transition from sole breastfeeding to supplementary feeding.[12]

A role for hunger in malaria lethality is also suggested in sex differentials in mortality in Punjab. In much of the subcontinent, as elsewhere in the world, recorded death rates during famine periods typically were greater amongst males than females, a pattern Maharatna has shown for southern and western regions of India. However, northwest India, he points out, was a notable exception to this general pattern.[13] Even in non-famine years, female death rates in Punjab province were higher than for males at most age levels, a reversal of the normal biological pattern. In years of frank famine, these differentials widened further, reflected in greater widening of the sex ratio (males per 100 females).[14]

Colonial authorities had long noted higher mortality rates among female children compared with male levels in a number of Punjab districts. A 'local enquiry' by Civil Surgeons in 1888, prompted by the central government, concluded that 'among the Rájpúts and Muhammadan Jats' of Jullundur district, female infanticide was practiced, particularly among 'the superior families.'[15] The practice was believed to involve 'deliberate starvation of the female infant . . . with the object of escaping marriage expenses in the future.'[16] In the course of the severe malaria epidemic of 1890, officials noted a doubling in the excess of female deaths over male deaths in worst affected districts,[17] observing that 'female children usually do not receive the same care as boys. . . . In times of scarcity, girls are the first to suffer. . . . The consequence is that female children are not usually so robust as boys are: they are more liable to be attacked by fever and other diseases than the better cared for and stronger boys, and a larger proportion of those attacked fall victims to disease.'[18] In 1908, the female fever death rate among infants was recorded as 7 per cent higher than that among males, a difference that increased to 14 per cent among young children 1 to 4 years of age, and up to 40 per cent higher in females 10–15 years old.[19]

It is difficult to explain these sex differentials in fever mortality among children in terms of differential exposure to malarial infection, nor access to quinine, given extremely low per capita availability.[20] A more likely explanation is cultural female disadvantage with respect to food entitlement, further exacerbated by heightened subsistence insecurity.[21] Though such mortality differentials were small relative to the overall mortality toll among both sexes in epidemic years such as 1908, they are consistent with the view of acute hunger underlying malaria lethality in epidemic years.

Hunger and recovery rate

The many clinical accounts of 'exalted' malaria in the British Indian famine records thus support the view of a direct relationship between acute hunger and malaria lethality, mediated through impaired immune capacity. Malaria's selective sensitivity to acute hunger relative to lesser degrees of undernourishment appears to distinguish it from many other common endemic diseases such as tuberculosis and whooping cough. Modern nutritional science research lends support perhaps for a causal link to this association. 'Many of the body's generalized defenses against infectious disease,' Nevin Scrimshaw details,

> are reduced by relatively mild degrees of nutritional deficiency. These include, among others, cell-mediated immunity, phagocyte function, complement function, and delayed cutaneous hypersensitivity. . . . With the more severe deficiencies of famine [(semi-) starvation], *specific humoral* antibody defenses and capacity to produce phagocytes are also weakened.[22]

As principally a bloodstream infection, malaria could perhaps be expected to manifest greater lethality under starvation conditions where the humoral (bloodstream) immune mechanisms are also suppressed. Certainly, undernourishment rose within South Asian populations during periods of famine,[23] expressed in increased 'nutritional stunting.'[24] But what distinguished famine conditions was a greater proportionate rise in acute hunger – those already chronically undernourished readily slipping into semi- or frank starvation.

Further indications of the impact of hunger-compromised immune capacity on malarial morbidity can be seen in relation to clinical illness 'relapses.' In his 1911 Bombay malaria study, Bentley documented the effect of food deprivation on malaria recrudescence among adult labourers. '[A]mong troops and bodies of labourers infected with malaria,' he noted, 'abstinence from food, prolonged only a few hours beyond ordinary meal-times, is sufficient to bring about many relapses of malaria a few days afterwards.' Sudden fluctuations in foodgrain prices, he suggested, had a similar impact, in turn triggering increased local transmission.[25] Christophers also documented clinical relapse in relation to heavy physical labour.[26] In his 1911 study of malaria among the convict population on the Andaman Islands, he concluded that malarial fevers were largely due to relapses of quartan malaria (P. malariae) rather than active transmission of new infection, as evidenced in very low prevalence rates of falciparum or vivax malaria.[27] '[C]ertain kinds of convict labour . . . [involving] arduous physical exertion' such as road making and excavation work were observed to be 'more associated with malaria than others': hard labour was associated with a three-fold greater number of fever admissions compared with 'ordinary' labour.[28] He also documented a much higher prevalence of 'very large spleen,' typically seen among the undernourished, amongst those dying of pneumonia, with the latter a major cause of death among the inmate population.[29]

Christophers may well have specifically sought out the Andaman study, anticipating the 'unique' opportunity the penal colony offered for further research into malaria intensity, a setting where 'not only is every member of the community under close observation, but in the case of death an autopsy is performed as a routine practice.'[30] He went on to hypothesise that the presence of quartan malaria (P. malariae) in a population suggested the kind of debilitating conditions where 'transmission is low but factors favouring relapses high.'[31] His recommendations emphasised 'the necessity of attending to everything affecting the general condition of the convicts.'

[A]n abundant dietary and comforts are not altogether a matter of mere luxury, but under peculiar conditions may be a medical necessity if a reasonable death rate among the community is aimed at.

Economy under these circumstances should not be short-sighted and a saving on a dietary, estimated to be just sufficient, may well lead to ultimate loss when hospital expenditure and labour efficiency with all that this means is taken into account.[32]

In subsequent writing, Christophers continued to stress the epidemiological significance of recovery rate, concluding in a 1914 analysis of splenic enlargement that prevalence rates in a population appeared to be a function not simply of infection (transmission) rates but also of 'a greatly lengthened recovery period the result of some racial or physiological diathesis.'[33] The impact of starvation on recovery rate was reflected also in the generally poor response to malaria treatment among the famished. 'It is well known,' Hehir also noted in his 1928 malaria text, 'that starved and overworked people with chronic malaria require something more than quinine to cure them,' explaining the disappointing results for quinine in terms of 'lowered natural resistance due to unfavourable conditions of life.'[34]

Microbiologic aspects to malaria intensity

The introduction of unfamiliar, potentially more virulent, strains of the malaria parasites into a non-immune population frequently is cited in historiographical accounts of epidemic malaria to explain heightened lethality from the disease. For Punjab, however, the appearance of new *plasmodium* strains was an unlikely explanation of the regional epidemics, given near-simultaneous appearance of intense epidemic fever across the province. In theory, highly favourable entomological conditions in 1908 may have allowed an earlier shift to the more severe, falciparum form of malaria infection. Yet falciparum parasite rates of over 40 per cent continued to be documented in young children in mid-1930s Karnal district in years of minimal autumn fever mortality[35] – such levels suggesting near-universal infection given characteristic intermittency of parasitaemia (parasites visible in blood smears). Such high falciparum rates were also documented in the 1980s with the rebound in transmission in the Lahore region, but apparently were associated with little mortality.[36] Moreover, it is difficult to see why such qualitative microbiologic aspects would have altered substantially after 1908 to explain epidemic decline in the absence of major changes in rainfall.

As seen in chapter 2, Christophers did consider variation in dose of infection as also contributing to malaria intensity during fulminant epidemics, with 'intensity in this sense being an expression of the *quantum of sporozoites* inoculated per unit of the community.'[37] He hypothesized, in turn, a direct relationship between residual infection among the physiologically weakened and dose of infection transmitted in subsequent successive cycles of transmission.[38] The relationship between recovery rate, 'residual' infection, and intensity (dose) of malaria transmitted would be further explored in 1914 by Acton and Knowles, Directors of the Pasteur Institute at Kasauli. Working on avian malaria, they observed that,

> when heavily infected pigeons were . . . brought into the laboratory from outside, into better conditions of feeding, watering, warmth, etc. . . . the intensity of gamete infection present steadily dropped. Within ten days or so the crescent counts [gametocytes] had fallen to half . . . [whereas in] those pigeons kept in the open under less favourable conditions the reduction is less marked and occurs more slowly.[39]

Their observations were made 'during the cold weather' when active transmission had ceased, and thus were unlikely to be confounded by continuing re-infection among the latter group. They also observed that the pigeons 'which had been kept for several months in good conditions' showed little evidence of parasites in the lungs, whereas those without such care, 'shewed numerous young gametes . . . in the peripheral blood. . . [and] mature schizonts of the asexual cycle . . . in the lung.'[40] The latter observation held potential significance regarding the well-recognised association between intense malaria and subsequent predilection to pulmonary pneumonia. But they also bore potential import for subsequent transmission dose.

Acton and Knowles hypothesised that two factors were concerned 'in initiating an epidemic of malaria':

> One factor is the number of gamete carriers present in the human population – this determines the *numerical extent* of the epidemic. The other is the intensity of the infection in these gamete carriers, and upon it depends the *character* of the epidemic that ensues, as to whether it is fulminant or mild. It will be seen that both factors are very considerably influenced by the allied factors of plentiful feeding and good hygienic environment.[41]

As in the case of Christophers's avian malaria experimental work, these observations were not assessed in modern statistical terms.[42] They nevertheless convey the seriousness with which leading scientists at the time considered a relationship between physiological debility, lethality of malarial infection, and also ensuing dose *(intensity)* of malarial transmitted in general in a population.

Among the range of factors affecting gametocyte infective 'quality' and 'effective dose' of infection transmitted to the human host in subsequent cycles of malaria transmission, it seems probable that the immune response of the human host would have an influence.[43] This is suggested by very high gametocyte numbers observed in non-immune young children, and conversely, low numbers in older age-groups with prolonged exposure.[44] It is suggested as well with subsequent observations in the 1920s and early 1930s that anopheles fed upon previously unexposed (non-immune) malaria patients showed a much greater number of oöcysts in the mosquitoes' stomach walls than those fed on previously malaria-exposed patients.[45]

But is there empirical evidence linking hunger-related compromised immune response to sporozoite dose and malaria intensity? Immunological response to malaria infection is, of course, a subject central to present-day malaria vaccine research efforts. Yet the question of how pre-existing immune suppression in the human host may affect gametocyte infectivity is one that appears to remain unclear to date. Determinants of gametocyte infectivity are considered 'extraordinarily variable,' their analysis viewed to be amongst the most elusive endeavours in modern malaria research.[46] In some forms of non-human malaria, anti-gametocyte antibodies ingested in the mosquito's blood meal have been observed to reduce or 'neutralise' subsequent infectivity of gametocytes in the mosquito vector and, in turn, dose of infection (sporozoites) transmitted.[47] A comparable effect in human malaria, however, is unconfirmed.[48] If future research in the area of gametocyte infectivity shows a similar 'neutralising' effect of human antigamete antibodies to be at play, this could help to explain the *generalised* increase in severity of infection observed during epidemics such as 1908 among famished sub-populations.

Yet even assuming increased dose of malarial infection in epidemic years, other questions remain. Higher doses of infection might help to explain more severe infections from the earliest stages of an epidemic, as in 1908. But it is difficult to see how it could explain the recurring pattern of class differentials in mortality. One would expect, instead, to see an impact of dose on lethality distributed more or less randomly among the population rather than selectively among the poor. Interior resting of a 'high-dose' infected mosquito could undoubtedly lead to multiple 'intense' cases in a single household, and thus a clustering of severe cases. But there is perhaps less reason to expect mosquitoes initially feeding on a high-gametocyte human host to return selectively to the most destitute households, after egg-depositing on exterior water sites and the 10-day period of parasite development – particularly in the highly compact villages of Punjab – to explain such consistent differentials in mortality in a rural population as a whole.[49] Indeed, the generalised pattern of enhanced intensity, but not lethality, of infection in populations under epidemic conditions, documented also in 1943 Bengal,[50] also suggests otherwise.

Thus, though the question of dose of malaria infection remains an important biological and epidemiological question, a role in explaining differential mortality appears likely to have been secondary to the direct effect of starvation on capacity to survive an attack of malaria. And, even here, higher dose would itself be a secondary consequence of hunger-induced debility.

Malaria-induced hunger

Because of the strong temporal association between malaria transmission and rainfall, increased prevalence of malaria infection in Punjab coincided with peak agricultural labour demand.[51] Malaria thus could exact a relatively greater impact on a rural economy compared with other seasonal diseases. In the course of the severe 1890 epidemic, Punjab sanitary officials described a village in Sialkot district where 'there were several square miles of rice-fields in which the crops were breaking down from being over-ripe, and the villagers were so weak that they could not reap them.'[52] Malaria historiography offers many other dramatic accounts of the economic impacts visited upon populations under epidemic conditions. Christophers and Bentley describe the vicious cycle thus:

> Once sickness, debility and anaemia become rife the pressure and frequency of individual hardship becomes enormously increased. Pay cannot be earned by the sick, who may suffer actual starvation. Nor is it only the workers who suffer . . . their relatives and dependents are exposed to greater hardship and increasing liability to sickness; and the greater the number of sick the more intense becomes the general infection, until as a result an immunity that may protect under ordinary conditions is broken down under exposure to more virulent and intense malaria, so that even those originally the strongest and most healthy become involved also.[53]

This account describes conditions observed among indentured labourers on large construction sites where destitution was endemic. But

Christophers relates a similar sequence in 1908 Punjab towns under the combined effects of post-famine flooding conditions where pre-existing acquired immunity amongst the adult population appears to have been readily overwhelmed.

> For many weeks labour for any purpose was unprocurable and even food vendors ceased to carry on their trade. Thus not only was ordinary food difficult to obtain and the prices excessive, but, owing to malaria among the cowkeeper class, milk, a necessity for the very young and the sick, was practically unprocurable even at the exorbitant rate of 8 to 12 annas per seer.[54]

Simultaneous debility meant few adults able to work, or to feed one another, a situation that deepened and extended the period of economic collapse, destitution, and starvation. 'Babies die,' Christophers would later describe, 'not only from the direct effects of malaria but from lack of milk and attention from their prostrated mothers. Crops are left standing in the fields and everywhere there is pestilence and death.'[55] Such accounts also bear more than passing resemblance to descriptions of conditions among non-immune entire populations suddenly exposed to unfamiliar infectious diseases, referred to in its classic form as 'virgin-soil' epidemics.[56]

Often overlooked, however, in the citing of historical accounts of epidemic-related socio-economic collapse is the fact that such instances were exceptional events. In Punjab, simultaneous malarial fever on its own, in the absence of prevailing hunger-induced debility, did not trigger the drastic levels of social and economic paralysis evident in 1908. Nor, it seems, did flooding. Rapid increase in malaria prevalence was the norm in Punjab in years of even average monsoon rainfall, as evidenced in the 'normal' autumnal fever curve. But in non-scarcity years, morbidity generally was much less severe, of shorter duration, associated with lower 'relapse' rates, and unaccompanied by mass breakdown in previously acquired immunity protection.

There can be little question that the seasonal timing of malaria transmission itself could interfere with timing of agricultural operations. But this impact was very much greater – reaching disastrous levels – when universal infection was visited upon an already severely debilitated (sub-)population. After 1920, one sees few references in the administrative records to crop loss on account of malarial fever, in spite of similar levels of monsoon rain and recurring episodes of severe flooding and high levels of seasonal malarial infection.

Famine and malaria exposure

Within modern epidemic historiography, there has been a tendency to categorise infectious diseases in terms of their exceptional form: virulence observed in particular epidemic instances assumed to be an inherent aspect of each specific mircro-organism. In the case of malaria, this perhaps helps to explain its recent categorisation along-side smallpox and bubonic plague.[57]

In recent South Asian epidemic historiography, explanations of malaria epidemicity have also turned increasingly towards the micro-biological domain. In the case of Punjab, the relationship between epidemic malaria and famine has been interpreted in germ-transmission terms as driven substantially by entomological conditions such as prodigious proliferation of anopheline mosquito vectors with return of the rains, or deviation of vector feeding to humans consequent upon drought-related cattle mortality. 'Deprived of cattle,' it has been suggested,

> [t]he vector population, swollen by the enhanced rate of proliferation . . . fed almost exclusively on humans. . . . Cattle mortality in all probability contributed significantly to human morbidity and mortality in these catastrophic years.[58]

A 'crucial part of the explanation' of the 1908 Punjab epidemic, it is suggested, 'lies not in "famine" as such, but rather in the peculiar climatic character of the famine years.'[59]

The 'vector-deviation' thesis of malaria epidemicity appears to have originated in the malaria research literature of the early 1920s with identification of the different feeding habits of anopheline mosquitoes.[60] With confirmation that the major South Asian malaria vector, *An. culicifacies*, was a zoophilic species – preferentially feeding on livestock[61] – the thesis was soon advanced that famine-associated 'loss of cattle [was] a factor of the first importance in the causation of the great epidemics of malaria in India.'[62] Though unexamined empirically, the postulate was rapidly embraced within the discipline of tropical medicine through to the post-Independence era.[63]

Heavy loss of cattle, of course, was common during periods of prolonged drought, particularly in southeastern Punjab. Bhattacharya notes that well over half the cattle in Hissar district perished in the famine period of 1866–1869. 'When grass and fodder were scarce, supplies were reserved for calves. Older animals were allowed to die of starvation, or slaughtered if they could not be sold.' During the recurring famines in the district between 1896 and 1904, he estimates total cattle population fell by 35 per cent.[64]

After 1908, enhanced provision of 'fodder relief' undoubtedly reduced cattle mortality and distress sales in this region in years of drought, policy timing that corresponds to beginning decline in epidemic malaria in the province. However, livestock census figures pre-1910 do not suggest marked decline in total numbers over the major famine periods, even in Hissar district. Total livestock numbers in the district declined from 549,598 in 1896 to 506,809 in 1897, and to 449,173 by 1901–1902.[65] Moreover, livestock loss during famine years elsewhere in the province was more limited still, though fulminant malaria was experienced through much of the province in 1900: autumn fever deaths soaring, for example, in the north-central district of Ludhiana to 24.1 per 1,000 despite very limited reported livestock mortality.[66] Loss of cattle unquestionably was a marker of extreme economic hardship for households affected. But there appears to be little general relationship across the province between epidemic fulminancy and the extent of such losses.

Christophers, at the time, would urge caution regarding the cattle deviation thesis, noting that 'close association with cattle does not always prevent a human epidemic. In the Punjab epidemic of 1908 the cattle zone of Amritsar city was one of the worst epidemic areas.'[67] Moreover, malaria mortality was consistently greater in urban centres in epidemic years, he observed, than for the rural population although vector breeding sites were generally fewer.[68] As we have seen, the urban fever death rate in the famine year of 1879 in Punjab rose 250 per cent over the 1870–1879 mean, to 53.7 per 1,000, compared with 36.6 per mille in the rural population (Table 6.1). Higher urban malaria mortality is consistent, instead, with greater prevalence of destitution in the towns, urban migration often a strategy of last resort for the destitute during both famine and non-famine times.[69]

Punjab exceptionalism?

Finally, to what extent was Punjab's propensity to 'fulminant' malaria a function of the region's distinctive ecology: the combination of its continental climate, agricultural economy, topography, geology, and soil hydrology? Certainly, in the eyes of the early colonial malaria workers, Punjab malaria epidemicity was seen as exceptional. In drawing up a map of malaria endemiology of the Indian subcontinent, Christophers and Sinton in the 1920s designated malaria in the northwest Indo-Gangetic plains by a distinctive dark red colour.[70] A major contributing factor in this potency was the region's flood propensity, the severe economic impacts of which continued to be documented well after 1920. 'Owing to inundation of rivers and exceptionally heavy rainfall,' Punjab Public Health Commissioner, K.A. Rahman, observed in relation to the severe floods of 1933,

> [t]he intensity of malaria . . . was greatly aggravated . . . by the debilitating conditions due to floods, exposure to chills and accentuated by anxiety caused by extensive loss of property, falling of a very large number of houses and by scarcity of food as a sequel to the soiling and decomposition of hoarded grain in the homes and destruction of crops in the fields.[71]

And yet actual fever mortality levels in 1933 were less than one-quarter the level experienced in heavy rainfall years such as 1908, the latter preceded by famine (Table 6.2).[72] The 1933 epidemic, in other words, once again suggests the contingent effect of flooding on malaria lethality. When combined with pre-existing mass destitution, flooding exacerbated malaria lethality in a manner that seems to have had little parallel in other regions of the subcontinent. Flooding on its own, however, did not.

This suggests, then, that the fulminancy propensity of malaria in Punjab derived more from the pronounced *economic* variability that low and highly variable rainfall ordained than from changing entomo-immunological conditions year-to-year. Low monsoon rainfall was accompanied by marked variability in annual rainfall, thus a greater frequency of both drought and flooding, and pronounced harvest variability in turn. Across the 1871–1984 period, one in four years in Punjab were drought-afflicted (rainfall deficit 25 per cent or greater), and years of severe flooding (rainfall 25 per cent in excess) were almost as frequent.[73] By contrast, over the same 114-year period, lower Bengal experienced a single year of comparable drought and only eight flood years. It is possible, then, that epidemic propensity – the 'exceptionalist' character to the 'notorious' malaria epidemics of Punjab – reflected the *economic* fine line the region's rainfall and physiography prescribed between agricultural prosperity ('normal' rains) and economic paralysis (too little rain *or* too much).[74]

Such a conclusion is suggested also in the context of post-1908 epidemic trends. As we shall consider in the following chapter, drought and severe flooding continued after 1920, though fulminant epidemics did not. As will become apparent in the second portion of the study, there appears to have been little if any change in the region's ecology after 1920 to affect substantial levels of malaria transmission. What did change after 1908 was the British Raj's response to both.

Table 6.2 Oct.–Dec. fever death rate (per 1,000), nominal and 'corrected' for non-malaria fever deaths,** 23 plains districts, Punjab province, 1933, 1908

District	Oct.–Dec. FDR (per 1,000)		Oct.–Dec. FDR 'corrected' for non-malaria fever deaths		Estimated** non-malaria Oct.–Dec FDR
	1933	1908	1933	1908	
Southeast:					
Hissar	7.7	19.9	2.6	14.8	5.1
Rohtak	9.4	21.0	4.1	15.6	5.4
Gurgaon	9.3	35.0	4.2	29.9	5.1
Karnal	9.5	30.8	6.3	27.6	3.2
Amballa	6.8	14.8	5.1	13.1	1.7
Central:					
Hoshiarpur	6.2	29.8	1.6	25.2	4.6
Jullundur	5.4	20.5	1.1	16.2	4.3
Ludhiana	4.2	22.1	0.0	17.9	4.2
Ferozepur	6.6	26.1	1.6	21.2	4.9
Lahore	3.2	25.7	0.0	22.4	3.3
Amritsar	5.4	34.7	1.5	30.7	4.0
North:					
Gurdaspur	7.4	27.1	3.4	23.2	3.9
Sialkot	10.0	38.6	5.6	34.2	4.4
Gujrat	12.3	36.6	8.1	32.4	4.2
Gujranwala	17.8	21.3	13.6	17.2	4.1
Jhelum	9.5	32.3	5.3	28.1	4.2
West/Southwest:					
Shahpur	11.1	10.9	8.0	7.8	3.1
Jhang	5.9	30.6	2.4	27.2	3.4
Montgomery	6.9	22.7	2.7	18.5	4.2
Multan	10.6	8.0	7.2	4.5	3.5
Dhera Ismail Khan	10.1	9.0	4.3	3.2	5.8
Muzaffargarh	11.8	7.1	7.4	2.7	4.4
Dhera Ghazi Khan	9.9	5.8	5.2	1.1	4.7
23-district Mean	**8.6**	**23.1**	**4.4**	**18.9**	**4.2**

Source: See Table 4.1.

** Based on the Oct.–Dec. FDR for 1938, a severe drought year (third-quarter rain, 7.5 inches). See note 72.

Notes

1 W.R. Cornish, *Report of the Sanitary Commissioner for Madras for 1877* (Madras: Government Central Branch Press, 1877), 11, 142, xxviii [hereafter *MSCR*].
2 *MSCR* 1877, 141.
3 *MSCR* 1878, 4–6. See also, *PSCR* 1884, 10; *PSCR* 1890, 8.

4 PSCR 1892, 3, 16.
5 G.C. Geddes, Administrative Experience Recorded in Former Famine Times (Calcutta: Bengal Secretariat Press, 1874), cited in MSCR 1878, 141.
6 'Note on the Results of the Enquiries Made into the Mortality in the North-Western Provinces and Oudh,' Government North-Western Provinces and Oudh, 596, Mar. 17, 1879, in Report of the Famine Commission, Part 3, Famine Histories (London: HMSO, 1885), 243–249 [hereafter Famine Histories].
7 Famine Histories, 243–249. Leela Sami notes a similar caste profile to mortality in the 1876–1877 South Indian famine; 'Starvation, Disease and Death: Explaining Famine Mortality in Madras 1876–1878,' Social History of Medicine, 24, 3, Nov. 2011, 700–719.
8 See ch. 11, at note 61.
9 PSCR 1880, 40.
10 The 1907 fever death rate among European and native troops was 1.3 and 3.0 per 1,000, respectively; for prisoners, 5.1 per 1,000; J.T.W. Leslie, "Malaria in India," Proceedings of the Imperial Malaria Conference, Simla, October 1909 (Simla: Government Central Branch Press, 1910), 4 [hereafter Simla Conf.].
11 S.R. Christophers, 'Malaria in the Punjab,' Sci. Mem. Off. Med. San. Dep., 46 (Calcutta: Superintendent Government Printing Office, 1911), 12–14 [hereafter MP].
12 R. Shrimpton, et. al., 'Worldwide Timing of Growth Faltering: Implications for Nutritional Interventions,' Pediatrics, 107, 2001, 1–7.
13 A. Maharatna, The Demography of Famines: An Indian Historical Perspective (New Delhi: Oxford University Press, 1996), 77.
14 Ibid., 29, Table 2.1.
15 'The civil authorities . . . are of the opinion that actual violence is not resorted to. . . . It is strongly suspected that in some villages mothers abstain from suckling their female children, who soon become so weak as to be unable to suck – death follows, and the cause is entered in the Police Returns as "Adam Shír Noshi"'; PSCR 1889, 3.
16 PLGP, 1, in PSCR 1887.
17 PLGP, June 25, 1891, 1, in PSCR 1890.
18 PSCR 1890, 3. The 1911 Punjab Census report explained higher female child mortality in terms of 'early weaning of girl children in order that a male child may be conceived'; Census of Punjab, 1911, 224, 231. I thank Leela Sami for this reference; 'Gender Differentials in Famine Mortality: (1876–1878) and Punjab (1896–1897),' EPW, 37, 26, June 29, 2002.
19 PSCR 1908, 13. A 2 per cent relative increase over 1903–1907 levels is seen in total mortality in 1908 among female children 1–4 years of age over males. This compares with a 30 per cent increase for both sexes in the epidemic year of 1908.
20 See ch. 9.
21 For discussion of continuing sex differentials in child mortality in north/north-west India, see for example, J. Drèze, A. Sen, 'Gender Inequality and Women's Agency,' in India: Development and Participation (New York: Oxford University Press, 2002); M. Das Gupta, 'Selective Discrimination Against Female Children in Rural Punjab,' Population and Development Review, 13, 1, Mar. 1987, 77–100; M. Bhalla, 'The Land of Vanishing Girls,' in M. Rao, ed., The Unheard Scream: Reproductive Health and Women's Lives in India

(New Delhi: Zubaan, 2004), 259–278. For historical factors underlying cultural patterns of female disadvantage in the region, see B. Miller, *The Endangered Sex* (Ithaca, NY: Cornell University Press, 1981); P. Bardhan, 'On Life and Death Questions,' *EPW*, 9 (Special Number), Aug. 10, 1974.

22 N. Scrimshaw, 'The Phenomenon of Famine,' *American Review of Nutrition*, 7, 1987, 1–21; [emphasis added]. 'Humoral' refers to antibodies circulating in the bloodstream.

23 Reduced food consumption has been documented across much of affected populations even in mid-20th-century South Asian famines; J. Drèze, 'Famine Prevention in India,' in J. Drèze, A. Sen, eds., *The Political Economy of Hunger*, Vol. 2 (Oxford: Clarendon Press), 1990, 13–122, at 83.

24 A.M. Guntupalli and J. Baten have found a decline in adult stature in those cohorts born during years of famine in 1917–1918 and 1943; 'Inequality of Heights in North, West, and East India 1915–1944,' *Explorations in Economic History*, 43, 2006, 578–608.

25 C.A. Bentley, *Report of an Investigation into the Causes of Malaria in Bombay and the Measures Necessary for its Control* (Bombay: Miscellaneous Official Publications, 1911), 86.

26 Technically, the term 'relapse' is used to refer to reactivation of a dormant form of the parasite seen only in vivax malaria, clinical illness reappearing months or even years after initial infection. More immediate recurrence of clinical symptoms and parasitemia following initial recovery in falciparum malaria has been termed 'recrudescence'.

27 Quartan malaria generally results in a milder illness and is much less prevalent than either vivax or falciparum malaria.

28 S.R. Christophers, 'Malaria in the Andamans,' *Sci. Mem. Off. Med. San. Dep.*, 56, 1912, 24.

29 Ibid., 31, 35–40.

30 Ibid., 30.

31 Ibid., 31.

32 Ibid., 42.

33 S.R. Christophers, 'The Spleen Rate and Other Splenic Indices: Their Nature and Significance,' *IJMR*, 2, 1914, 823–866, at 851–852. Christophers's reference to racial difference in recovery rate here is puzzling, having earlier cited data indicating little such difference.

34 P. Hehir, *Malaria in India* (London: Humphrey Milford, 1928), 281. Recent research into immune response to malaria in undernourished children, though limited, appears to support the view of compromised immune capacity; F. Fillol et al., 'Impact of Child Malnutrition on the Specific Anti-*Plasmodium Falciparum* Antibody Response,' *Malaria Journal*, June 2, 2009; B. Genton, 'Relation of Anthropometry to Malaria Morbidity and Immunity in Papua New Guinean Children,' *American Journal of Clinical Nutrition*, 68, 1998, 734–741.

35 E.P. Hicks, S. Abdul Majid, "A Study of the Epidemiology of Malaria in a Punjab District", *RMSI*, 7, 1 (1937), 1–43; M.F. Boyd, 'Epidemiology: Factors Related to the Definitive Host,' in M.F. Boyd, ed., *Malariology*, Vol. 1 (Philadelphia: W.B. Saunders, 1949), 551–607, at 555.

36 G.T. Strickland et al., 'Endemic Malaria in Four Villages of the Pakistani Province of Punjab,' *Transactions of the Royal Society of Tropical Medicine and Hygiene*, 81, 1, 1987, 36–41 [hereafter *TRSTMH*]; __,

'The Interrelationship of *Plasmodium Falciparum* and *P. vivax* in the Punjab,' *TRSTMH*, 83, 4, 1989, 471–473.

37 MP, 129.

38 Simla Conf., 45.

39 H.W. Acton, R. Knowles, 'Studies on the *Halteridium* Parasite of the Pigeon,' *Haemoproteus Columbae, Celli & San Felice*,' *IJMR*, 1, 4, 1914, 663–690, at 674, Tables 2, 3.

40 Ibid., 675. A schizont is a form of the malaria parasite that develops in an organ of the human or animal host after vector inoculation from which numerous merozoites develop and are released into the bloodstream.

41 Ibid. '[O]ur results establish the converse of [Christophers's] proposition. If food be plentiful and hygienic conditions be good, the infective feeding ground will be small and we may, therefore, expect this fact to diminish the next season's epidemic'; ibid., 674.

42 Mean parasites level among the 50 open dove-cot pigeons was 43,750 and 22,000 among those housed under laboratory conditions; ibid., 673–674.

43 Margaret Humphreys has also raised this question, one that appeared frequently in earlier literature as well; *Malaria: Poverty, Race, and Public Health in the United States* (Baltimore: Johns Hopkins Press, 2001), 55; W.A.P. Schuffner, 'Two Subjects Relating to the Epidemiology of Malaria, Part 1. The Importance of Determining the Spleen Rate and the Limits of its Usefulness,' *Indian Journal of Malariology*, 1, 1938, 221–256; G. Macdonald, 'Community Aspects of Immunity to Malaria,' in L.J. Bruce-Chwatt, V.J. Glanville, eds., *Dynamics of Tropical Disease: The Late George Macdonald* (London: Oxford University Press, 1973), 81.

44 Interestingly, it has been suggested that extremely high immunity levels in holoendemic populations may lower *effective* gametocyte dose transmitted, thereby offering some ultimate protection to the non-immune infant sub-population; I.A. McGregor, R.J.M. Wilson, ch. 20, 'Specific Immunity: Acquired in Man,' in W.H. Wernsdorfer, I.A. McGregor, eds., *Malaria: Principles and Practice of Malariology* (London: Churchill Livingstone, 1988), 559–619, at 563.

45 S.P. James, Commentary, in R. Briercliffe, 'Discussion on the Malaria Epidemic in Ceylon 1934–1935,' *Proceeding of the Royal Society of Medicine*, 29, 1936, 537–562, at 559–560. It is suggested indirectly also by recent observation that human immunodeficiency virus infection is associated with 'greater malignancy' of malarial infection; E.L. Korenromp et al., 'Malaria Attributable to the HIV-I Epidemic, Sub-Saharan Africa,' *Emerging Infectious Diseases*, 11, 9, 2005, 1413.

46 R. Carter, P.M. Graves, ch. 7, 'Gametocytes,' in *Malaria: Principles and Practice of Malariology* (London: Churchill Livingstone, 1988), 253–306, at 292. 'Under controlled laboratory conditions,' gametocyte density of the blood meal ingested by a mosquito appears to predict severity of subsequent infective "oocyst load" per mosquito. This relationship is apparent also in the case of human malaria but is less predictable, suggesting other factors at play; ibid.

47 McGregor and Wilson, 'Specific Immunity: Acquired in man'; V.S. Moorthy, M.F. Good, A.V.S. Hill, 'Malaria Vaccine Developments,' *Lancet*, 363, 2004, 150–156.

48 McGregor and Wilson, 'Specific Immunity: Acquired in Man.'
49 The centripetal progression of malaria mortality from periphery to central core of Amritsar in 1908 suggests, Christophers concluded, that vector anophelines responsible came mainly from breeding sites outside the town, which was likely also the case for the compact rural villages of Punjab; MP, 31–32, 38–41.
50 See ch. 12.
51 This timing of transmission with agriculture demands is common beyond Punjab and South Asia. See, for example, R. Chambers, R. Longhurst, A. Pacey, eds., *Seasonal Dimensions to Rural Poverty* (London: Frances Pinter Publishers, 1981).
52 *PSCR* 1890, 9, 5.
53 S.R. Christophers and C.A. Bentley, 'The Human Factor: An Extension of our Knowledge Regarding the Epidemiology of Malarial Disease,' in W.E. Jennings, ed., *Transactions of the Bombay Medical Congress* (Bombay: Bennett, Coleman & Co., 1910), 78–83 at 78–79. This paper appears to be the single instance Christophers used the term 'starvation'.
54 MP, 9.
55 S.R. Christophers, 'Measures for the Control of Malaria in India,' *Journal of the Royal Society of Arts*, Apr. 30, 1943, 285–295, at 291.
56 A.W. Crosby, *The Columbian Exchange: Biological and Cultural Consequences of 1492* (Westport, CT: Greenwood, 1972).
57 R.I. Rotberg, 'Nutrition and History,' *Journal of Interdisciplinary History*, 14, 3, 1983, 199–204.
58 E. Whitcombe, 'Famine Mortality,' *EPW*, 28, June 5, 1993, 1169–1179, at 1178.
59 Ibid., 1177.
60 E. Roubard, 'La Differenciation des Races d'Anopheles et la Régression spontanée du Paludisme,' *Bulletin de la Société de pathologie exotique*, 14, 9, 1921, 577–595.
61 Delhi studies in the 1930s and 1940s found over 90 percent of *An. culicifacies* feeding on livestock rather than human blood; T. Ramachandra Rao, *Anophelines of India*, 1st ed. (New Delhi: Malaria Research Centre, ICMR, 1984), 374.
62 F.W. Cragg, 'The Zoophilism of *Anopheles* in Relation to the Epidemiology of Malaria in India: A Suggestion,' *IJMR*, 10, 3, 1923, 962–964, at 964.
63 A. Balfour, H.H. Scott, *Health Problems of the Empire: Past, Present and Future* (New York: Henry Holt, 1924), 238; G. Macdonald, 'The Analysis of Equilibrium in Malaria,' *Dynamics of Tropical Diseases*, 142. See also, Famine Inquiry Commission, *Report on Bengal* (New Delhi: Government of India Press, 1945), 122.
64 N. Bhattacharya, 'Pastoralists in a Colonial World,' in D. Arnold, R. Guha, eds., *Nature, Culture, Imperialism: Essays on the Environmental History of South Asia* (New Delhi: Oxford University Press, 1998), 48–85, at 67, 65, 62. Total livestock declined from 549,598 in 1896 to 506,809 in 1897 and to 449,173 by 1901–1902; *PLRA* 1896–1897, 26; *Report on the Season and Crops of the Punjab* (Lahore: Civil and Military Gazette Press, 1901–1902), xiii.

65 In 1896, livestock was estimated at 368,623; in 1901–1902, 372,557; *PLRA 1896–1897*, 26; *Season and Crop Report*, 1901–1902, xiii.

66 *PLRA 1896–1897*, 26; *Season and Crop Report*, 1901–1902, xii.

67 As recounted in A.B. Fry, 'The Role of Cattle in the Epidemiology of Malaria,' *Indian Medical Gazette*, Jan. 1922, 1–2.

68 MP, 29, 38.

69 Such urban:rural differentials in fever death rates are all the more notable given greater male urban migration, hence proportionately fewer infants and elderly, those subgroups typically most vulnerable to malaria.

70 S.R. Christophers, J.A. Sinton, 'A Malaria Map of India,' *IJMR*, 1926, 14, 1, 173–178; reproduced in P. Hehir, *Malaria in India* (London: Humphrey Milford, 1928), 441–443. Hehir would describe East and North Punjab as 'subject to overwhelming and appalling outbursts of epidemic malaria – *it is the home of this latter form of the disease*'; ibid., 16 [emphasis in original]. Such malaria epidemicity extended to the neighbouring region of Rajasthan and western UP.

71 *Report on the Public Health Administration of the Punjab* (Lahore: Government Press, 1933), 15.

72 Non-malarial autumn fever deaths are estimated on the basis of Oct.–Dec. fever death rates recorded in the severe drought year of 1938 (mean third-quarter rain, 7.5 inches) when malaria transmission across the province could be expected to be virtually negligible. This rate (4.2 per 1,000) is subtracted from those recorded in 1933 and 1908, giving a 'corrected' mean for the 23 districts of 4.4 and 18.9 per 1,000, respectively.

73 B. Parthasarathy, N.A. Sontakke, A.A. Monot, D.R. Kothawale, 'Droughts/Floods in the Summer Monsoon Season over Different Meteorological Subdivisions of India for the Period 1871–1984,' *Journal of Climatology*, 7, 1987, 57–70.

74 One further entomological question relating to Punjab epidemic propensity is recent recognition of 'sibling' subspecies of *An. culicifacies*, each associated with differing levels of transmission efficiency. Sibling species A that dominates in Punjab and western Uttar Pradesh appears to be a more efficient malaria vector than subspecies in southern India; V.P. Sharma, 'Determinants of Malaria in South Asia,' in E.A. Casman, H. Dowlatabadi, eds., *The Contextual Determinants of Malaria* (Washington, DC: Resources for the Future, 2002), 110–132. Such differences are considered to explain higher vector infection rates in the northwest, and thus present greater challenges in present-day efforts to control malaria transmission in the region. But the relevance for historical malaria *mortality* patterns is less clear.

Part II

Colonial malaria control

Policy and practice

7 Malaria policy in British India

Within South Asian public health historiography, it has generally been assumed that the British Raj undertook little in the way of systematic malaria control work in the subcontinent: that despite many major research contributions to understanding malaria as a vector-borne disease, practical measures were few, limited to desultory efforts to distribute quinine.[1] At the same time, the task of malaria control in India has often been viewed as inherently at odds with agricultural and health development due to the 'malariogenic' effects of canal irrigation. With the British administration continuing to pursue expansion of canal irrigation as their principal policy for rural economic growth through the early decades of the 20th century, any prospect of malaria control is thought to have receded even further, above all in Punjab.[2]

Yet autumn fever mortality in Punjab declined in the final decades of colonial rule in all regions of the province, those with widespread canal irrigation, and those without, and in districts where foodgrain prices pre-1910 were a significant predictor of malaria epidemics, and in those where they were not. And it did so though monsoon rainfall remained unchanged and flooding continued, as we will consider in more detail ahead. This rapid decline in malaria epidemicity in Punjab in the years following release of Christophers's inquiry report on the 1908 epidemic presents two key questions. To what extent were his recommendations – those explicitly delineating flood control and quinine measures, and those implicit in the economic realm – acted upon? And in each case what was their potential contribution to malaria mortality decline?

Assessment of malaria control efforts inevitably hinges on the meaning intended by the term 'control.' Central to the 1911 Punjab inquiry was recognition of the distinction between malaria infection (transmission) and malaria mortality, between 'normal' seasonal malarial fever and regional epidemics of high malaria lethality. Narrative accounts of morbidity portray enormous variation, from a week or so of intermittent fever on the one hand, to prostration, coma, and death on the other. Applying either definition of 'malaria control' – transmission or mortality – to the pre-1900 period, the perception that colonial efforts were negligible is largely apt. While malaria deaths among the British Indian military declined rapidly after army 'sanitary' reforms[3] in the 1860s, highly lethal epidemics continued to afflict the general population in Punjab for another half-century.

For the post-1908 period, however, the assumption that malaria control was negligible misses a good deal. The commissioning of the Punjab malaria inquiry in late 1908, and eventual release of Christophers's report as a public document in 1911, points to a very different level of imperial engagement in the malaria problem in the early 20th century – albeit propelled by imperial interests and constrained in important ways. Certainly from 1908 on, the Government of India took seriously the public health cost of the 'exalted' form of malaria seen in various regions of the country, and was attempting to decipher, and at some level grapple with, the spectrum of causal factors underlying that lethality.

That engagement, and a critique of its practical effects and limits, is the subject of this second portion of the study. The scope of official concern over the malaria toll, and its political 'optics,' is evident in the proceedings of two key medical conferences of the period, the Bombay Medical Congress convened in February 1909, and the Imperial Malaria Conference held at Simla eight months later.[4] The emergence of concerted malaria policy can be traced in large part to the epidemiological research presented at these two medical gatherings, findings that laid the basis for malaria policy for the remainder of the colonial period. Though subject to undoubted editing, the proceedings from these conferences open up for historians much more complex aspects to the malaria debate than the 'extirpationist' (vector sanitation) versus 'ameliorationist' ('quininist') framework that had come to characterise public malaria policy discussion of this period. They provide, in turn, an essential base for interpreting malaria policy formulation and practice across the final decades of colonial rule, policy directed explicitly to malaria's *mortality* burden.

At the Bombay Congress, with epidemic plague still raging, a substantial portion of the three-day medical meet was devoted to the subject of malaria. Among the presentations, two papers would come to shape all subsequent malaria policy in British India. The first, presented by Indian Medical Service (IMS) researcher S.P. James, offered an account of the preceding seven years of intensive anti-mosquito operations undertaken at the Mian Mir military cantonment in central rural Punjab. It concluded that the program had failed to eliminate, or even substantially limit, prevalence of malaria, with the cantonment swept up in the autumn regional epidemic of 1908 along with much of the rest of the province. Sickness rates of European troops at Mian Mir in 1908 were recorded at 576 per 1,000.[5] Autumn death rates for the military were minimal, whereas for the cantonment civilian population, they closely paralleled those in villages outside the experimental area.[6]

The second major malaria paper presented was co-authored by Christophers and C.A. Bentley (1873–1949), former chief medical officer of the Empire of India and Ceylon Tea Company. Entitled 'The Human Factor: An Extension of our Knowledge regarding the Epidemiology of Malarial Disease,' it offered a frank distillation of the findings from their recently concluded inquiry into the syndrome of blackwater fever on the northeastern Duars tea plantations, conclusions, the investigators suggested, that bore direct implications for understanding malaria mortality patterns across the subcontinent.[7] Blackwater fever was a generally uncommon but serious medical syndrome involving sudden red blood cell destruction (hemolysis), triggered, it appeared, by repeated quinine use for recurrent malarial infection, and thus seen typically in areas of very high malaria endemicity. In India, blackwater fever was considered to occur mainly among non-immune European and Bengali managerial staff of the northeastern tea plantations. More problematic for the imperial administration, the association of blackwater fever with quinine was increasingly undermining public confidence in the therapeutic safety of quinine, and by extension, in the principal anti-malarial policy that the government then had at hand.

The two authors of the 'Human Factor' paper concluded that human destitution amongst the labour populations on the Duars plantations played an overriding role in the highly prevalent and exceptionally 'intense' form of malaria seen on the estates. Constant re-infection in turn of the managerial staff and their repeated resort to quinine led to the high incidence of blackwater fever among them. The central emphasis of the 'Human Factor' paper, however, extended well beyond the Duars plantations. The authors went on to articulate a more general relationship between hunger (economic stress), malaria intensity, and its lethality, pointing to endemic destitution in the labour camps across much of the subcontinent and in regions of agricultural decline.

The questions raised in Bombay by the Mian Mir and 'Human Factor' papers would go on to inform discussions at the Imperial Malaria Conference at Simla the following October, a six-day gathering where

Christophers's presentation of his Punjab inquiry findings formed the basis of deliberations.[8] Together, the three reports ushered in a period of remarkable epidemiological research on malaria in South Asia, work that would make a seminal contribution to the understanding of malarial transmission, and of malaria mortality patterns in human populations. Within a decade and a half of Ross's confirmation of malaria as a vector-borne disease, India would become a leading centre of malaria research with regular conferences and journals devoted solely to the subject, work which contributed very substantially to modern understanding of malaria epidemiology, endemiology, and medical entomology.[9]

The malaria policies that emerged in India in these opening years of the 20th century, based upon this research, can be seen to have taken shape in four stages. The first, spanning the decade leading up to the Bombay Medical Congress in February 1909, was a period during which the colonial administration was coming to terms with mounting expectations for vector control amongst both the colonial and metropolitan medical professions – expectations triggered in 1897–1898 by Ross's identification of the developmental stages of the malaria parasite in mosquitoes.[10] Mian Mir had made it clear that there was no ready vector extirpation 'fix' on the horizon for the control of malaria transmission in the vast rural areas of the subcontinent where the disease took its principal toll. The technical and fiscal difficulties revealed at the cantonment, combined with growing notoriety of malaria in its epidemic form as manifested in the 1908 epidemic, only served to intensify the crisis of sanitary legitimacy already facing the British Raj with the outbreak of plague a decade earlier. In the final days of 1908, the colonial administration thus had little choice but to acknowledge the broader economic dimensions to the malaria problem.

The second stage of malaria policy formulation extended from the Bombay Medical Congress in February 1909 to the Simla malaria conference convened the following October, a period of crisis management. Imperial strategy centred on taking into confidence senior sanitary officials and members of the Indian Medical Service (IMS) regarding the economic determinants underlying malaria's 'exalted' form. The goal was to achieve consensus on where government priorities should lie: directing public effort primarily to areas of 'intense' malaria, and their causes, rather than to transmission *per se* and general mosquito reduction. 'If we could prevent the mortality from epidemic fulminant malaria,' Christophers argued at Simla, 'we should have removed the most urgent and distressing effects of this disease and those manifestations which the people themselves are most impressed by.'[11] Redefinition of the 'malaria problem' required convincing leading sanitary and medical officials as to the soundness of the assessment of the malaria problem as primarily economic, and of the government's commitment to institutional malaria research; to policies of malaria mortality – and famine – control; and to expansion of quinine access to those most at risk, the latter premised on re-establishing medical confidence in the drug's general safety. In effect, the GOI, through Christophers and colleagues, were proposing adoption of a strategy for malaria 'control' similar to that being pursued in Italy at the time through the work of Angelo Celli,[12] arguably at least as ambitious as that of abolishing the Italian latifundia.

A third stage followed in the months after the October 1909 Simla conference, a period in which the administration was coming to terms with the irresistible momentum posed by the sanitary ideal of mosquito extirpation. Reclaiming legitimacy in the sanitary realm in India, and in Britain, required some formal embracing of the anti-mosquito stance on the part of the colonial administration. Official malaria policy would now take two tracks. First, a handful of high-profile urban or industrial enclave anti-mosquito programs would be initiated, while behind the scenes the administration began to address the worst levels of epidemic and endemic destitution underlying the 'exalted' forms of the disease amongst the vast rural population through fundamental changes in famine relief (prevention) and labour law reform.

Post-World War I fiscal retrenchment ushered in the fourth stage, which would see marked reductions in malaria research funding, with research now channelled primarily to anti-malarial treatment. In terms of practical measures, epidemic control took the form of flood and drought relief efforts and surface drainage programs undertaken by the irrigation and public works departments, measures seen as anti-malarial primarily for their economic rather than entomological effects. Provincial sanitary departments (in 1922 renamed 'public health') were left with the role of quinine distribution and forecasting epidemic occurrence. Vector control activities increasingly were offloaded to industrial and plantation ('estate') interests and interested municipalities or left to off-shore institutions as 'demonstration projects' undertaken by the Rockefeller Foundation and Ross Institute in selected tea plantations.

This four-stage malaria policy trajectory is not readily evident in the medical and administrative annals of the period, no doubt due to imperial sensitivities with escalating political tensions and resistance to colonial rule. But it can be traced indirectly in the scientific research and administrative deliberations recorded in the published reports and

Indian scientific journals of the period. This trajectory is essential to investigating the determinants of post-1920 epidemic decline, providing an exceptional vantage point for tracing the fundamental shifts taking place at this time in both economic theory and imperial governance as well as in modern medical thought.

Underlying the tactical manoeuvring in early 20th century malaria policy formation were the findings of the Mian Mir and Duars reports, presented at the 1909 Bombay Medical Congress. Because of their central role in colonial malaria policy, and the relative invisibility of the Duars report, in particular, within contemporary malaria historiography, these two Congress papers are considered here in some detail. First, however, we turn briefly to consider pre-1908 malaria policy, and the larger challenges the colonial regime faced at the turn of the century in struggling to retain some semblance of political legitimacy in the sanitary and economic spheres.

Pre-1908 colonial malaria policy

Through much of the 19th century, the British colonial administration paid little attention to malaria as it affected the general population of the subcontinent. Historically, malarial fever in Britain and much of Europe had long been associated with stagnant water and poor drainage, and viewed as resulting in 'air tainted by injurious emanations from decomposing animal or vegetable matter.'[13] The miasmic theory, applied to India, was considered to fit generally with the manifest association of malarial fever with the annual monsoon rains, with the notable exception that malarial fever was not limited to marshes or low-lying tracts but endemic across much of the South Asian plains. With little possibility of draining the vast rural tracts of the subcontinent, the scope for preventing autumnal fevers was deemed limited, and little action was undertaken.

For the British Raj, this *laissez-faire* stance amounted to simple pragmatism. Although malaria was a cause of considerable seasonal sickness in the military, measures of control within the army and European administration based on quinine and residential segregation were straightforward, relatively inexpensive, and logistically feasible independent of the general (native) population. In the immediate aftermath of the 1857 Indian Rebellion – with memories still fresh of autumnal malaria having compromised East India Company military efficiency – the new imperial government had moved quickly to ensure adequate local supplies of quinine for British Indian troops, establishing the first cinchona plantations in the Nilgiri Hills in the Madras Presidency in

1860. Over subsequent decades, limited quantities of quinine began to be supplied to urban medical departments as well, but non-military distribution otherwise remained largely restricted to government employees and estate managerial staff.[14] To the extent that malaria merited attention from the later 19th-century colonial administration, it did so as an incidental cost or economic hindrance in industrial or plantation labour camps and in railway construction through certain highly malarious tracts such as those along the Bengal-Nagpur line. Elsewhere, malaria was overshadowed by attention to those epidemic diseases of special strategic military and trade concern to the British imperial administration: cholera and, by the turn of the 20th century, plague.[15]

In Punjab, however, one notable exception was realignment of the Western Jumna Canal. Constructed in the 14th century Mughal period, the canal cut across natural drainage lines in the southeastern region of the province and had led to extensive waterlogging in Karnal district northwest of Delhi. Malaria concerns had arisen initially in the 1840s regarding the 'salubrity' of the military cantonment located in the region. This had prompted an investigation that included a spleen survey of the surrounding rural population, the first recorded use in the colonial records of spleen enlargement as a measure of malarial fever prevalence.[16] Of wider interest, the Baker-Dempster report documented the association between the infertile waterlogged tracts and intense malaria amongst the 'the poor ill-fed,' and recommended realignment of the canal explicitly as a malaria control measure,[17] work ultimately completed in the 1880s.[18]

With delegation of administrative powers to municipal councils beginning in the 1870s, attention shifted to urban drainage measures. Renewed interest in rural drainage occurred under the Dufferin vice-regal administration in the later 1880s, and surveys of local drainage conditions were undertaken in Punjab. Few resources ultimately were allocated however, and accounts of such work, both urban and rural, disappeared from the annual sanitary reports in the later 1890s.[19]

This picture of relative neglect changed dramatically with Ross's confirmation of the role of mosquitoes as vector in malaria transmission in 1897–1898.[20] Overnight, the odium associated with a disease seen by European colonialists as a sign of 'oriental backwardness' shifted to the shoulders of the British Raj itself. Malaria, 'a disease of waste land, waste water and waste men,'[21] was fast becoming a sign of imperial neglect. Malaria, Harrison notes, was 'one of the most important signifiers in the moral and medical topography of the Indian subcontinent . . . symbolis[ing] the wild, unconquerable and hence "uncivilised" spaces of British India.' By the late nineteenth century 'this rhetoric was turned on its head by Indian critics of the British regime.'[22]

Within the administration itself, concern over malaria was fuelled by growing recognition of the economic cost of rail disruption associated with epidemics such as that in 1908.[23] But by this point, pressure for government action was coming from another direction as well. In the wake of the 1857 Mutiny, the ensuing Royal Commission of Inquiry into sanitary conditions in the British Indian army had recommended the new imperial government establish a system of vital registration as a means of monitoring general epidemic conditions across the entire territory, rural as well as urban, a policy initiated in the mid-1860s. The disease of central concern to imperial trade interests at this point was cholera.[24] But the monthly mortality data recorded all deaths, and within a decade, the annual sanitary reports were providing graphic evidence of the far greater impact of scarcity (famine-level foodgrain prices) on death rates across the subcontinent and the enormous and recurring role played by malaria in mortality tolls of the later 19th-century Indian famines.[25] More damning still, the entire toll of 'fever' deaths was now coming under scrutiny as malarial and laid at the feet of the government sanitary establishment as preventable, only one-quarter or less of which were actual malaria deaths.[26]

Meanwhile in Europe, response to Ross's 1897–1898 vector findings was even more immediate: British commercial trade interests founded the Liverpool School of Tropical Diseases in 1898. The following year, the Royal Society established a special Malaria Committee, and deputed three medical scientists, C.W. Daniels, J.W. Stephens, and a 26-year-old Rickard Christophers, to investigate malaria transmission and blackwater fever in British Central Africa (Blantyre, Malawi), the Gold Coast (Ghana), and Lagos.

Blackwater fever was a syndrome seen in areas of extremely intense falciparum malaria transmission. The acute pathological process was poorly understood but was associated with limited acquired immunity and with repeated and often irregular quinine use. Derived initially from Peruvian cinchona bark, quinine had been recognised by European powers by the mid-19th century as an effective anti-malarial drug. Subsequent global expansion of its cultivation had transformed European imperial access to malarious regions where extremely intense ('holoendemic') transmission prevailed such as in much of West Africa. With increased use of the drug in the later 19th century, however, blackwater fever, once considered a rare side effect, had become in some areas of West Africa as frequent a cause of death among non-immune colonials as malaria itself.[27]

By the turn of the 20th century, concern was rising as well over the growing incidence of the syndrome among the managerial staff in the hyperendemic malarial conditions on the plantations of northeastern India. In 1900, Stephens and Christophers would be reassigned to India to investigate blackwater fever in the Duars tea plantations of northern Bengal, with the two investigators soon reporting an incidence even greater than that observed in West Africa.[28] Concern over blackwater fever soon led the Royal Society to investigate the possibility of controlling malaria transmission itself, based on the new entomological understanding of vector transmission.

Mian Mir

Within a year, the Royal Society's Malaria Committee initiated an experimental mosquito control program at the rural military cantonment at Mian Mir in the Lahore district of Punjab province, its purpose to assess the feasibility of interrupting malaria transmission in a specific locale employing anti-mosquito and anti-larval brigades. Much has been written about Mian Mir in the annals of colonial malaria historiography, and the intense public controversy generated between Ronald Ross, then a lecturer at the Liverpool School, and senior colonial sanitary officials in India over the unsuccessful outcome of malaria control efforts at the rural cantonment.[29] Ross would attribute the failure to technical incompetence and government disinterest.[30] And subsequently the trial would come to be viewed as a 'premature' and 'misguided' effort that set back malaria control activities in South Asia for the remainder of the colonial period.[31] The intraprofessional acrimony generated in the trial's wake unfortunately has tended to overshadow many of the epidemiological insights gained, and their importance in understanding subsequent malaria policy in India. Hence, it remains an important starting point for interpreting the region's malaria mortality history under British rule.

Mian Mir was a major British military cantonment in the strategic northwest of the Indian subcontinent four miles outside Lahore. The region was typical of much of the Punjab alluvial plains. With 18.1 inches of annual rainfall, the agricultural economy was highly dependent on inundation and canal irrigation, the latter developed from the early years of the colonial period. Well known for intense seasonal malarial fever, the cantonment was selected for the malaria control trial in consultation with Ross as a co-member of the Royal Society

Malaria Committee;[32] the chances of success at this site were assumed to be greater relative to regions with higher rainfall.

Anti-malaria operations aimed to reduce anopheline breeding sites by clearing and straightening irrigation channels in and around the cantonment, draining pools of standing water, filling depressions, oiling of ponds, and so on – work carried out by 'mosquito brigades.' Ross saw the project as a practical demonstration of the new, and presumed less costly, method of malaria control through localised anti-mosquito operations, compared with earlier large-scale drainage operations, the 'method of the ancients,' such as realignment of the West Jumna canal undertaken in the 1880s.[33] However, those directly involved in the work saw the project in experimental terms as an investigation into the feasibility of replicating the 'minor-works' model on a larger, public health scale.

Preliminary survey work conducted by J.W.W. Stephens and Christophers in October 1901 under the auspices of the Royal Society had shown *An. culicifacies* to be the main, likely sole, vector of malaria in the area, and irrigation channels as prolific sources of this anopheline species.[34] In April 1902, the Government of India then took over the project under the direction of S.P. James, a senior officer in the Indian Medical Service. Intensive anti-larval operations were undertaken in a four-square mile area of the cantonment, a decision based on earlier survey work that suggested a half-mile flight range for the vector.[35] Fifty coolie labourers cleared undergrowth from the irrigation ditches and another four were permanently assigned to 'mosquito brigade' work in and around the military barracks and local bazaar. Anti-mosquito work was supplemented by quinine administered to all military and administrative personnel, and in subsequent years to 'bazaar children' to further reduce the parasite load in the resident 'native' cantonment population.[36] In early 1903, Christophers, now a Lieutenant in the Indian Medical Service, took over control of the project for a further year of anti-larval operations.

Despite the ease with which millions of anopheline larvae could be destroyed by such measures, it was clear by the end of this second year of intensive work that malaria transmission had not significantly diminished. In the autumn months of 1903, fever rates among British and native troops were higher than the previous year. More disconcerting still, fever admission rates among troops in the section where intensive anti-mosquito operations had been undertaken remained double the rate of those elsewhere in the cantonment. Christophers surmised from these 'startling' results, as had James a year earlier, that the area of operations was insufficient, and that likely 'infiltration of adults [anopheles] from outside the area . . . could not be prevented by any means in our power.'[37] But he also had begun to contemplate that post-monsoon malaria vector breeding occurred not just in irrigation channels, but also in collections of rainwater over the expanse of the surrounding plains.

> It was found that the heavy rain filled many of the pits to over-flowing, and washed the larvae out over the land. Such larvae were then found in shallow puddles among grass and it was frequently very difficult to destroy them. Unless, then, all breeding-places were destroyed prior to a shower of rain, complete destruction of larvae could not be carried out.[38]

In their presentation to the British Medical Association annual meeting, back in Britain in July 1904, James and Christophers observed:

> It is easy enough to destroy larvae in millions and to do away with hundreds of breeding places. It by no means follows that malaria is diminished or adult *Anopheles* banished, and the success of operations *on a large scale* is still very doubtful. . . . Perhaps the most valuable result of the Mian Mir operations was that they gave an insight into the difficulties which are almost certainly to be encountered in most really malarious places. . . . [T]he difficulty of keeping up with the ever-changing situation of breeding places under different degrees of rainfall was very great. We found that . . . local destruction was utterly futile.[39]

In the face of these disappointing results, a senior military medical officer was asked to review the 'causes of failure.' E.P. Sewell, a captain in the Royal Army Medical Corps, concluded that though anti-mosquito operations had been 'in the right direction,' they needed to be applied on a far larger geographic scale, and in conjunction with 'the entire abolition of the irrigation systems and the clearing off of all watered crops in the cantonment, and around it for the distance of at least one mile.'[40] Not surprisingly, the Government of India was unwilling to take on this much more 'radical' approach, not only because of the enormous recurring expense entailed, but also due to the added long-term economic losses associated with the elimination of irrigation and the district's agricultural base. The trial project, in other words, was manifestly no longer one with broad applicability. Christophers would be reassigned to assume the directorship of the King Institute of Preventive Medicine in Madras, on special duty to investigate kala azar, and the formal status of the Mian Mir experiment as a special GOI investigation came to a close.

This would hardly be the last word on Mian Mir, however. Interest in the project in Britain had grown sufficiently by this point to have merited an entire section of the 1904 British Medical Association (BMA) annual meeting, where papers presented by James, Christophers, and Stephens detailed results of the work at the cantonment.[41] Ross, also invited, did not attend personally. In an article published a month earlier in the *Journal of Tropical Medicine*, Ross had attributed the Mian Mir 'failure' to 'defective . . . organisation.'[42] In a paper submitted in advance to the BMA meet, he again criticised the competency of the work undertaken at Mian Mir, dismissing the troop hospitalisation data as 'almost worthless'[43] and urging continuation of the operations under more rigorous scientific direction.

Had there been the opportunity to discuss Ross's criticisms in person, many aspects of the Mian Mir controversy might have been resolved at the 1904 meeting itself. As it was, the charges contained in Ross's submission remained unexamined, and the debate was left with Ross's resolute assertion, based on efforts at Ismailia,[44] that

> [t]he logical basis of the great measure of mosquito reduction is absolute. There is no doubt whatever that in any locality we can reduce mosquitos [*sic*] to any percentage we please, provided that we arrest their propagation to a sufficient degree and within a sufficient radius. . . . [I]f local authorities wish to clear the malaria in a large town or cantonment they must be prepared to spend money on the work, just as they would for a new water supply or sewerage system. The example of Ismailia is always before them. The road leads straight forward.[45]

Yet Ross's 'example of Ismailia' was hardly an apt model for comparison with Mian Mir.[46] Ismailia was a model town built in the 1870s by the Suez Canal Company in the Sinai desert, a region with less than two inches of annual rainfall, sandy rather than impervious soil, and where malaria transmission was minimal with only three or four severe cases since 1877 and no deaths. It was unclear, moreover, what anti-larval work had contributed to the project's success relative to that of quinine.[47]

Nevertheless, the publicity which the conference had attracted in Britain, heightened by Ross's 1902 Nobel laureate prominence, made it difficult for the colonial government to be seen as entirely abandoning the Mian Mir project. It would neither fund radical mosquito reduction operations at Mian Mir in subsequent years, but nor would it interfere. Preoccupied with plague, and with senior military figures eager to continue with vector extirpation, the project was now left entirely under military funding and direction. In 1905, the entire irrigation system within a 12-kilometre area of the cantonment was filled in, and expanded anti-larval operations extended for a further four years.

In the autumn of 1908, the limitations of even these measures would be dramatically confirmed. The whole of Lahore district was swept up in the vast regional epidemic of 1908, and with it the Mian Mir cantonment as well. James, returning in October of that year, would find, mid-epidemic, few mosquito breeding sites but anopheles 'exceedingly numerous' and near-universal rates of infection among the stationed troops.[48] This, despite 10 grains of quinine provided twice weekly for the previous three years to all troops and their families and to the children of the village market. The 1908 epidemic reaffirmed the importance of rainfall in enabling seasonal transmission in the province and thus raised fundamental questions regarding the feasibility of vector control as a general approach to rural malaria control in the region. Thus, Mian Mir threw the logistics of rural anti-larval operations into question well beyond Punjab. At the very least, much more research was required at local levels. But the experience also triggered sobering reflection with regard to where vector eradication advocacy was leading sanitary thinking. The cantonment had been reduced to its former near-desert condition, prompting the acting Sanitary Commissioner with the GOI, C.J. Bamber, to openly ponder in a 1908 memorandum the '[a]bsurd prospect' of sacrificing food supply in the name of public health. 'We cannot ask people to starve, so that they may not suffer from malaria.'[49]

In retrospect, it is easy to see how the attention of military sanitation officers in these early years had come to focus on irrigation. From the beginning of the Mian Mir project, irrigation channels had been identified as a major, nearly year-round, site for *An. culicifacies* larvae.[50] In his 1904 report, it appears Christophers still considered this species was breeding primarily in irrigation canals, and that it was only *An. rossii* (later renamed as *An. subpictus*, the second of the two main anopheline species found in the region) that flourished in the surface waters brought with the monsoon rains, a species already recognised as one that did not transmit malaria.[51] Moreover, a link between irrigation and fever had long been recognised: troop fever admission rates at the cantonment, for example, had doubled following opening of the Bari Doab canal nearby in 1868, due in part perhaps to its effect in extending the active transmission season beyond the immediate post-monsoon period. So it was an easy step to direct anti-larval work to clearing, oiling, and ultimately eliminating these channels.

In the course of his investigation of the 1908 epidemic, earlier conjectures regarding the entomological importance of surface water led Christophers to conclude that *An. culicifacies* bred also in 'temporary . . . shallow accumulations of rain water.'[52] The importance of the monsoon rainwaters as a vector breeding site was also the only interpretation consistent with observed epidemiological patterns: namely, simultaneous and near-universal post-monsoon malarial fever across large expanses of the province in epidemic years irrespective of proximity to irrigation canals or river inundation tracts. In effect, the monsoon rains potentially converted the plains into an almost unbounded *An. culicifacies* breeding surface.[53] It was the coincident increase in atmospheric humidity associated with such surface water collections, however, that by extending vector lifespan was key to effective *transmission*. In other words, abolishing irrigation channels may have reduced malaria transmission and fever admissions during the dry, non-monsoon portion of the year. But it could do little for seasonal post-monsoon transmission.[54]

Given the enormous expectations, it was perhaps inevitable that Mian Mir would come to be seen as a failure. Yet as James observed in his February 1909 paper at the Bombay Congress, it was so only to the extent that it confirmed there was no ready technique for interrupting malaria transmission in the vast rural tracts of Punjab and indeed the subcontinent. The seven years' work had, in fact, brought many 'extremely important' insights into malaria transmission and the larger dimensions of the malaria problem. And, it was precisely because there was no ready technique for vector extirpation that the experience ultimately would force the colonial government to face, and to address to some substantive degree, the larger dimensions to the malaria 'problem,' dimensions already evident in Punjab in the autumn months of 1908 and on the Duars tea estates. Moreover, conditions of human destitution were influencing not only mortality from the disease, but they were also contributing directly, the 1909 Christophers-Bentley Bombay presentation contended, to malaria transmission levels as well. The 'path,' in other words, was not simply 'straight forward.'

Imperial legitimacy and malaria control post-Mian Mir

Mian Mir laid the basis for subsequent malaria control policy in several ways. In addition to highlighting the generally prohibitive recurring costs of anti-larval measures, it demonstrated the importance of distinguishing policies feasible for the largely rural population from those appropriate for urban or small industrial or plantation ('enclave') populations. But Mian Mir also left quinine, by default, as the sole publicly visible measure upon which the colonial government could base a malaria policy: in terms of public 'optics,' amounting to 'business as usual.' Thus, in the public sphere, it brought only increasing frustration and acrimonious dispute, for it was clear also by this time that quinine had its own limitations, and access to it remained woefully inadequate. At the same time, Ross remained a vocal, long-distance critic of the malaria work undertaken in India, his prominent advocacy for abolishing canal irrigation at Mian Mir touching upon the even more sensitive question of the 'malariogenic' impacts of rail, road, and canal construction on surface drainage. With canal irrigation a pre-eminent guarantor of fiscal security as a source of growth in tax and irrigation revenues for the British Raj, the implications extended far beyond the domain of sanitary policy.

Moreover, malaria was not the only epidemic disease, at this point, with which the Government of India had to contend. Already it was reeling from intense criticism and alarm, both international and domestic, over the 1896 outbreak of plague in the subcontinent, an epidemic that had followed grain and cotton export routes through Punjab and the Bombay Presidency.[55] Increasingly, global commercialisation of the Indian subcontinent's foodgrain production was seen to be associated with major late 19th-century famines. Now, to the imperial debit sheet was added plague mortality, also linked to the grain-export economy. Plague had pushed the colonial government in 1904 to set up and fund a small network of laboratory services in India. The epidemic nonetheless continued to rage, claiming 10 million lives across the first three decades of the 20th century, with Punjab as its epicentre.[56]

The relationship between colonial attention to malaria and to plague at this time is open to interesting conjecture on a number of levels. In the year preceding the 1908 malaria epidemic, plague mortality in Punjab had reached the catastrophic peak level of over 600,000 deaths. Fear of plague may well have deterred many in Punjab from resort to famine relief 'test' works through the severe drought of 1907–1908, thereby precluding declaration of famine and initiation of relief measures.[57] Moreover, by this time it was clear that the British Raj had few effective plague control measures to offer, and continued to face extreme opposition to the measures initially attempted to control the epidemic.[58] As it became apparent that plague mortality was affecting primarily the poor, government policy shifted to one of letting the epizootic run its course.[59] Then in 1907, confirmation of the rat flea as plague vector led to a policy of rat 'extirpation,' a politically visible and acceptable 'sanitary' policy response, if one unlikely to substantially hasten elimination of the disease. By contrast, for malaria, the government post-Mian Mir could offer no comparable 'vector sanitation' program.

In the summer of 1908, an outbreak of malarial fever amongst Bombay dock labourers debilitated much of the crew on an outgoing P. & O. vessel and malaria would be added to the list of epidemic diseases haunting British Indian shipping lines.[60] Within weeks, the Bombay dock outbreak was followed in September and October by the paralysing epidemic in Punjab. By late 1908, the administration was facing a crisis of 'sanitary' legitimacy of imperial proportions, one that was rapidly spreading to the popular press.

Yet the crisis facing the British Raj by this point was limited neither to epidemic disease, nor international *cordons sanitaires*. These were years also of escalating political unrest. Labour riots had broken out in the textile factories of Bombay earlier in the year over 'scandal[ous]' working conditions.[61] In Punjab, deeply unpopular, top-down agricultural policies in the canal colonies had triggered rioting and virtual rebellion, leading to the imposition of even tighter press censorship.[62] Across the subcontinent the growing nationalist movement was critical of recurring famines, taxation policies, and 'unBritish' rule, popular discontent taking expression ultimately in an assassination attempt on the Viceroy in Ahmedabad in November 1909. Mohandas K. Gandhi was just an emerging political figure in South Africa in 1908, returning to India only in 1915, but a hint of the powerful resistance to come was already foreshadowed with his first *satyagraha* jailing to protest pass laws in January of that year.[63] To this explosive mix would be added yet another famine. Severe drought in 1907 in the northwest had triggered frank famine conditions in the United Provinces within the year, with much of the mortality toll expressed, typically, in soaring malaria deaths in the autumn months of 1908 with return of the rains. But the epidemic, and scarcity prices preceding it, had extended further west into neighbouring Punjab province, sweeping across the heart of rebellion country – in a province ostensibly the breadbasket, economic development showcase, and principal military recruitment grounds, of the British Indian empire.

Thus, if epidemic conditions at Mian Mir in 1908 had inversely vindicated James and Christophers's conclusions with respect to the difficulties of anti-mosquito operations there, the fact of the wider malaria epidemic across the province that claimed 300,000 lives in Punjab in three brief months would hardly bring the government respite. With the GOI still reeling from the devastating famine of 1899–1900, the larger public message from the 1908 epidemic was a transparent reminder of the deadly impact of foodgrain prices and hunger (scarcity), one that could only further ratchet up criticism of colonial governance in the economic realm.

Meanwhile, medical concern with the malaria toll in India was growing in Britain as well, most trenchantly in the pages of the *Journal of Tropical Medicine and Hygiene*, the medical journal of the newly established London School of Tropical Medicine. G.M. Giles, a prominent retired IMS researcher and entomologist, had described the malaria control policy of the Indian Government as 'one of masterly inactivity,' with the colonial 'bureaucracy' viewing Ross's appeals for vector eradication as 'an unmitigated nuisance.'[64] Adding fuel to the 'sanitary bugbear' fire,[65] Ross in July of 1908 published his proposed plan for mosquito extirpation in Mauritius, a report in which he confidently predicted successful malaria control in the plantation estates on the island based on anti-larval methods. Reviewed in the British medical press, the book was immediately lauded as 'a striking illustration of the application of modern methods to the scientific investigation of tropical medicine.' 'Professor Ross recommends the organizing of "moustiquiers,"' the *Lancet* review noted, and urged that 'no expense should be spared' in following the encouraging example Ross had set.[66] The contrast between the optimism of the mosquito-extirpationist Ross – Nobel laureate and public 'man of action' hero – and the seeming 'defeatism' of Mian Mir was too stark to be missed by even a politically preoccupied colonial administration.

Then came the October 1908 Punjab epidemic. By this point, the medical community in Britain was attuned to the malaria toll in the subcontinent – if not to its underlying economic dimensions. As the former health officer of Calcutta, W.J. Simpson -- editor and co-founder of the *Journal of Tropical Medicine and Hygiene* -- had been a prominent critic of the British Raj's plague control policies and of the government's failure to exploit the potential of medical research. In a scathing December 15, 1908, editorial he attributed malaria's toll in part to 'the lethargy of the Government of India, or its absolute unwillingness to utilize recent advances of medical knowledge,' and derided the proposed Punjab inquiry by a single investigator (Christophers) as amounting to 'cheap' public relations. That 'the land where Ross worked out the problem of malaria is still far behind the rest of the world in taking advantage of his discovery,' the editorial lamented, was the classic example of 'the proverbial lack of home appreciation for prophets.'[67]

In the absence of a coherently articulated malaria policy, the government had left itself fully open to the charge. The need to decipher and deal with the factors underlying the malaria 'death storms' of Punjab was inescapably urgent. Nájera observes that the pressure on the British Indian colonial regime to emulate the U.S. anti-malaria campaign in the Panama Canal zone was such that the term 'God-Sakers' had been coined to describe officials desperate to appease mosquito-extirpation advocates who urged 'for God's sake let us do something.'[68]

Quinine and blackwater fever

It is in this context that the dilemma posed by blackwater fever takes on its larger implications. Concern over the syndrome had not gone away since Christophers's and Stephens's initial Duars investigation in 1901. That study had found the syndrome to be limited to a small number of areas where malaria was peculiarly intense, primarily the northeastern tea plantations.[69] This had done little, however, to allay medical or public concern, with a September 1907 letter to the *Indian Medical Gazette*, warning that 'the matter has reached the columns of the lay press . . . adding to the difficulties already experienced by the unfortunate medical man in malarial countries.'[70] Thus, quinine as the government's primary response to the malaria problem was already under serious shadow well before the 1908 epidemic, and with it any semblance of an overall control strategy. To make matters worse, it recently had become apparent that quinine was ineffective against gametocytes, the sexual form of the malaria parasite, and thus unable to interrupt the chain of transmission.[71]

In early 1908, Christophers was deputed back to the Duars. This time, in addition to a detailed account of the incidence of blackwater fever among the managerial staff, published in the prestigious *Scientific Memoirs* series as an official report,[72] the inquiry included an in-depth investigation of labour conditions on the tea estates, undertaken in collaboration with Bentley. This latter portion of the study, *Malaria in the Duars*, was left unpublished, however, until its appearance as a one-off document in 1911.[73]

The Duars was a hill tract of the eastern Himalayas wrested from Bhutan in 1865, and subsequently making up much of Jalpaiguri district of the Bengal Presidency. Situated between Nepal and the Darjeeling tea plantations on the west, and Assam to the east, the region encompassed approximately 100 labour camps that were considered notoriously unhealthy, the seat of malaria 'in its . . . most perni-cious form.'[74] This intensity was related in part to the anopheline vector primarily responsible for malaria transmission in the region, *An. minimus*, a highly anthropophilic species (feeding preferentially on humans)[75] in contrast to the zoophilic species, *An. culicifacies*, in much of the plains.[76] The two investigators concluded, however, that the 'peculiar'[77] pathogenicity of malaria observed on the Duars labour lines could not be explained primarily in entomological terms. Villages adjacent to the tea estates, where transmission conditions were similar, or even more favourable with widespread rice culti-vation, did not exhibit the same fever lethality.[78] Marked intensity of malarial infection appeared to stem instead from an inability of the plantation labour populations to throw off infection, a situation that kept rates of re-infection extremely high. This state of persistent parasitemia they termed 'residual infection,'[79] and concluded that widespread '[p]hysiological misery' underlay the phenomenon.[80] Physical hardship broke down immunity, leading to a vicious cycle of 'continuous infestation' amongst the labour population, constant re-infection spilling over secondarily to managerial staff.[81] Repeated and irregular quinine use by staff triggered, in turn, episodic haemo-lytic crises (blackwater fever).

Labour 'camp conditions,' Christophers and Bentley concluded, 'play into the hand of malaria more than any others known to us.'[82] Wage levels below famine relief levels were insufficient to meet mini-mum energy requirement,[83] leaving nothing for periods of illness and incapacity. One-third of labourers, they judged, were too morbidly ill to be capable of any work. The complete absence of vital registration made estimating mortality rates difficult, but among the several labour lines of new recruits studied, they estimated that 12 per cent of adults died annually. Over the course of the six-month study period, 43 per cent of infants had died. In other lines, they observed an 'almost com-plete absence of children, . . . every child dying within a year or two of its birth.'[84]

Extreme mortality levels necessitated constant immigration, new recruits often with limited acquired immunity thus adding 'fresh fuel upon an already glowing fire.' But non-immunity, they concluded, was a consequence of the morbid cycle rather than its principal cause.[85] Arriving destitute, often as famine migrants, and highly indebted, the newly arrived immigrant labourer was exposed to continuous malaria infection at a time 'when all his resources [were] necessary to enable him to combat malaria successfully.'[86] The 'hostile' conditions faced coming on to the estates dramatically conspired against recovery and acclimatisation to the malaria endemically present.

> [O]ften originally possessed of poor physique and little stamina, living under conditions of depression, privation, and hardship pushed to their extreme, it is obvious that these form a soil far more suitable for the continued existence of malaria, *and the problem therefore becomes an entirely different one.*[87]

Concluding that 'anti-larval operations offer no hope of even partial success,' the report advised 'adoption of active measures to ascertain all malign influences affecting the new coolie in his new home, and the taking of steps to combat these and to ensure the general prosperity and comfort of the new coolies.'[88]

What was being documented in the pages of *Malaria in the Duars* was a condition of endemic semi-starvation – a state where life expectancy was so low that the population was in continual decline, save for mass in-migration. Had vital registration data been available, they likely would have shown annual death rates approaching levels associated with some of the most severe epidemic malaria years in Punjab. In effect, 'normal' mortality levels in the labour camps were at what might be considered a state of continuous or endemic famine: what the investigators themselves termed 'a permanent condition of epidemic malaria.'[89] And the underlying driver of the vicious cycle, they concluded, was the recruitment system. Though not formally 'indentured' labourers as in Assam, Duars recruits were effectively owned, through debt bondage, by the recruiting agents *(sardars)*, who in practice held full penal powers over them, with no State oversight.[90]

Labour conditions under the *sardari* system of the Duars, the investigators observed, resembled 'very closely [those under] the class of "*caporali*" described and condemned by Celli in his account of malaria among the labourers in the Roman Campagna.'[91] According to Celli, improvement in malarial conditions following drainage of a country was not due primarily to entomological changes in malaria transmission but 'largely secondary in nature and bound up to a great extent with the permanent settling of populations and other conditions favourably affecting the human host.'[92]

'Tropical aggregation of labour'

The larger significance of the Duars inquiry, then, lay in linking the 'exalted malaria endemicity' on the Duars estates to labour conditions more broadly across South Asia. Up to this point, European colonial observers had interpreted the intense malaria seen in tropical labour camps in miasmatic terms: the release of damp vapours (miasma) associated with 'opening up of the soil.' 'So long as the soil remains undisturbed, agues and the severe forms of fever are comparatively rare,' Patrick Manson observed, 'but so soon as building, roadmaking, and other operations implying soil disturbance commence, then severe malarial fevers appear.'[93] With identification of mosquitoes as malaria vector, sanitary attention turned correspondingly to anopheles breeding sites on construction sites:[94] in particular, excavations ('borrow-pits') formed where large quantities of soil were removed in the process of creating rail, road, and canal embankments. But here, too, a purely entomological view of the malaria problem was 'quite an inadequate conception of the true state of affairs,' the authors of the Duars malaria report argued.

> It is not the soil disturbance . . . but the occurrence of labour camp conditions, or what we shall call for convenience of description THE TROPICAL AGGREGATION OF LABOUR in association with these enterprises which has given them their evil reputation. . . . [It] is not solely, or even mainly, the result of special facilities for the breeding of anopheles, or of the existence of a particular species but on the contrary is bound up in what we shall call the 'human factor'. . . . [W]e have, then, to deal not alone with the formation of borrow-pits and the interference with surface drainage, but with a peculiar set of conditions mainly associated with the human host . . . which it is impossible to dismiss without serious thought if we wish to understand the natural history of great outbreaks of malaria.[95]

Christophers and Bentley went on to challenge much of the recent malariology literature where economic dimensions had been disregarded in interpreting epidemic conditions, beginning with the infamous 'Burdwan fever' in lower Bengal.[96] From the mid- and later 19th century, 'exalted' malarial fever had appeared in much of the once 'salubrious' western Burdwan division, associated with construction of rail, road, and canal embankments north and west of Calcutta, and with it, large temporary labour camps. Subsequent analysis by Bentley, as Bengal Sanitary Commissioner, would show that economic immiseration was not limited to the labour population and immediate period of construction, but extended to the rural population, triggered by obstruction of the naturally occurring deltaic inundation patterns by railway infrastructure embankments.[97] Agricultural productivity in the now 'dying' river tracts declined rapidly, and as in the Duars, endemic semi-starvation was reflected in an endemically 'exalted' form of malaria lethality, 'destroy[ing] an estimated two million people.'[98]

Punjab does not appear explicitly in the Duars inquiry's survey of 'malariogenic' labour conditions in British India, much of the inquiry investigation having preceded the 1908 epidemic. But Christophers, in his Simla malaria conference presentation the following year, pointedly identified levels of destitution among the Kashmiri weaver community as underlying the severe malaria epidemic in Amritsar city in 1881.[99] Though the most notorious excesses of the indentured labour system took place in the northeastern tea plantations, the system was applied variously across the subcontinent, a 'spectacular increase' in penal contracts occurring in Punjab after 1904, attributable to increased canal construction and subsequent building of New Delhi.[100] Contrary to Gandhi's idealisations, Anderson suggests, labour 'conditions in small-scale production were often worse than in larger undertakings, and frequently assumed the character of semi-slavery.'[101]

The 1909 Duars report extended their 'The Human Factor' analysis to malaria conditions beyond India as well, openly questioning Ross's recent interpretation of the 1866–1867 Mauritius malaria epidemic as caused by the introduction of *An. gambiae* to the island at this time.[102] They pointed instead to severe drought conditions on the island and coincident famine in India leading to increased transport of indentured labourers to the island's sugar plantations. The Mauritius epidemic was 'a typical example[of tropical aggregation of labour,' they suggested.[103] Even more controversial perhaps, the Duars report challenged prevailing views of malaria control in the Panama Canal zone, at the time lauded as the pre-eminent mosquito-extirpation triumph. Malaria control measures were not limited to anti-mosquito measures, they pointed out. Citing an 'abstract' from the canal project's administrative records, they suggested a key ingredient to success under U.S. Army Colonel Gorgas – in addition to unlimited quinine – lay in a well-fed labour force: workers were 'compelled to eat' through provision of cooked food, the cost of which was deducted from their wages, an arrangement adopted expressly to limit labourers remitting earnings back to families and skimping on their own nourishment. 'This abstract is quoted,' they added, 'because we wish to make it absolutely clear that the question of alimentation cannot be neglected if malaria is to be dealt with.'[104]

Christophers and Bentley's 1909 Duars report thus was challenging an entire body of recent malaria literature where interpretation of malaria conditions, among labour camps and elsewhere, had increasingly been reduced to microbiologic explanations that overlooked predisposing economic determinants. In effect, the report was countering, in nascent form, the emerging reading of malaria *per se* as a 'block to development,'[105] and countering the views of many of the most prominent malaria scientists in the process. These were conclusions that could not but have had official imprimatur. In the case of the Duars tea estates, they offered support for challenging private tea company operators who continued to oppose changes to the 1859 indentured labour act. It was evident by this point that, even with vast supplies of cheap labour thrown up by the subcontinent with each recurring famine,[106] an unregulated plantation recruitment system was too inefficient, and bore too large added costs in the form of blackwater fever amongst managerial staff and larger imperial interests, to continue to ignore.

But the Duars study can also be seen as a way of countering the growing tendency among medical scientists to interpret malaria epidemicity exclusively in microbiologic terms of malaria transmission, a stance that was fuelling public expectations of mosquito control programs. It seems likely that only the highest echelons of the government and sanitary administration would have had access to the actual contents of the *Malaria in the Duars* report. However, by early 1909 in the wake of the 1908 Punjab epidemic, there was little option but to place its core economic conclusions on view for senior medical and sanitary officers for there to be any prospect of redeeming medical confidence in its malaria policies and in quinine safety. To achieve this, of course, it was essential first to convince them of the human destitution determinants underlying blackwater fever prevalence in the Duars. And second, to convey that the State was committed to remedying at some level the destitution that underlay malaria's fulminant form. Precisely how the British Raj manoeuvred across this diplomatic and political mine-field offers a fascinating story, one that begins with the release of the conclusions of the Duars study in the form of a paper, delivered by Christophers and Bentley at the February 1909 Medical Congress in Bombay.

Notes

1 S. Watts, 'British Development Policies and Malaria in India 1897-c.1929,' *Past and Present*, 165, 1999, 141–181; I. Klein, 'Development and Death: Reinterpreting Malaria, Economics and Ecology in British India,' *IESHR*, 38, 2, 2001, 147–179.

2 M. Harrison, '"Hot Beds of Disease": Malaria and Civilization in Nineteenth-Century British India,' *Parassitologia*, 40, 1–2, June 1998,

11–18 at 17; W. Bynum, 'Malaria in Inter-War British India,' *Parassitologia*, 42, 1–2, June 2000, 25–31, at 31.

3 *Report of the Commissioners Appointed to Inquire into the Sanitary State of the Army in India, PP*, Vol. I (London: HMSO, 1863).

4 *Proceedings of the Imperial Malaria Conference held at Simla in October 1909* (Simla: Government Central Branch Press, 1910) [hereafter Simla Conf.].

5 S.P. James, 'Malaria in Mian Mir,' in W.E. Jennings, ed., *Transactions of the Bombay Medical Congress* (Bombay: Bennett, Coleman & Co., 1910), 84–93, at 87 [hereafter *Trans. Bombay Congress*].

6 Ibid., 87; R. Nathan, H.B. Thornhill, L. Rogers, *Report on the Measures Taken Against Malaria in the Lahore (Mian Mir) Cantonment* (Calcutta: Government Printing, 1910), 37.

7 S.R. Christophers, C.A. Bentley, 'The Human Factor: An Extension of our Knowledge regarding the Epidemiology of Malarial Disease,' in Jennings, ed., *Trans. Bombay Congress*, 78–83 [hereafter 'The Human Factor'].

8 S.R. Christophers, 'On Malaria in the Punjab'; Simla Conf., 29–47.

9 William Bynum provides an important overview of much of this research in 'Malaria in inter-war British India.'

10 R. Ross, 'On some Peculiar Pigmented Cells Found in Two Mosquitos Fed on Malarial Blood,' *British Medical Journal*, Dec. 18, 1897, 1786–1788.

11 Simla Conf., 43; A. Celli, 'The Restriction of Malaria in Italy,' in *Transactions of the Fifteenth International Congress on Hygiene and Demography, Washington, September 23–28, 1912* (Washington, DC, 1913), 516–531.

12 Simla Conf., 44.

13 Ibid., 2.

14 See ch. 9.

15 R. Ramasubban, *Public Health and Medical Research in India: Their Origins under the Impact of British Colonial Policy*, SAREC report R4 (Stockholm: SIDA, 1982); __, 'Imperial health in British India, 1857–1900,' in R. Macleod, M. Lewis, eds., *Disease, Medicine and Empire* (London: Routledge, 1988), 38–60; D. Arnold, 'Crisis and Contradiction in India's Public Health History,' 335–355 at 339–340, in D. Porter, *The History of Public Health and the Modern State* (Amsterdam: Rodopi, 1994).

16 W.E. Baker, T.E. Dempster, H. Yule, *Report of a Committee assembled to report on the causes of the unhealthiness which has existed at Kurnaul,* (1847), in Collected Memoranda on the Subject of Malaria, *RMSI*, 1, 2, Mar. 1930, 1–68; T.E. Dempster, 'Notes on the Application of the Test of Organic Disease of the Spleen as an Easy and Certain Method of Detecting Malarious Localities in Hot Climates (1848),' *RMSI*, 1, 2, Mar. 1930, 69–85.

17 Dempster, 'Notes on . . . disease of the spleen,' 55.

18 G. Macdonald, J. Abdul Majid, 'Report on an Intensive Malaria Survey in the Karnal District, Punjab,' *RMSI*, 2, 3, Sept. 1931, 423–477, at 426.

19 Christophers noted that '[t]o fill in a small fraction of the . . . great depressions around the city of Amritsar. . . (197 acres) took 8 years (1884–1892) and cost Rs 2,56,568'; MP, 133.

20 For an account of Ronald Ross's identification of the malaria parasite in the anopheline mosquito vector and preceding contributions of other scientists to the elucidation of the complex life cycle of the malaria parasite, see G. Harrison, *Mosquitoes, Malaria and Man: A History of the Hostilities Since 1880* (New York: E. P. Dutton, 1978).

21 V. Venkat Rao, 'Review of Malaria Control in India,' *IJM*, 3, 4, Dec. 313–326, at 322. In Jan. 1908, the *Indian Medical Gazette* devoted four pages to an anonymous review of W.H.S. Jones's, *Malaria, a Neglected Factor in the History of Greece and Rome* (Cambridge: Macmillan & Bowes, 1907), published the year before with an introduction by Ronald Ross; anon., 'Malaria and Empire Decay,' *IMG*, Jan. 1908, 23–26.

22 Harrison, 'Hot Beds of Disease,' 11.

23 Simla Conf., 66; MP, 18.

24 M. Harrison, *Public Health in British India: Anglo-Indian Preventive Medicine 1859–1914* (Cambridge: Cambridge University Press, 1994), 61.

25 *Report of the Sanitary Commissioner for Madras for 1877* (Madras: Government Central Branch Press, 1878).

26 Simla Conf., 14–15.

27 Blackwater fever, Stephens and Christophers concluded, is 'pre-eminently the cause of death among Europeans in tropical Africa . . . a preventable and avoidable disease,' quinine deemed the 'proximate cause'; 'Blackwater Fever: Summary and Conclusions,' *RMCRS*, 5, 1901, 12–27.

28 Four cases of blackwater fever were reported within a fortnight on the Duars estates, a number 'never encountered by us either in British Central Africa or West Africa'; J.W.W. Stephens, S.R. Christophers, 'The Occurrence of Blackwater Fever in India,' *RMCRS*, 8, 1902, 3–13, at 7.

29 Bynum gives a comprehensive account of the initial organisation, findings, and personality dynamics of those involved in the Mian Mir trial; W. Bynum, 'An Experiment that Failed: Malaria Control at Mian Mir,' *Parassitologia*, 36, 1–2, 1994, 107–120, at 109.

30 R. Ross, 'The Anti-Malarial Experiment at Mian Mir,' *Journal of Tropical Medicine*, vii, Aug. 15, 1904, 255 [hereafter JTM].

31 M. Watson, 'The Lesson of Mian Mir,' *Journal of Tropical Medicine and Hygiene*, July 1, 1931, 183–189, at 185 [hereafter *JTMH*]; D. Bradley, 'Watson, Swellengrebel and Species Sanitation: Environmental and Ecological Aspects,' *Parassitologia*, 36, 1–2, 1994, 137–147, at 139, 142.

32 Bynum, 'An Experiment that Failed,' 109–110.

33 James, 'Malaria in Mian Mir,' 85; R. Ross, *Mosquito Brigades and How to Organize them* (London: George Philip and Son, 1902).

34 Among 259 dissections of *An. culicifacies*, Stephens and Christophers had found 11 positive for malaria parasites but none in *An. rossii* (later renamed *An. subpictus*); J.W.W. Stephens, S.R. Christophers, 'Relation Between 'Species' of Anopheles and the Endemicity of Malaria,' in *Transactions of the Malaria Conference Held at Nagpur in January* (Nagpur: Central Jail Press, 1902), 85–88, at 86; S.P. James, 'Malaria in India,' *Sci. Mem. Off. Med. Sanit. Dep.*, 2, 1902, 78.

35 Stephens and Christophers, 'Relation Between 'Species' of Anopheles and Endemicity,' 33.

36 S.P. James, 'First Report on the Anti-Malaria Operations in Mian Mir, 1901–1903,' *Sci. Mem. Med. Sanit. Dep.*, 6, 1903.

37 '[D]estruction of larvae was enormous. A single oiling of a canal . . . must have destroyed millions, since it was not unusual to remove fifty or more specimens in a single dip of the dipping can. In the pits also, . . . larvae were often so abundant as to the give the appearance of a scum'; S.R. Christophers, 'Second Report of the Anti-Malarial Operations in Mian Mir, 1901–1903,' *Sci. Mem. Med. Sanit. Dep.*, 9, 1904, 16, 19–21, 5.

38 Christophers, 'Second Report of the Anti-Malarial Operations in Mian Mir,' 11.

39 S.P. James, S.R. Christophers, 'The Success of Mosquito Destruction Operations,' in 'Discussion on the Prophylaxis of Malaria,' Annual meeting of the British Medical Association, Oxford, July 26–29, 1904. Section of Tropical Diseases, Sept. 17, 1904, *British Medical Journal*, ii, 629–642, at 631–632.

40 E.P. Sewell, 'The Results of the Campaign Against Malaria in Mian Mir,' *British Medical Journal*, Sept. 1904, 635–636.

41 James and Christophers, 'The Success of Mosquito Destruction Operations'; J.W.W. Stephens, 'Discussion on the Prophylaxis of Malaria,' *British Medical Journal*, Sept. 2904, 629–631.

42 R. Ross, 'The Anti-Malarial Experiment at Mian Mir,' *British Medical Journal, ii*, 1904, 632–635. See note 30, above.

43 Ross's critique was based largely on the format of Christophers's 1904 report (no date, table of contents, index, nor map of surrounding country) and insufficient funding. Criticism of anti-mosquito methods related to frequency and area of oiling surface water pools, Christophers choosing intervals of 12 days, a decision based on observed larval development, and limited to a half-mile radius; 'The Anti-Malarial Experiment at Mian Mir,' 633–635.

44 R. Ross, 'The Extirpation of *Culex* at Ismailia,' *British Medical Journal*, July 18, 1903, 173.

45 Ross, 'The Anti-Malaria Experiment at Mian Mir,' 635.

46 'At Ismailia the . . . operations of the mosquito brigade were very largely devoted to treating cesspits which were the breeding grounds of *Stegomyia*, a process which of course could not affect malaria one way or another'; Stephens, 'Discussion on the Prophylaxis of Malaria.' Other anti-mosquito projects undertaken by Ross, in Freetown, Sierra Leone in 1899 and 1902, had private funding withdrawn for lack of success; C.M. Poser, G.W. Bruyn, *An Illustrated History of Malaria* (New York: Parthenon Publishing Group, 1999), 142.

47 Nathan et al., *Report on the Measures Taken Against Malaria,*' 6–7.

48 James found 7 out of 10 troops infected in late Oct. 1908; 'Malaria in Mian Mir,' 87.

49 C.J. Bamber, (Offg. Sanitary Commissioner with the GOI), 'Collected Memoranda on the Subject of Malaria,' 1908; reprinted in *RMSI*, 1, 2, Mar. 1930, 86–87.

50 W.W. Stephens, S.R. Christophers, 'An Investigation into the Factors Which Determine Malarial Endemicity,' *RMCRS*, 7th series, Aug. 15, 1902, 23–45, at 38.

51 Christophers, 'Second report,' 3. From the attention Christophers directed in his 1904 report to the difficulty of detecting *An. culicifacies*, it appears

he was considering surface rainwater as a possible breeding site. 'In the case of *A. culicifacies* . . . [t]his species is extremely careful to secrete itself, and . . . it may very easily be considered absent when in reality it is abundant'; ibid., 17.

52 MP, 83–84.

53 This conclusion appears in a subsequent paper; S.R. Christophers, 'A Revision of the Nomenclature of Indian Anophelini,' *IJMR*, 3, 2, 1916, 454–488, at 463; T. Ramachandra Rao, *Anophelines of India*, 1st ed. (New Delhi: Malaria Research Centre, ICMR, 1984), 397–398.

54 Within senior military echelons, a focus on irrigation channels continued, with Sewell offering a highly convoluted argument to explain what Bynum has referred to as 'the vexed question of why malaria incidence so closely followed rainfall levels'; 'Anti-Malarial Operations at Mian Mir,' *Journal of the Royal Army Medical Corps*, 5, 1905, 132–134; Bynum, 'An Experiment that Failed,' 113. Elsewhere in India, without the distinctively flood-prone soils and physiography of Punjab, the role of irrigation-induced waterlogging in enabling transmission may have been more important; P.F. Russell, 'Malaria Due to Defective and Untidy Irrigation,' *JMII*, 1, 4, 1938, 339–349.

55 Hirst suggested a 'far more important seasonal factor in the spread of plague [was] the *effect of agricultural operations* [emphasis in original], the ripening of crops and their movement after harvest' through the now dense network of rural grain depots; L. Fabian Hirst, *The Conquest of Plague: A Study of the Evolution of Epidemiology* (Oxford: Clarendon Press, 1953), at 264, In Punjab, Mar.–May plague seasonality corresponded to both conducive climatic conditions and the *rabi* harvest and transport of wheat through storage 'go-downs.'

56 In Punjab, the cumulative plague death toll between 1897 and 1918 reached 122.3 per mille (2,992,166 deaths); in Bombay, 87.4; UP, 49.5; Madras, 3.45; and Bengal, 1.49; *GOI-SCR* 1918, 66, 68. Punjab plague deaths across this decade exceeded those from malaria, and occurred largely among adults.

57 Provincial officials noted 'the problem of the supply of labour [had] become even more acute than formerly owing to the ravages of plague and to general economic conditions such as the rise in prices'; *PLRA* 1907–1908, 10.

58 I. Catanach, 'Plague and the Tensions of Empire, 1896–1918,' in D. Arnold, ed., *Imperial Medicine and Indigenous Societies* (Manchester: Manchester University Press, 1988), 149–171; Harrison, *Public Health in British India*, 117–138; B. Pati, M. Harrison, *Health, Medicine and Empire: Perspectives on Colonial India* (London: Sangam Books 2001), 18; I. Klein, 'Plague, Policy and Popular Unrest in British India,' *Modern Asian Studies*, 22, 4, 1988, 723–755 [hereafter *MAS*].

59 R. Chandravarkar, 'Plague Panic and Epidemic Politics in India, 1896–1914,' in T. Ranger, P. Slack, eds., *Epidemics and Ideas* (Cambridge: Cambridge University Press, 1992), 203–240.

60 C.A. Bentley, *Report of an Investigation into the Causes of Malaria in Bombay* (Bombay: Miscellaneous Official Publications, 1911), 55. See also, M. Ramanna, 'A Mixed Record: Malaria Control in Bombay

Presidency, 1900–1935,' in Deepak Kumar, Raj Sekhar Basu, eds., *Medical Encounters in British India* (New Delhi: Oxford University Press, 2013), 208–231, at 212.

61 Lovat Fraser, *India Under Curzon and After* (Bombay: Times of India, 1911), 331–335.

62 N. Gerald Barrier, 'The Punjab Disturbances of 1907: The Response of the British Government in India to Agrarian Unrest,' *MAS*, 1, 4, 1967, 353–383; ———, *Banned: Controversial Literature and Political Control in British India, 1907–1947* (New Delhi: Manohar, 1976).

63 Fraser, *India Under Curzon*, 28–29.

64 G.M. Giles 'Cold Weather Notes on Mosquitoes from the United Provinces, India,' *JTM*, May 16, 1904, 149–152, at 151–152.

65 Giles, 'Cold Weather Notes,' 151.

66 R. Ross, *The Prevention of Malaria in Mauritius* (London: Waterlow, 1908); Leader, 'The Story of Malaria in Mauritius,' *Lancet*, Mar. 27, 1909, 926–928.

67 Editorial, 'The Epidemic of Malaria in India,' *JTMH*, Dec. 15, 1908, 377–379, at 378.

68 *Report of the Civil Medical Service from 1911 to 1918*, 1920 (English Summary). Mededeelingen van den Burgerlijken Geneeskundigen Dienst in Nederlandsch-Indie, as cited in J.A. Nájera, 'Malaria Control: Achievements, Problems and Strategies,' *Parassitologia*, 43, 1–2, 1–89, 2001, 26.

69 Blackwater fever was reported less frequently also in the Jeypore hills and Western ghats, both areas with highly anthropophilic vectors. In the Punjab plains, the syndrome was considered 'excessively rare – even if it occurs at all'; C.A. Gill, 'Epidemic or Fulminant Malaria Together with a Preliminary Study of the Part Played by Immunity in Malaria,' *IJMR*, 2, 1, July 1914, 268–314, at 305.

70 W.A. Murray, 'The Etiology of Black-water Fever,' *IMG*, Sept. 1907, 353–354.

71 Simla Conf., 9.

72 S.R. Christophers, C.A. Bentley, 'Black-Water Fever: Being the First Report to the Advisory Committee Appointed by the Government of India to Conduct an Enquiry Regarding Black-Water and Other Fevers Prevalent in the Duars,' *Sci. Mem. Med. Sanit. Dep.*, 35, 1908 [hereafter BWF].

73 S.R. Christophers, C.A. Bentley, *Malaria in the Duars: Being the Second Report to the Advisory Committee Appointed by the Government of India to Conduct an Enquiry Regarding Blackwater and Other Fevers Prevalent in the Duars* (Simla: Government Monotype Press, 1911) [hereafter MD].

74 *MD*, 22. Following the 1833 abolition of slavery in Britain, alternate means of labour control in the empire entailed 'indenturing' workers. The1859 Indian Workman's Breach of Contract Act XIII was modelled on British master-servant labour legislation where the penal contract (indenture) committed labourers to a number of years' labour on threat of criminal prosecution, imprisonment and/or punishment (flogging), but differed in offering no protection whatever for Douglas Hay, Paul Craven eds., *Masters, Servants and Magistrates in Britain and the Empire, 1562–1955* (Chapel Hill/London: University of North Carolina Press, 2004), 432. For further discussion see also E. Kolsky, 'One Scale of Justice for the Planter and Another for the Coolie': Law and Violence on the Assam Tea Plantations,' in *Colonial Justice in British India* (New York: Cambridge University Press,2010), 142–185.

75 T. Ramachandra Rao, *The Anophelines of India* (New Delhi: Malaria Research Centre, ICMR, 1984); J. Nandi et al., 'Anthropophily of Anophelines in Duars of West Bengal and other regions of India,' *Journal of Communicable Disease*, 32, 2, 2000, 95–99.
76 BWF, 29; Stephens and Christophers, 'Blackwater Fever: Summary,' 20.
77 *MD*, 1.
78 Ibid., 62.
79 Ibid., 5; BWF, 29.
80 *MD*, 5.
81 BWF, 29; *MD*, 8.
82 BWF, 22.
83 *MD*, 48–49, 53.
84 Ibid., 77, 24. See also, R.P. Behal, P. Mohapatra, 'Tea and Money Versus Human Life: The Rise and Fall of the Indenture System in the Assam Tea Plantations 1840–1908,' *Journal of Peasant Studies*, 19, 3/4, 1992, 142–172, at 160–161.
85 *MD*, 3–5.
86 Ibid., 49, 90.
87 Ibid., 5 [emphasis added].
88 Ibid., 90, 80.
89 Ibid., 26 [emphasis added]. See note 46.
90 Ibid., 88. '[I]n the Duars the regulations applying to Assam have never been enforced, and the recruitment of labour under the "voluntary" or "*sadari*" system . . . which, since it entails no legal binding of the coolie, is generally considered as not necessitating measures for his protection'; ibid., 42–43.
91 Ibid., 48, 4.
92 Ibid., 19.
93 P. Manson, *Tropical Diseases: A Manual of the Diseases of Warm Climates* (London: Cassell and Co., 1898), 98.
94 *MD*, 13–14.
95 Ibid., 9, 1–2 [emphasis added].
96 Ibid., 12–19.
97 C.A. Bentley, 'Some Economic Aspects of Bengal Malaria,' *IMG*, Sept. 1922, 321–326; __, *Malaria and Agriculture in Bengal* (Calcutta: Government of Bengal, 1925).
98 *MD*, 13.
99 Simla Conf., 38–39.
100 Anderson, 'Illusion of Free Labour.'
101 Ibid., 434.
102 R. Ross, *Report on the Prevention of Malaria in Mauritius* (London: Churchill, 1909), 49.
103 *MD*, 12, 14. Christophers continued to question Ross's entomological explanation of the 1867 Mauritius epidemic, suggesting it was 'probable that the conditions in Mauritius, sometimes ascribed to introduction of *A. gambiae* from the African continent, were really due to large-scale importation of labour from India which occurred about this time'; 'Endemic and Epidemic Prevalence,' in M.F. Boyd, ed., *Malariology* (Philadelphia: W.B. Saunders Co. 1949), 698–721, at 715. For similar critique of environmental determinism, see H.F.G. Floate, 'The Mauritian Malaria Epidemic 1866–1868: Geographical Determinism one Hundred Years Ago,' *Journal of Tropical Geography*, 29, 1969, 10–20.

104 *MD*, 56–57.
105 P.J. Brown, 'Malaria, *Miseria*, and Underpopulation in Sardinia: The "Malaria Blocks Development" Cultural Model,' *Medical Anthropology*, 17, 1997, 239–254.
106 P. Mohapatra, 'Coolies and Colliers: A Study of the Agrarian Context of Labour Migration from Chotanagpur, 1881–1920,' *Studies in History*, 1, 2, n.s., 1985, 247–299, at 266–269.

8 The 'Human Factor' articulated

The 1909 Bombay Medical Congress

Even before word of the autumn 1908 malaria epidemic in Punjab had reached senior officials, it was certain that malaria would figure prominently at the Bombay Medical Congress in February 1909. Moreover, if the implications of the Mian Mir trial were to be successfully grappled with, the colonial government's most internationally prominent malaria policy adversary could hardly be excluded from the Bombay proceedings – though it was clear there was little prospect of bringing Ronald Ross on side after the personal acrimony on display at the 1904 British Medical Association meet.[1]

Up to this point, Ross had largely avoided open debate, offering criticism of malaria policy in India from the distance of prepared statements, or in publications. Quite possibly the Government of India came to see the Bombay Congress as an opportunity for senior sanitary officials to hear the actual content of Ross's criticism, and to contend with the larger policy questions it left unaddressed. Still, it was no small gamble: the need to be frank about the economic dimensions to the malaria problem balanced against the risks of public notoriety associated with the same. It was a gambit that would preoccupy the administration for the next three years, a period of intense diplomatic juggling as the British Raj struggled to regain control of the sanitary and larger imperial agenda.

Four major malaria papers were presented at the Congress: one by Ross offering a general account of his malaria control theory and anti-mosquito brigade organisation; the second, a report by S.P. James on epidemic conditions in Mian Mir in October 1908 in the context of the previous vector extirpation operations at the cantonment; and two papers by Christophers and Bentley: one a purely technical account of the physiology of blackwater fever, and the second, their paper entitled

'The Human Factor: An Extension of our Knowledge Regarding the Epidemiology of Malarial Disease' which summarised the broader economic insights from the Duars investigation and their implications for understanding malaria lethality elsewhere in the subcontinent.

In his presentation, Ross outlined his mathematical 'theorems' explaining the priority of anti-larval operations ('small works') in malaria control strategy: '[m]alaria must decline if mosquito numbers are reduced below a critical level. . . [and] nearby breeding places are [the] most dangerous ones.' Major works (requiring an engineer), he conceded, might be necessary in some circumstances, but their cost was often prohibitive; thus, it was best to begin with 'the cheapest' measure, 'mosquito brigades,' a detailed account of which followed. He concluded by urging immediate action. The basic facts were known:

> there is no reason to hold up mosquito reduction until . . . researches are complete . . . we may assume that one of the local Anophelines is the culprit, and the method of dealing with all are broadly similar.[2]

This was a position that the seven years of effort at Mian Mir had shown to be scientifically, and practically speaking, unwarranted in the northern plains of the Indian subcontinent. The results at Mian Mir, James concluded in his own presentation, were 'as unequivocal as [they were] disappointing': intensive anti-mosquito operations had 'proved ineffective' in breaking the chain of autumn malaria transmission despite 'reconverting the Cantonment into the arid desert which it was fifty years ago.'[3] The two papers were a universe apart.

Ross in his own presentation had avoided any reference to Mian Mir, or indeed even to India, citing instead anti-mosquito work at Ismailia, the Panama Canal, Federated Malay States, and Ceylon, all illustrations of enclave anti-malaria operations with ample funding and quinine.[4] Thus, missing also was acknowledgement of the central distinction between policy appropriate for limited enclave areas, and policy appropriate for whole populations. In discussion that followed, Christophers questioned Ross's embrace of 'all methods,' which, left at a general level, skirted practical constraints and the need for policy prioritising.

> Attention being so much confined to anti-larval operations had hindered in India a proper amount of attention being given to quinine . . . . The Italians who had conditions to deal with like those

in India, *ie.* a population mainly rural, had practically abandoned anti-larval operations in favour of quinine prophylaxis.[5]

Christophers and Bentley's paper on 'The Human Factor' in malaria[6] distilled the findings of the as-yet unpublished *Malaria in the Duars* report. Graphic accounts of labourers' wages, the labour recruitment system, household illness, and starvation were omitted, but the central economic insights were lifted almost in their entirety. Blackwater fever amongst the managerial population on the Duars plantations was at root a product of the larger morbid process of pervasive destitution and 'residual infection' amongst much of the labour population. It was not a problem that mosquito extirpation could solve.[7] Solutions lay instead in the realm of addressing the 'physiological misery' among the labour lines. 'Hardship, exposure, bad housing, poor and insufficient food supply. . . [and] overcrowding of dwellings,' the paper urged, 'all require attention.'[8]

As in their *Duars* report, the focus of the paper was on destitution associated with labour conditions well beyond the northeastern tea plantations: 'conditions that in our experience are practically always associated with the existence of malaria in its most intense form.'[9] The vicious cycle of residual infection and 'exalted' malarial transmission, they argued, meant that 'an immunity that may protect under ordinary conditions is broken down under exposure to more virulent and intense malaria . . . so that even those originally the strongest and most healthy become involved also.'[10] It meant, as well, the insufficiency of policy directed primarily to mosquito extirpation.

These were conclusions which in the anti-vector enthusiasm of the day bordered on the heretical. Here, it was probably only Christophers's scientific stature at this point that allowed a non-entomological explanation to be heard and convincingly argued, with a level of frankness in a public document that also reflected just how politically vulnerable the government viewed itself in the final days of 1908. And once again, the two investigators concluded by pointing to the Italian experience: Celli's observation that 'improvement' in malarial conditions 'following such [drainage "bonification"] works must often be largely secondary and bound up to a great extent with the *permanent settling of populations* and other favourable conditions affecting the human host.'[11]

The prominence accorded the economic interpretation of the malaria problem in India presented at the Bombay Congress did not necessarily mean abandonment of anti-mosquito measures altogether. Here, the government was quick to depute Bentley to investigate malaria in

Bombay city that same year, a study that recommended highly specific anti-larval measures alongside improved dock-worker labour conditions.[12] But the feasibility and appropriateness of mosquito extirpation in a given area could not be assumed, it had to be tested. What was being urged was a more pragmatic approach to malaria control: a channelling of limited resources to areas worst affected by malaria mortality, and a shift to mitigation of these worst effects. It was a prescription also for much more research into local conditions, research which at the same time encompassed 'the widest possible view. . . . Each district of India is probably a problem requiring study in itself: a study whose object is not in one sense scientific research but simply the getting of information absolutely necessary to action.'[13] The malaria problem in India, they urged, went beyond mosquitoes alone.

Lead-up to Simla

Did the strategy of hunger-disclosure work? It is interesting to ponder how Bombay conference delegates came to terms with the disparate views of the malaria problem presented by Ross and by Christophers and Bentley. Not surprisingly, ensuing discussion was left unrecorded in the published proceedings, an account of the conference in the *Indian Medical Gazette* later describing the session as having generated 'a considerable amount of heat and even personal warmth.'[14] More significantly, the *IMG* report quoted extensively from the 'Human Factor' paper, including explicit reference to 'starvation.' As for quinine, however, no hint of the blackwater fever controversy surfaced either in the proceedings themselves, or in the *IMG* report. And in the days that followed, blackwater fever as a 'dreaded' public health concern would largely drop out of sight from the Indian malaria literature.

This suggests that the Bombay Congress did succeed in bringing onside, or into line, the higher echelons of the Indian Medical Service with respect to the underlying economic dimensions to the blackwater fever problem in India. But the question remained, how to convince those members of the sanitary and medical establishments, already committed to the vector control paradigm, as to the wisdom of a policy directed primarily to malaria mortality – much less the medical establishment in Britain where public acknowledgement of hunger was as politically problematic for the British Raj as in India. Even with medical confidence in quinine reclaimed, 'quinine prophylaxis' hardly presented the semblance of a galvanizingly new 'malaria control' strategy. Clearly, there was need for a much more substantial display of imperial engagement and intent. Before the ink was dry from the February 1909 Congress proceedings, a follow-up conference devoted exclusively to malaria policy had been set for the following October, under the aegis of the viceregal office itself.

In the intervening months, acrimonious debate would play out however in the pages of the leading British medical journals. Declaring James's Mian Mir conclusions as 'groundless,' Ross called for an 'impartial inquiry' into 'the fiasco.'[15] The *Journal of Tropical Medicine and Hygiene* followed with an editorial denouncing 'the fallacies of [James'] Jeremiad on anti-mosquito work,' claiming Mian Mir was a 'pronounced success' based on 'diminution of malaria' in the years preceding the 1908 epidemic, and defending abolition of irrigation as 'well worth the sacrifice of a few peas and cabbages.'[16]

To this, the GOI responded in the form of a letter to the editor of the *Lancet* penned by Christophers and James in late June 1909, simultaneously published in the *Indian Medical Gazette*, explaining their emphasis on reducing malaria mortality rather than on mosquito extirpation.[17] The question facing public health officials in India was not primarily one of technique, they argued, but rather where and for what part of the population malaria government control efforts were to be undertaken. Should the State, they asked, 'restrict itself to the mitigation of the disease in the large cities. . . [and] cantonments, or ought it seriously to attempt to reduce mortality in the villages [where] the vast majority of the population of India live?'

> [D]emonstrations of success in anti-larval operations cease to be of value when their cost is such as to prohibit their general employment in India. . . . Unless the State then is prepared to leave rural India altogether out of account, it must turn its attention and its chief expenditure in systematically endeavouring to extend the benefits of quinine.[18]

This was not an argument against anti-mosquito measures *per se*, as Bentley's Bombay city malaria inquiry, then in progress, would show, but rather, one of priorities. 'India as a whole is not intensely malarious,' Christophers and James pointed out. '[T]here are wide tracts of country where the disease, though present, is not markedly interfering with the prosperity and natural increase of the population.' '[A]ttention should be first concentrated,' they urged, where the disease is 'acting as a pestilence.'[19] To that end, access to quinine had to be vastly expanded. No serious attention, they averred, had been given to making quinine widely available – the number of pice packets of quinine sold annually, James had pointed out at Bombay, was less than the number of vaccinations performed each year[20] – though it was the only strategy capable of reaching a significant portion (*viz.* rural) of the population.

Yet in this much more public forum of the *Lancet*, Christophers and James only obliquely referred to economic dimensions to malaria lethality revealed at Bombay:

> We need not here describe the events and conditions that are concerned in causing epidemics of malaria . . . nor need we mention other examples in which recent work has revealed what are the really important factors concerned. It suffices if we emphasize the fact that the prevalence of anopheles, though always important, is by no means in every case the most important factor to be considered.[21]

Those 'really important factors' would remain unenunciated, the 'Human Factor' paper cited quietly and unadorned in a small-font footnote at the close of the paper.

In effect, Christophers and James were battling the medical opinion battle with one arm tied behind their backs: arguing the case for addressing malaria mortality, but without the political manoeuvring room to explain the key factor they saw as determining much of that mortality. Instead, the Italian experience once again would be called up as proxy. '[I]n Italy, anti-larval operations have been abandoned,' they pointed out, 'in favour of measures . . . in *practical malaria sanitation* (especially in that dealing with agrarian conditions) . . . reforms [which have been] carried on with such excellent results.'

> It is not without due reason that Professor Celli lays such stress on legislative amendment of agrarian laws and so on, that he emphasises the fact that in the Roman Campagna malaria is not a result of want of drainage, and that it is one of the diseases to be surveyed from the outlook which will give the widest possible view if we ever hope to control it.[22]

Here, finally, was a concrete glimpse, if from the vantage point of another continent, of the other measures in addition to quinine that the Indian researchers were advocating.

Undeterred, Ross would counter again, this time intimating wilful sabotage of the Mian Mir project by Christophers. Appended to his letter was a note by a Colonel Forman of the Bombay Brigade who charged that James and Christophers were

> guilty of a very grave scientific crime in thus unwarrantably attacking proven prophylactic measures. . . . [I]t is certain that with the prevalent procrastination of the East, the [sanitary] awakening which we had fondly hoped was at hand, will now be indefinitely postponed.[23]

Thus, the Simla conference would convene in a cloud of public controversy.

The imperial malaria conference at Simla, October 1909

Though generally recognised as forming the cornerstone of all subsequent malaria policy of the British colonial government in India, the Imperial malaria conference held at Simla in October 1909 has attracted surprisingly limited historiographic attention. Where cited, the empirical content of Christophers's presentation on epidemic malaria in Punjab – analysis that framed the proceedings – has received arguably even less attention despite the epistemic questions raised. Among medical historians, William Bynum has most clearly recognised the scientific and historical importance of the extensive malaria research literature from the South Asian colonial period and concludes that 'Christophers emerges as the most sophisticated of the Indian malariologists of the period, especially in his attempts to understand the wider features of the disease.'[24] Yet these 'wider features' remain unexplored and at times misread. Sheldon Watts's analysis of early 20th-century colonial malaria policy highlights the importance of the Simla conference, but interprets it as 'a campaign to disprove and deny that irrigation was an important causal factor in [the] creation' of the malaria problem in India, and Christophers, as a 'hoodwink[ing]' apologist thereof.[25]

Certainly, one can agree that there was much to criticise regarding the deleterious ecological effects of the vast canal irrigation network in northwest British India. But such a critique aims ironically at the wrong target: Christophers and C.A. Bentley authored the few malaria studies in these early years in which the larger economic contradictions inherent to colonial rule were precisely documented and, however diplomatically, brought to public light. Here, we turn to consider the content of the conference proceedings in some detail, recognising inevitable limitations to the transparency of an officially vetted document.

A 'predetermined agenda'

The Imperial malaria conference at Simla was convened on October 11, 1909, to fill the policy vacuum around this latest epidemic disease to be acknowledged as 'disastrously' afflicting British India.[26] That six days were allotted for the conference highlights the balancing act anticipated by the administration in bringing onside senior sanitary and Indian Medical Service officials with the conclusions of the Punjab and Duars inquiries. By this point, however, frustrations within India over malaria policy were no longer limited to advocates of anti-mosquito campaigns. Urging more circumspection and less panic, exasperated army officials were now appealing to the government 'to stem the devastating flood of recommendations. . . [for] ill-founded, half-digested schemes' of mosquito extirpation and irrigation abolition.[27] What was needed was clarity with respect to the problem, to the goals pursued, and to the effectiveness of the methods employed.[28]

But there was confusion over basic biological questions as well. Many aspects of the malaria transmission cycle had yet to be thoroughly delineated, a task of some complexity in light of the major differences in malaria epidemiology and entomology being documented from region to region. Complicating policy discussion further was the imprecision with which much of the new malarial terminology was framed and employed. The decade of renewed malaria writing had thrown up a panoply of new technical terms. Many, such as 'mitigation,' 'radical versus palliative' measures, permanent versus non-permanent works, were poorly defined, though already in common usage.[29] The term 'prophylaxis' was routinely applied to quinine, for example, both as a preventive measure (in jails and among British and Indian troops) and as curative treatment (therapeutic quinine), but with the intended meaning often unclear.[30] Other terms such as 'drainage' held multiple meanings, variously referring to surface water flows, subsoil water levels, natural inundation irrigation conditions, and so on, each bearing very different and largely unresearched implications for malaria transmission depending on local topography and methods of agricultural production.

Confusion abounded, above all, over basic epidemiological concepts fundamental to interpreting the 'burden' of malaria across the continent. By the early 20th century, most sanitary officials came to malaria deliberations with a vocabulary and conceptual framework derived from the later 19th-century British sanitary movement, one where the distinction between infection, disease, and mortality had been largely set aside. Ross's focus on mosquito reduction was addressing malaria infection (transmission); Christophers and others by this time, by contrast, recognised that the major epidemics of malaria they were being called upon to investigate were 'epidemics of death'[31] and represented quite a different form of malaria, far more intense, lethal, and epidemiologically and economically detrimental than ordinarily seen with seasonal transmission. Younger members of the Indian Medical Service would have had limited direct experience with famine, fewer still with the destitution seen in the Duars plantations, and thus little opportunity to observe the distinction between ordinary and 'exalted' malaria. This made for debate fraught with ambiguity and incomprehension, with medical and sanitary officials often speaking past each other in discussions of malaria 'control.' Many questions remained even in the realm of therapeutics regarding suitable forms of quinine and effective distribution agencies.

Thus, while the goals of the Simla conference encompassed political containment at the top of the unofficial agenda, a broad range of basic scientific goals and tasks also demanded urgent attention. As Sanitary Commissioner with the Government of India, J.T.W. Leslie's (1861–1911) role at Simla was pivotal. Responsible for initiating the first serious expansion of medical laboratories and research facilities in India five years earlier, Leslie's scientific and administrative credentials were impeccable.[32] Paramount among scientific priorities was the need for establishing the size of the malaria problem as a public health (mortality) issue in varying regions of the subcontinent.

Among political goals, that of restoring medical confidence in the safety of quinine appears to have been achieved already in the wake of the February 1909 Bombay Congress. The other side of the containment strategy, however, still remained: that of convincing medical delegates of the limits to mosquito extirpation, and the primacy of addressing the 'fulminant' form of malaria. Regaining political and fiscal control thus also meant convincing all parties of the central role of destitution in its epidemiology, and of the government's commitment to addressing the economic conditions giving rise to it.[33] Little surprise, then, that the malaria conference convened at Simla in October 1909 took an 'imperial' format with proceedings officially opened by the Viceroy, presided over by the Home Secretary, with senior officials of the British India army, Indian Medical Service, the Central Research Institute, Civil Hospitals, and medical colleges in attendance, and several 'native Indian' representatives added on.

Nestled in the Punjab Himalayan foothills, Simla was the summer seat of the colonial government, a setting conducive to imperial persuasion through the week-long meet.[34] Much undoubtedly went unrecorded. What discussion did find its way into the 107 pages of official published proceedings, nevertheless, offers more than a glimpse into the internal political challenges, and contradictions, of an imperial power in concerted effort to contain political crisis.

From the outset, the conference tone was one of some candour. In his opening address, the Viceroy pronounced malaria to be 'a problem of Imperial Magnitude,' one exacting a 'dismal' toll across the country estimated at 1,130,000 malaria deaths annually, one-quarter of all recorded fever deaths, doubling in number in epidemic years, a 'death-roll' acknowledged as largely preventable.[35] This was followed with the announcement of the commissioning of a permanent Malaria Bureau within the Central Research Institute at Kasauli, a hill station near Simla. The Bureau's role was three-fold: ongoing epidemiological, entomological, and biomedical malaria research; training and assisting counterpart provincial malaria committees; and the convening of annual conferences for dissemination of research findings and field experience. Here, the government was appropriating the seemingly activist stance of the extirpationists, but framing policy in a tone of conciliation towards the warring sides of the malaria control debate. Ronald Ross would be included as an advisory member to the Scientific Advisory Board of the Malaria Bureau,[36] his appointment no doubt intended to soften the absence of an invitation to the conference.

In the lead-up to the conference, Ross had conveyed that he viewed his exclusion as a personal slight. Yet arguably there were few scientific reasons to include him. Having retired from the Indian Medical Service in 1899, Ross had had no practical malaria control experience in India, and at Bombay eight months earlier had declined to address the key public health policy issues raised by the seven years' vector control experience at Mian Mir.[37] An even more serious consideration for the government was political, Ross having already forfeited the confidence of the crown by stoking public concerns of a possible 'quinine conspiracy.'[38]

Yet if physically absent from the Simla conference, Ross's mosquito extirpation views permeated the deliberations, with a number of delegates openly sympathetic to his advocacy of general anti-mosquito campaigns. Among them was J.A. Turner, the highly respected Bombay Medical Officer of Health, already pursuing energetic efforts of municipal mosquito control. Another was William King, former

Sanitary Commissioner for the Madras Presidency, for whom the recently established King Institute of Preventive Medicine in Madras had been named. King was an ardent 'drainage' advocate, and in the days that followed he would continue to criticise the calibre of anti-mosquito operations at the Mian Mir trial in the pages of the *Journal of Tropical Medicine and Hygiene*, published from the newly established London School of Tropical Medicine. For both men, and other local sanitary officials, limiting government malaria control action largely to areas of 'intense' malaria mortality was not what they had set their sights upon. If an image of serious intent were to prevail, Ross and supporters could not be dismissed out of hand. Containment of advocacy for mosquito extirpation as a general approach to malaria control would have to come by other means.

With the delegates cloistered at Simla, the weight of viceregal officialdom no doubt lent persuasive pressure. But the GOI also based its hopes, it appears, on the ability to persuade through clarity of analysis. In his opening remarks, Leslie had set the stage, framing the central question for the conference: what determines the epidemic form of malaria 'when the disease becomes not only much more common, but enormously more fatal than in ordinary years.'[39] He would go on openly to incriminate human destitution as underlying that transformation, graphically describing 'people who lead a hand to mouth existence.'

> [I]ll-housed, ill-clad and ill-fed, they pick up a precarious livelihood . . . have unsuitable food at the best of times; and they have no savings, so that when anything occurs to check the demand for such work as they can do, the scanty coarse food becomes scantier and coarser and they and those dependent on them offer little resistance to malarial infection and readily succumb to its effects.[40]

Contrasting prisoner and general population death rates, he acknowledged that

> if we could place all the people in fairly good hygienic conditions, give them prophylactic dosage of quinine during the fever season and provide them with suitable food and skilled attendance when they are attacked, we should prevent three-fourths of the deaths.[41]

Acknowledgement that 1 million fever deaths a year in British India were 'preventable' was an extraordinary admission under any circumstances. Here it was offered no doubt as a sign of the administration's confidence in Christophers's conclusions with respect to larger economic factors underlying the phenomenon of 'exalted' malaria, the latter's presentation framing the conference proceedings. Ross was entirely correct to have suggested a pre-determined agenda.

'On Malaria in the Punjab'

Christophers prefaced his 22-page presentation with an account of his use of *thana*-level vital registration data for estimating epidemic mortality across the province.[42] Such quantitative methods, S.P. James pointed out, made it possible to identify where malaria control efforts 'are advisable, in what parts they are essential, and in what parts they are not only essential but urgent.'[43] What followed in Christophers's main presentation, 'On Malaria in the Punjab,' was a detailed account of his assessment of the relative roles of rainfall and destitution in predicting autumn mortality across the province in 1908.[44] Throughout, Christophers maintained a marked reserve in portraying the human face of destitution so delineated, deferring to Leslie for details. His focus instead was on the biological mechanisms underlying that human 'face' to epidemic lethality. It was at Simla that he first presented the results of his experimental work on intensity of malarial infection in sparrows, calling for much further investigation into 'the whole subject of endemic malaria which by supplying the gamete carriers may be an underlying cause of epidemic conditions.'[45] It was at Simla also where he implicated harvest failure ('particular areas subject to adversity') as underlying the distinctive geographical pattern of epidemic foci, pointing to differences in regional agricultural economies and, by implication, differing harvest vulnerabilities in any given rainfall year.[46] Phrased tangentially, this was, nevertheless, the core epidemiological insight of the study.

Response of conference delegates

Quite apart even from his economic conclusions, the range of questions Christophers was exploring in his Simla presentation was immense, and the technical aspects correspondingly complex. Not surprisingly, much of the content was lost on some, the acting Director-General of the Indian Medical Service, C.P. Lukis, asking 'whether [Christophers] had dealt with rural areas' at all.[47] Moreover, his detailed attention to Punjab soils and physiography could only fan expectations of engineering solutions, leaving many of the delegates unprepared for what they saw as his counsel of 'drainage' futility: that drainage could not address the *general* phenomenon of flood propensity across the region. Thus, in terms of modern anti-malarial methods, the paper appeared to offer little, the delegates' frustration was summed up by Colonel King, now Inspector-General of Civil Hospitals, Burma. 'Christophers,' he suggested,

> had treated the matter in an exceedingly scientific manner, but it was necessary to remove oneself from the glamour of his methods and to test his results from a practical point of view. Captain Christophers' paper led one to think that the question of drainage was going to have a happy ending, but in the manner of some novelists he had killed off his hero.[48]

Christophers, of course, was *implying* a great deal in terms of economic reforms. But such measures apparently were too sensitive for overt articulation and were lost on some delegates, leaving little in the way of ameliorative policies visible – except quinine.

'Bonification' in Punjab

Conference organisers appear to have anticipated this reaction. Slotted into the proceedings at this point was a very different voice, that of a former Punjab Irrigation official, L.M. Jacob, now Secretary to the Public Works Department, GOI, his testimony likely an attempt to reassert an activist image. Though not listed among official delegates, Jacob presented 'an account of remedial action taken to reduce waterlogging associated with the Western Jumna Canal,'[49] and duly reported on a 'vast' improvement in local fever conditions in the absence of specific anti-mosquito operations: a 'classic' example of beneficial drainage 'improving both the health of the people and of the soil.'[50]

The intervention appears to have succeeded. Discussion veered away from general soil drainage and mosquito extirpation, and instead to the Italian strategy of 'bonification,' where the goal was economic not entomologic.[51] But Jacob's intervention may also have been timed as a foil to the subsequent item on the agenda: reports on mosquito control work to date in India. Scheduled to speak first, King could only report that despite 'toil[ing] incessantly to promote anti-malarial measures' in both Burma and in his previous Madras Presidency posting, his results were 'undefinable.' 'I cannot to-day point to any locality,' he ultimately acknowledged, 'in which it may be said malarial fever has been absolutely extirpated.'[52] Similar results were reported for anti-mosquito efforts in the Central Provinces where systematic anti-mosquito brigade efforts had been undertaken.[53] The juxtaposition of these results with the 'vastly improved' health in the West Jumna canal realignment tracts described moments earlier by Jacob could hardly have been more stark.

Yet as beneficial as canal realignment (unblocking natural drainage) could be for specific waterlogged tracts, the practical relevance of Jacob's testimony was limited in terms of the problem Christophers had been deputed to Punjab to investigate. *Malaria in the Punjab* was an inquiry into *epidemic* conditions in 1908: analysis of the general phenomenon of regional epidemic malaria in the province, the factors that transformed endemic 'ordinary' malaria into its intense form. Though particular waterlogged tracts would often be included in epidemic foci, the problem of fulminant epidemics was not limited to areas of obstructed surface drainage, or indeed to tracts where subsoil water levels were high. At the same time, much of the flooding which so strongly predicted the worst affected tracts within an epidemic area could not be prevented. The economic hardship and malarial debility, however, could be relieved. Here, Christophers turned to urge ready access to quinine treatment and an organisational system for its rapid distribution in areas where severe epidemics threatened. But, of course, 'relief' for inundated, famished populations required food as well. And here he fleetingly, and tangentially, alluded only to other 'special ameliorative measures.'

> [W]ith a more detailed knowledge of the physical features of the country and of the *economic conditions of the people* as they related to malaria, that we could predict epidemics *with certainty and accuracy* is I think very probable. . . . [W]ith a proper organisation we [can] . . . know in which year *special ameliorative measures* were most required and could as a result bring these measures to bear from the very beginning of the epidemic with *special urgency* in areas likely to be most severely affected.[54]

These economic 'recommendations' were as unequivocal as were those for quinine. But tucked into the general text of his paper they were easy to overlook.

Quinine conundrums

Regarding quinine policy,[55] some candour also prevailed, with numerous accounts of 'failures,' and a range of serious questions still needing urgent investigation. Officials openly acknowledged the dire insufficiency of supply. Current production in India was sufficient to treat, at most, 3 million of the estimated 100 million malaria cases each year, treatment for all requiring three times the total world quinine production. Cultivation in South Asia, begun in 1861, amounted to scarcely 3 per cent of world production, the remainder mostly coming from Dutch plantations on Java. Though considered 'desirable' to increase production in India, no commitment was forthcoming.

The only option, beyond government medical institutions and dispensaries, was one of targeted distribution to priority areas of endemically intense malaria and impending epidemics. Here, Leslie reminded the administration that distribution of quinine could not be made 'self-supporting,' that the cost of quinine remained an absolute barrier to those who needed the drug the most, even where sold at the cost of production.[56] At the same time, delegates reported widespread reluctance to make use of quinine, related to side effects of nausea, diarrhoea, and ringing in the ears. What was needed was mass education, James urged, in a paper on 'Experimental [quinine] demonstration camps.'[57]

Recommendations

Through the interstices of six days' discussion, initial dismay with Christophers's analysis had given way to agreement on at least some basic 'practical measures.' 'Mosquito extirpation' would be accorded notional prominence in the two pages of formal recommendations, the phrase heading the entire section of recommendations dealing with drainage. Yet in content, most drainage recommendations, such as removing obstructions to surface water flows, had little to do with mosquito control. Specific anti-mosquito measures were limited to urban areas, and there, to methods 'not prohibitive' in cost, and only where standing water could be directly linked to malaria transmission. Prohibition of wet (rice) cultivation in the vicinity of towns was recommended, but again only where 'it is established that malaria in a town is due to anopheles mosquitoes breeding in wet cultivation in the immediate vicinity.'[58]

With regard to drainage, efforts to lower subsoil water were limited to specific 'highly malarious localities' and only where 'financially practicable.'[59] Throughout, Christophers was quietly reinforcing the need for local studies and flagging pre-conceived or unwarranted assumptions as they surfaced in discussion: noting, for example, that the notoriously malarial Punjab town of Palwal was 'splendidly drained.'[60] For Christophers, all policies needed to be based on local conditions and testing – in modern parlance, 'evidence based.'

As for quinine, no targets for government production or distribution were offered. Nor does discussion of quinine price subsidies appear in the published proceedings despite ardent pleas by several delegates for price reduction in view of charges in the lay press of a government profiteering 'conspiracy.'[61] Free distribution would be available 'only in the case of severe epidemics.'[62] Expansion of outlets for the sale of quinine beyond the existing post office system was recommended, to include distribution by local officials and 'all available agencies.' But details were few, presaging the difficulties of distribution that were to plague quinine access over the ensuing decades.

As for economic measures, not a word would appear in the list of final recommendations – though implicit in Leslie's opening remarks, in Christophers's presentation, and in repeated references to the Italian experience.[63]

Containment achieved?

Did the Simla conference succeed in shifting opinion on malaria policy away from general mosquito extirpation? As was the case for the Bombay 'Human Factor' paper, all discussion of economic dimensions following Christophers's Punjab presentation was omitted from the published Simla proceedings. One can surmise from the final recommendations that many delegates had come to accept limited, rather than open-ended, mosquito extirpation, and by extension a malaria policy directed primarily to the highly lethal forms of the disease and to the factors underlying that form of malaria. Certainly, in the years immediately following, senior Indian Medical Service and sanitary officials took seriously the role of hunger in the malaria toll across India, as we will consider in chapter 9, with the human factor clearly informing policy at the highest levels. By this time too, Bentley's coterminous inquiry and subsequent report on malaria in Bombay city offered an example of targeted vector 'sanitation.' Bentley identified the source of the chief malaria vector, *An. stephensi*, in the city to be domestic wells and cisterns and concluded that its highly specific breeding habits offered the possibility of ready interruption of transmission, a concept subsequently termed 'species sanitation.' His report served to demonstrate that the government was not rejecting anti-mosquito measures out of hand.[64]

Within the higher echelons of the colonial administration, then, it appears the Simla meet succeeded in bringing about some appreciation of the role of economic hardship underlying the malaria problem, while keeping the politically explosive dimensions of that factor largely away from public gaze. Sanitarian compliance was backed up by a non-recurring grant of Rs 57 lakhs for town drainage and flood control schemes then 'under consideration,' to be allocated in 1910–1911.[65] As to the sensitive topic of irrigation malaria, the Simla meet appears to have quietly defused the issue. Christophers's mapping of epidemic patterns suggested a limited role for canal irrigation in epidemic patterns.[66] 'Malariogenic' canal irrigation was a serious problem, but it was a different one from the vast regional epidemics the province had experienced in 1908 and recurringly before.

Yet the question remained how to convince the wider medical establishment of the colonial government's commitment to dealing with 'malaria control.' Government officials had come to recognise by this point that some kind of extirpation-friendly public image was unavoidable. The British Raj had resolved itself, in other words, to policy doublespeak: nominally championing mosquito extirpation, while behind the scenes attempting to tackle the underlying causes of extreme mortality from the disease. Such a strategy, however, was unlikely to succeed with the most ardent advocates of mosquito extirpation who continued to view official efforts at Mian Mir as flawed. And here, the government agreed to Ross's call for a review of James's assessment of the adequacy of anti-mosquito operations undertaken at the cantonment.[67] But even before the Nathan report's release in December 1909 which largely confirmed James's conclusions, highly embarrassing questions were being raised in the British parliament with public health spending in India compared starkly with that directed to military expenditures.[68] The Simla conference, in other words, had yet to dampen criticism of colonial India sanitary policy in the British medical press. Two weeks later, the entire text of Leslie's opening address to the Simla conference appeared in the November 20 issue of the *Lancet*, with much of his frank depiction of the economic dimensions to the problem of intense malaria in India unexpunged.[69]

The decision to disseminate sensitive colonial records would bring a truce of sorts from the *Lancet*. But there would be no let up elsewhere. A January 1910 editorial in the *Journal of Tropical Medicine and Hygiene* lamented lack of anti-malaria measures on engineering works in India, and 'the petty economy of . . . our Indian authorities on all sanitary questions. . . [which] too often wrecks their sanitary ship for the lack of a pot of paint.'[70] This was followed by scathing criticism of the work done at Mian Mir:

> No attempt whatever [was] made to prevent the establishment of breeding-places within the courts of the houses, each of which contains a number of large water-jars seldom or never completely

emptied, besides the usual accessories of broken crockery, empty tins, and other malarial facilities.[71]

In light of the primacy of monsoon rainfall in ensuring vast vector breeding sites in the region, the latter critique was clearly misplaced. But its inappropriateness was unlikely to be understood by a British audience unfamiliar with rural malaria entomology in the subcontinent. Then, in June 1911, the *British Medical Journal* published an acerbic letter from King, now retired, trashing not just the anti-malaria work conducted at Mian Mir and the Simla conference, but also the 'autocratic' Central Malaria Committee set up, post-Simla, to coordinate ongoing malaria research in India.[72] More, clearly, was required in the way of containment strategy than the six-day Simla conference.

The Lukis Memorandum

In January 1910, C.P. Lukis had been appointed as Director-General of the Indian Medical Service. As one of the senior members of the IMS most sympathetic to King's mosquito-sanitationist advocacy, the Lukis appointment may well have been an attempt to mollify vector sanitation advocates. One year later, Lukis also took over as officiating Sanitary Commissioner for the Government of India with the sudden death of Leslie in March of 1911. Six months later, he released a formal Memorandum on the 'Suppression of Plague and Malaria' in India.[73] In it, he reviewed medical research and malaria and plague control programs to date, reminding readers of the major Indian research accomplishments for both diseases, and highlighting Bentley's Bombay city 'species sanitation' recommendations and projected town drainage projects. Reprinted in full in the *British Medical Journal*,[74] and excerpted in the *Indian Medical Gazette*, the memorandum's purpose appears to have been primarily public relations, the *Indian Medical Gazette* version noting the memorandum's wide circulation in the lay press, 'commend[ing the] document to . . . critics in Europe' and praising 'the good work being done by the Government and the Medical Dept in India.'[75]

In terms of practical content, however, there was little new. Most of the research and training commitments referred to in the Memorandum had already been announced two years earlier at Simla. Tucked away in the final paragraphs, however, was new territory. Here, for the first time, anti-mosquito policy was placed within the domain of personal responsibility,[76] admonishing 'individuals [who] persist in . . .

furnish[ing] breeding places for mosquitoes,' mirroring almost verbatim the reproach delivered by the *Journal of Tropical Medicine and Hygiene* editorial one year earlier. The pendulum, in other words, was swinging away from economic determinants and back to vector sanitation, but now with emphasis directed in and around the household,[77] a shift mirrored administratively with the transfer of the sanitation (public health) portfolio from Home Affairs to a newly instituted Department of Education.

The second General Malaria Committee meeting, November 1911

Lukis's vector control sympathies would be expressed more prominently two months later in his Presidential address to the second General Malaria Committee meeting at Bombay in November of 1911. In his opening remarks, he openly warned against

> sole reliance [on quinine] in Indian villages, . . . [that] quinine prophylaxis should go hand in hand with general sanitation and with the destruction of anopheles breeding grounds wherever this can be accomplished at reasonable expense. . . . [Y]ou cannot get away from the fact that if there were no mosquitoes there could be no malaria.[78]

'[P]reliminary investigation' into local aspects of malaria transmission 'must not be carried to extremes,' he urged.

> [W]e are perhaps too much inclined to pin our faith entirely on the scientific investigator to the detriment of the practical worker. . . . [I]f we wait until our experts have made a complete investigation of all the problems connected with the epidemiology and endemiology of the disease, there is the danger that India will remain for many years practically untouched.[79]

This view, of course, was the antithesis of the approach of Christophers and Malaria Bureau colleagues in their efforts to train and organise a cadre of malaria workers to conduct local malaria and entomological surveys. Moreover, it is unclear how enthusiasm for general anti-mosquito operations squared with his responsibilities for the 90 per cent of India where the main malaria problem was acknowledged to lie. Clearly, profound divisions in malaria control thought remained within the sanitary and medical services.

In attendance at the November 1911 Bombay meet, Christophers reminded delegates that Bombay city was 'a special case,' and warned 'that it would only lead to waste to draw conclusions for the whole of India from Bombay,' comments echoed by the Bengal Sanitary Commissioner, W.W. Clemesha.[80] Despite efforts by the Chairman to straddle the divide, however, the voice that ultimately reached the public ear was one advocating vector sanitation.[81] Within weeks, the *British Medical Journal* published Lukis's opening address to the 1911 meet. 'The work of Sir Ronald Ross has demonstrated the danger of anophelines as carriers of malaria,' the journal urged. '[L]ose no opportunity of preaching a crusade against the mosquito.'[82]

The Lukis appointment to head the Indian Medical Service at this time suggests it was clear within the higher echelons of the administration that the idea of mosquito eradication had attained irresistible medical momentum, and that it was politically untenable to respond otherwise.[83] Malaria control policy would now have two dimensions: a public face with limited but highly visible species sanitation projects (Bombay) where feasible, alongside emphasis on citizens' anti-mosquito responsibilities; and the other, a behind-the-scenes quiet grappling with the need for fundamental reforms in famine policy and labour conditions.

The colonial administration also appears to have realised by this point that limited 'enclave' mosquito control measures was enough – *was* sufficient to satisfy extirpationist expectations back in Britain as well as in India. There was, in fact, little political push from medical figures for extirpating mosquitoes in rural India where malaria transmission posed by far the greater public health problem. 'Demonstration' projects of urban mosquito reduction were sufficient to the purpose of regaining political legitimacy in the sanitary realm. And this could be done at relatively modest cost, while the expense of anti-mosquito operations in industrial or plantation enclaves would be assumed by the enterprises themselves. In effect, adoption of select, high-profile anti-mosquito trial operations would allow the administration political space to proceed, quietly, in the meantime to address the most severe forms of starvation underlying the fulminant forms of the disease. Thus, by the end of 1911, the British Raj had arrived, inadvertently perhaps, at political containment, of sorts, in the sanitary realm.

Tabling the 'Human Factor'

With prominent anti-mosquito policies, institutions, 'control' projects, and Lukis's Memorandum now in place, it had become politically 'safe' in the final days of 1911 to release Christophers's two major epidemiological reports.[84] In the weeks following, brief reviews of *Malaria in the Punjab* would appear in the British medical press, with the *Lancet* noting that, in addition to flooding, 'loss in stamina' due to 'scarcity' contributed to Punjab's epidemics. But here the significance of the finding was muted in attributing responsibility to 'rich zamindars' who blocked 'better economic conditions.' The *British Medical Journal* in its brief eight-sentence review would attribute epidemic malaria solely to flooding, leaving scarcity unmentioned.[85] No review of *Malaria in the Duars* of any description would appear in either British journal, quite likely because copies had never been received.

In contrast to epigraphic reviews of *Malaria in the Punjab*, accolades would flow in the same pages of the British medical press for the September 1911 Lukis Memorandum. In January 1912, the *Lancet* applauded inauguration of a 'new era' in malaria control in India with 'quinine being now reinforced by much-needed major and minor works instituted with a view of reducing mosquitoes and destroying their breeding places.'[86] As for the Duars report, it would quietly slip from public view in the colonial malaria literature. In his 196-page bibliographic review of literature on the economic dimensions of the malaria problem, 'What malaria costs India,' J.A. Sinton two decades later would fail to refer to the study.[87] Yet if fleeting in its visibility, the content of the Duars study, summarised in 'The Human Factor' paper at the Bombay Medical Congress, had already played a central role, alongside *Malaria in the Punjab*, in shifting the parameters of post-1908 malaria policy.

It had been a remarkable three years, a period of unparalleled epidemiological investigation that Christophers later would remember as a 'golden age of malaria research in India.'[88] It was also one of equally remarkable administrative transparency. In retrospect, it is perhaps surprising that the two reports, 'Malaria in the Punjab' and *Malaria in the Duars*, were published at all. That they were, with the Punjab study accorded prominence in the *Scientific Memoirs* series, undoubtedly reflects the depth of the political crisis perceived on the part of the British Raj.

One can also ponder a certain irony. Had it not been for the intense political embarrassment posed by Ross's highly public charges of government inaction on anti-mosquito programs, would the Duars study's economic conclusions have been expressed as openly? Or been published in any form at all? Ross in his prominent 1910 text, *The Prevention of Malaria*, dismissed Christophers and Bentley's 1909 'Human Factor' paper for its lack of 'scientific' analysis and clarity of 'their methods of enumerating the Anophelines.'[89] Quite possibly, it was this criticism that pushed Christophers in the Punjab inquiry to pursue detailed statistical foodgrain price analysis and precision mapping of epidemic patterns in the province.

Three years later, the Government's dual stance would frame its 'Indian Sanitary Policy' resolution. Malaria, the 1914 document's preamble set out, was 'in many tracts . . . a scourge far greater than either plague or cholera . . . caus[ing] more sickness, misery and death than any other single disease.' The statement emphasised the 'great value' of quinine, but also general anti-mosquito measures even where full extirpation and interruption of transmission was not possible or practicable. 'In anti-larval operations, it is not necessary to abolish all mosquito breeding grounds,' the statement suggested. '[M]arked amelioration in health conditions will ensue if the chief breeding grounds of the malaria-carrying mosquitoes are cleared.' Yet, at the same time, it urged that anti-malarial measures be 'permanent in their effects.'[90] It was a list, in other words, intended to keep all content. Sufficiently abstract, there was something for everyone – except any reference to prioritising action against the intense form of the disease.[91] It was as if the more that was understood with successive inquiries about the importance of human hunger in malaria lethality, the more veiled economic insights/recommendations became in published documents. Offered initially by the colonial administration in an effort to quell British medical criticism and insistence on anti-mosquito eradication, the earlier transparency would quickly fade with a rhetorical surrender to the general medical expectation of vector extirpation.

Quinine 'versus' vector control: a debate misconstrued

The heated and intensely public controversy over malaria policy which the Simla conference was framed to head off in the final days of 1909 has often been seen by historians in oppositionist terms as a debate between mosquito destruction 'versus' treatment (quinine).[92] This characterisation derives from the period itself, summed up most succinctly perhaps by Ross in his unpublished memorandum to the GOI in 1911.

> [T]he quininists, consisting of . . . Colonel Leslie, Major James, and Captain Christophers, urge the general adoption of quinine treatment and prophylaxis, and apparently nothing else. Is India to be treated for ever with quinine alone? [Or a]re we to see proper measures for mosquito-reduction, and other means of prophylaxis carried out in appropriate places?[93]

Phrased thus, it is a short step to viewing 'anti-mosquito' advocacy as the more activist and enlightened stance, as pitting 'progressive' preventive public health activism against imperial fiscal stone-walling.[94] In that contest, the quininists are generally assumed to have 'won,' with colonial malaria policy remaining little more than limited desultory quinine distribution.

So framed, the 'eradication versus palliation' characterisation of the debate fails to capture the central nature of the dispute being grappled with during these years. Both 'sides,' in fact, acknowledged the dual importance of quinine and mosquito reduction. In his presentation at the 1909 Bombay Medical Congress, Ross allowed that quinine was likely the only then-feasible measure for the rural population.[95] For their part, Christophers, James, and Bentley did not preclude vector control where appropriate, advising selective mosquito destruction in localised areas where feasible.[96] Nor was the more traditional 'sanitationist' drainage approach ignored, with anti-waterlogging measures appearing in the Simla conference's final recommendations, operations which, in Punjab, were pursued side by side with quinine distribution, as traced ahead.

The real debate – a profound one – involved quite different questions. The first related to the malaria burden: the morbidity and mortality inherent to malaria transmission (infection), on the one hand, versus the 'intense' form of malarial where mortality was so high it interfered with population growth, on the other. The second question addressed administrative responsibility: the obligation of the State to develop a malaria control policy for the population as a whole (i.e., rural population), versus 'enclave' efforts – a mandate that also entailed preventing the latter from absorbing inordinate attention and resources from the former.[97]

Ross, however, consistently declined to engage on either key policy question.[98] While he professed rhetorical concern about malaria mortality in general terms when appealing for government support for his views,[99] in practice he saw malaria *infection* and the public health burden of malaria *mortality* as one and the same, convinced, it seems, that getting rid of the mosquitoes made the question of case mortality rates irrelevant.[100] Breaking the chain of vector transmission meant no malaria for *any*one, including the physiologically impoverished 'coolie,' to die from.[101] With respect to administrative mandate, a gulf equally wide existed between the two men. For Ross, it was enough to be 'performing [one's] small quota of good' if others, presumably, were doing likewise.[102] The dispute between the two 'sides,' in other words, was inherently unresolvable because each was addressing different questions.

Ross's sole reference to 'social' factors appears in his 1910 *Prevention of Malaria* text in a passing reference to Christophers and Bentley's 'Human Factor' paper, where he acknowledged that transmission rates depend 'not only on the appetite, energy and enterprise of the mosquitoes, but also on the intelligence, social status and habits of their victims.' Yet, even here, his argument veered to a combination of entomological factors and racist stereotypes, suggesting that '[s]tupid, poor, lazy people, living in badly-made huts, without much clothing and without mosquito-nets, are sure to be bitten much more easily than more civilised races. . . [with] [a]lcoholism, opium, etc, lead[ing] to neglect of precautions.' This was a subject, he demurred, 'too complex for detailed examination here.'[103] But, of course, it was precisely the 'too complex' subject of destitution – the 'human factor' – that underlay the so-called palliationist analysis.

The 'eradication' versus 'palliation' characterisation of the malaria control debate was an easy one to fall into. In part, it reflected the power of the sanitationist's extirpation promise, kindled 10 years earlier with confirmation of a mosquito vector in malaria transmission, and one that rendered eradication as a transparently superior goal. But a simplistic oppositionist framework emerged also because there was little interest from either group in highlighting the underlying economic dimensions to the malaria problem. For the British Raj, the issue of hunger (starvation) was potentially more politically damaging even than inaction on mosquito destruction. And Ross, for his part, was not disposed to acknowledging limits to the benefits of Western medical science or the progress thereby imperially bestowed. Defining the malaria problem in more complex economic terms was seen as challenging belief in both the civilising mission of British economic policy *(laissez-faire)*, and Western ('sanitary') science as a major vehicle for that mission as well as Ross's personal role in that mission. Arguably, Ross's antipathy for the 'quininists' derived as much from the irritation he felt with their explicit articulation of economic dimensions to 'the malaria problem' – and later, James' designation of malaria as a 'social disease' – as it did from the specific limitations of quinine. That aversion would surface explicitly two decades later in the pages of the *Journal of Tropical Medicine and Hygiene* in his response to the 'absurd notion [that] has been ventilated in the lay press to the effect that the way to prevent malaria fever is to feed the natives more copiously.'[104]

Both the GOI and Ross, then, were very content to leave the core issue, hunger, unstated, though for different reasons. This left those researching the human factor caught in the middle. It meant that in public debate as 'quininists,' they were arguing, as we have seen, with one hand – the dominant one – tied behind their backs. What stood out on the 'palliationist' side of the debate, by default, was quinine 'alone.'[105] Thus framed, it was a debate which from the beginning the so-called quininists could not win.

This is not to suggest that some of the concerns of Ross and King over the 'palliationist' policy framework were unfounded. Even aside from questions of supply, quinine was not a perfect anti-malarial drug. Ross and King also were correct in questioning the financial commitment of the British Raj in areas relating to malaria. Undoubtedly, the alternate 'mitigationist' recommendations were fiscally convenient to the GOI, offering an escape from incalculable and open-ended financial commitments to species sanitation across the subcontinent with every monsoon rainfall. Yet if important concerns, these were different questions.

Were the mitigation proponents, then, simply inadvertent apologists for GOI stringency as Ross openly charged? The question was hardly so simple. For their part, Christophers and colleagues by this time were convinced that human destitution played a central role in the 'exalted' form of malaria they were being called to investigate. Presumably they also felt confident about the prospects for addressing extreme destitution and the fulminant form of malaria to which they gave rise: 'We can deal with malaria among labourers on a railway, canal, coal-mine, or tea-garden . . . [and] reduce . . . the otherwise inevitable scourge of exalted and intensified malaria,' Christophers and Bentley argued in their Bombay Congress paper, inferring fundamental changes in working conditions and price, drought, and flood relief.[106]

Historiographically, Christophers's economic conclusions have been read as simply serving imperial economic efficiency interests[107] – in the plantation economy and other industrial labour enclaves. Yet the Punjab study was moving the spotlight far beyond the industrial enclave. The 'Human Factor' paper at Bombay and *Malaria in the Punjab* were reports that formally extended the economic critique to the entire subcontinent, with scarcity and industrial destitution openly implicated, a direct indictment of *laissez-faire* and blow to economic orthodoxy. Furthermore, the fiscal implications of the wider view of malaria control – dealing with epidemic hunger and endemic destitution, in drought, flood relief, tax reforms, labour regulation – were hardly cheap remedies either. In hindsight, such measures would be recognised as 'cost-effective.' But to the government of the day, this was not necessarily apparent when these decisions were being taken. Nor was quinine distribution in the quantities envisaged as needed particularly cheap. Such policies were politically imperative at that point, but not necessarily fiscally so.

Ross's concerns over a quinine 'palliation' focus absolving government from adequate funding for other malaria work were real and important. But he was not alone in his concerns. Christophers for his part was acutely aware of the limited supplies of quinine and reluctance of the GOI to increase quinine expenditures. He was equally concerned with financial commitment to research, in coming years publicly criticising the government for subsequent funding cuts.[108] But he also saw that even with greater funds, there was no possibility of vector eradication for the general population: that whatever public health funds could be wrenched from imperial coffers ought to be directed as efficiently as possible, to high malaria mortality localities, and to broader economic reforms such as more effective famine relief.

The Sanitarian's dilemma: larger dimensions to the 'debate'

The interesting historical question here is not simply Ross's personal reluctance to address the public health obligations in regard to malaria policy, or the economic dimensions. Rather, it is the fact that the anti-mosquito framework could remain so persuasive despite being demonstrably impractical, indeed impossible, in relation to general public health policy. That it did so is testament to the compelling nature of the paradigm. But it also suggests an even larger dynamic at play. Identification of the specific vector of the human malaria parasite had set up an impossible professional dilemma for the sanitarian, one succinctly illustrated in the consternation expressed by a local British Indian sanitary officer in response to the heated debate at the 1909 Bombay Congress. In a letter to the *Indian Medical Gazette*, Major Hooton related:

> Working on a small scale I have personally achieved the best results in two district prisons . . . the almost complete disappearance of mosquitoes, which were previously present in swarms . . . I know one very malarious town . . . which is traversed by a nalah [stream-bed] containing for the greater part of the year almost stagnant water. . . . Can anyone doubt that under conditions such as these anti-mosquito operations would be of the greatest use? This is a state of things which is very common in India . . . yet the advocates of quinine prophylaxis appeared to leave it out of consideration. . . . [A] casual visitor . . . must have left the malaria

section of the Congress under the impression that the Ross school was without honour in this country. . . . Is there a Civil Surgeon in the country who does not – if only in his own compound – undertake anti-mosquito operations?[109]

Hooton's words of support for Ross are understandable in his specific context, and as such they highlight the larger dilemma accompanying the new 'germ theory' of disease. In the case of malaria, once vector information was available, individual sanitary officers in sight of potential breeding sites were presented with a compelling obligation to act. It was virtually impossible not to, because on their own they could not tell if the specific anopheline mosquitoes in sight locally were, or might be at some future point, actual transmitters. The 'risk,' post-1897, was now always there. And clearly *not* having malaria *infection* was preferable to malaria transmission, regardless of 'intensity' or vulnerability to that infection. The basic question of what was appropriate policy for limited (enclave) versus whole populations was not just inherently unresolvable *at the level of the individual public health officer* but also, practically speaking, irrelevant.

There was, of course, no intrinsic contradiction between local (enclave) and population efforts. They were simply different mandates. The problem was that the compelling 'handles' for action offered by the identification of germs and vectors in the late 19th century made it difficult for many to keep the larger population framework in perspective. It is hardly surprising, in other words, that intense contention would ensue amongst sanitary officers following confirmation of malaria as a vector transmitted infection, and that intense pressures would be directed to the administration to act. Ultimately, the British Raj would resolve the predicament of irreconcilable positions by adopting a two-track malaria policy: one for general public consumption (and take its lumps for not following through, which it had little intention of doing), and another for practical administration.

Yet one can step back further still. The controversy and acrimony over malaria policy that marked these years was about much more than individual sanitarian dilemmas, or even imperial debit accounting. The debate between quininists and eradicators in its essence was a clash between two historical disease paradigms: the modern reductionist germ theory of epidemic behaviour, and an earlier predispositionist understanding of epidemic disease which, alongside external 'agents' of infection, took account of underlying conditions of the human host, conditions which could – for most of the historically important diseases – so profoundly alter susceptibility to a morbid outcome.

Simla was, in effect, the professional stage upon which this conceptual contest in South Asia was being played out.

In pointing to 'scarcity' and 'physiological poverty,' Christophers was attesting to the insufficiency of the germ theory of disease for informing understanding of epidemic patterns, or action necessary. There was no inherent scientific contradiction between predisposition (human host) and germ/vector aspects of the malaria problem. For some, like Christophers and Bentley, it was essential to incorporate both, and they did so, seamlessly. For Ross and others, the human side of the epidemic equation was a distraction from the important task at hand, considered 'too complex,' unscientific and, ultimately, irrelevant. The collision of these two paradigms, one broad and the other narrow, inevitably triggered intense intra-professional, and ultimately personal, confrontation between those in the Indian Medical Service and larger medical establishments who now viewed malaria control in narrowed microbiological terms as a problem primarily of plasmodia and mosquitoes, and those like Christophers, James, and Bentley who openly advocated that the broader economic factors had also to be addressed.

Beyond its significance for imperial history, then, Simla was a forum where fundamental and conflicting concepts of disease were being grappled with and debated with rare transparency and breadth. As such, the Simla proceedings offer an exceptional vantage point onto a key epistemological moment of medical and health history. We will return to consider these larger dimensions in the conclusion of the study. Here, we turn to examine the content and policy decisions which emerged from the Simla meet, the degree to which these policies were implemented, and their likely impact on subsequent malaria mortality across the province. We begin, in chapter 9, by considering the response of the sanitary establishment to the attempt by leading Indian Medical Service researchers at Simla to reinsert the 'human factor' into medical understanding of and approach to epidemic disease.

Notes

1 James and Christophers argued at the 1904 British Medical Association meeting, with Freetown and Ismailia in mind, that the 'occasionally-reported cases where a brigade has rid a town of malaria we have no hesitation in challenging as absurd'; 'The Success of Mosquito Destruction Operations,' *British Medical Journal*, Sept. 17, 1904, ii, 631–632. Ross, in his prepared statement, had stated that Mian Mir mosquito-extirpation work 'must be . . . executed by means of rigid tests applied by the brain as well as by the hand'; 'The Anti-Malaria Experiment at Mian Mir,' *British Medical Journal*, Sept. 17, 1904, ii, 632–635.

2 R. Ross, 'The Practice of Malaria Prevention,' in W.E. Jennings, ed., *Transactions of the Bombay Medical Congress* (Bombay: Bennett, Coleman & Co., 1910), 67–74, at 72–73, 71, 74 [hereafter *Trans. Bombay Congress*].

3 S.P. James, 'Malaria in Mian Mir,' *Trans. Bombay Med. Congress*, 84–93, at 89, 86 (includes ensuing discussion).

4 Ross, 'Practice of Malaria Prevention,' 72, 74.

5 James, 'Malaria in Mian Mir,' Discussion, 91.

6 S.R. Christophers, C.A. Bentley, 'The Human Factor,' *Trans. Bombay Med. Congress*, 78–83, at 78.

7 Ibid.

8 Ibid., 83.

9 Ibid., 79.

10 Ibid., 81.

11 Ibid., 83 [emphasis added].

12 C.A. Bentley, *Report of an Investigation into the Causes of Malaria in Bombay and the Measures Necessary for its Control* (Bombay: Miscellaneous Official Publications, 1911), 86.

13 S.P. James, S.R. Christophers, 'Malaria in India: What Can the State Do to Prevent it?' *Lancet*, June 26, 1909, 1860–1862.

14 Supplement, *IMG*, Mar. 1909, 9.

15 Letter to editor, 'R. Ross, 'Mosquitoes and Malaria: A Campaign that Failed,' *Lancet*, Apr. 10, 1909, 1074–1075.

16 Editorial, 'Mosquitoes and Malaria – The Campaign that Is Said to Have Failed,' *Journal of Tropical Medicine and Hygiene*, Apr. 15, 1909, 117–118 [hereafter *JTMH*].

17 James and Christophers, 'What Can the State Do'; __, 'Malaria in India: What Can the State Do to Prevent it?' *Indian Medical Gazette*, July 1909, 272–274.

18 James and Christophers, 'What Can the State Do.' C.A. Bentley later noted that '[a]t Panama . . . the Americans spent Rs 6 per head of the population per annum on anti-mosquito measures. . . [whereas t]he total revenue of Bengal for all purposes does not amount to Rs 2 per head'; 'Dr. Bentley on Amelioration of Malaria by Irrigation,' *Indian Medical Record*, Feb. 1922, 41–43. See also Hehir, 8–9.

19 James and Christophers, 'What Can the State Do.'

20 Ibid; James, 'Malaria in Mian Mir,' 93. By this time as well, quinine prophylaxis had been instituted in Punjab jails in 1907 on an experimental basis, a trial which was quickly seen to support the view as to the drug's efficacy in reducing mortality from malaria during a severe epidemic such as that of 1908; *Proceedings of the Imperial Malaria Conference held at Simla in October 1909* (Simla: Government Central Branch Press, 1910), 66 [hereafter, Simla Conf.].

21 James and Christophers, 'What Can the State Do' [emphasis added].

22 Ibid.

23 R. Ross, 'Malaria Prevention at Mian Mir,' *Lancet*, July 3, 1909, 43–45.

24 W. Bynum, ' "Reasons for Contentment": Malaria in India,' *Parassitologia*, 42, 1998, 19–27, at 21, 26, 25.

25 S. Watts, 'British Development Policies and Malaria in India 1897-c.1929,' *Past and Present*, 165, 1999, 141–181, at 159, 176.

26 Simla Conf., 66; S.R. Christophers, 'Epidemic Malaria of the Punjab, with a Note on a Method of Predicting Epidemic Years,' *Paludism*, 2, 1911, 17–26, at 17.

27 Lieut.-Col. H.B. Thornhill, 'Malaria in Cantonments: Wanted a Policy'; Simla Conf., 54–55.

28 Ibid., 13.

29 For varying uses of the terms 'radical' and 'palliative', see Simla Conf., 6, 51, 63.

30 The *Lancet* in Sept. 1909 confusingly characterised the debate as between those advocating 'systematic destruction of mosquitoes' alongside quinine 'for carriers,' versus 'complete prophylaxis of the exposed populations by means of quinine administered systematically'; Anon., 'Malaria in India: Government Action,' *Lancet*, Sept. 1909, 942. But already in 1909 it was 'admitted by everybody that continuous consumption [of quinine was] . . . inconvenient and unpleasant' and impractical; Simla Conf., 6. Yet the term 'quinine prophylaxis' continued to be routinely employed.

31 I am grateful to the late Philip Curtin for this phrase.

32 J.T.W. Leslie, Obit., *British Medical Journal*, Apr. 8, 1911, 848–849 [hereafter *BMJ*].

33 On the timing of initial indentured labour legislation reforms, see S. Zurbrigg, 'Destitution and Malaria on the Duars Tea Plantations,' in preparation.

34 The Bombay Medical Congress, dealing with the full range of diseases in addition to malaria, plague, and sanitary organisation, was of three days' duration, by comparison.

35 Simla Conf., 2–4.

36 The Scientific Advisory Board of the Malaria Bureau (Central Committee) appointed by the GOI was made up of the Director of the Central Research Institute, Kasauli (D. Semple), Christophers, and S.P. James as secretary. Each autumn, provincial delegates attended a meeting of a General [Malaria] Committee.

37 Since his 1897–1898 research, Ross had not engaged in entomological or epidemiological research in India and successful mosquito sanitation experience was limited to Ismailia. By this time, the appropriateness of large-scale anti-mosquito operations was being questioned by leading figures in tropical medicine, including Patrick Manson under whose close tutelage in the late 1890s Ross had been directed to pursue plasmodia in mosquitoes in southern India; M. Worboys, 'Manson, Ross and Colonial Medical Policy: Tropical Medicine in London and Liverpool, 1899–1914,' in R. Macleod, M. Lewis, eds., *Disease, Medicine and Empire: Perspectives on Western Medicine and the Experience of European Expansion* (London: Routledge, 1988), 21–37 at 31.

38 Simla Conf., 87, 91–92.

39 Ibid., 5.

40 Ibid., 5–6.

41 Simla Conf., 4. Here, Leslie appears to have been using the term 'hygiene' in its earlier meaning of 'health' rather than absence of microbes. The Memorandum on malaria control policy in India, released by Leslie in advance of the conference, was a summarised version of his Simla paper. In the latter, 'suitable food' would be added to the list of items required to

prevent the 'fatal' form of malaria, and the introductory words suggesting the GOI were 'held up to obloquy' were not included; J.T.W. Leslie, Sanitary Commissioner with the Government of India, Memorandum: 'A Proposal for the Further Investigation of Malaria in India,' reprinted in 'Collected Memoranda on the Subject of Malaria,' *RMSI*, Mar. 1930, 88–93.

42 For details, see Christophers, 'A New Statistical Method of Mapping Epidemic Disease in India, with Special Reference to the Mapping of Epidemic Malaria'; Simla Conf., 16–21; __, 'Suggestions on the Use of Available Statistics for Studying Malaria in India,' *Paludism*, 1, July 1910.

43 Simla Conf., 13.

44 Simla Conf., 29–46. Christophers's presentation included 'a series of coloured maps and diagrams,' presumably those reproduced in the final 1911 report; ibid., 29.

45 Ibid., 43.

46 See ch. 2, at note 64.

47 Simla Conf., 46.

48 Ibid., 44.

49 Ibid., 46–47.

50 Ibid., 47.

51 Ibid., 99.

52 Ibid., 48.

53 Systematic anti-mosquito measures in district headquarters towns over the previous several years (filling in borrow pits and draining stagnant pools) had resulted in no improvement in dispensary fever cases in 3 of 4 districts; Simla Conf., 22–24, at 23.

54 Ibid., 43.

55 S.P. James, 'Experimental Demonstration Camps,' Simla Conf., 83–93, at 83 [emphasis added].

56 Simla Conf., 10.

57 James, 'Experimental Demonstration Camps,' 83–93.

58 Oiling surface water collections, for example, was to be limited to small collections of water which contained anopheles larvae and could not be drained; Simla Conf., 106.

59 Ibid., 106.

60 Ibid., 61–62.

61 Ibid., 87.

62 Ibid., 107. Here, the government faced a real conundrum of limited supply rendering quinine a highly lucrative commodity on the private market, making adulteration almost inevitable.

63 Ibid., 8, 44, 106.

64 Bentley, *Malaria in Bombay*, 104.

65 Some GOI funds (Rs 8.2 million annually) were directed to 'rural sanitation' in several provinces, 'grants [which] have rendered practical the execution of [drainage] schemes which a few years ago seemed beyond the limits of financial possibility'; *Indian Sanitary Policy, 1914: Being a Resolution issued by the Governor General in Council on the 23rd of May 1914* (Calcutta: Superintendent Government Printing Office, India, 1914), 3. Containment of open-ended mosquito brigade programs,

however, ultimately was achieved by off-loading costs to the provinces, for both anti-mosquito operations and quinine, further stringency guaranteed with the constitutional devolution of responsibility for public health to the provinces in 1919.

66 Simla Conf., 38. See ch. 2, at note 103.
67 R. Nathan, H.B. Thornhill, L. Rogers, *Report on the Measures Taken Against Malaria in the Lahore (Mian Mir) Cantonment, 1909* (Calcutta: Superintendent Government Printing, 1910). See also W. Bynum, 'An Experiment that Failed: Malaria Control at Mian Mir,' *Parassitologia*, 36, 1994, 107–120, at 116.
68 Medical Notes in Parliament, 'Deaths from Fever in India and Sanitary Expenditure' and 'Sanitation and Malaria in India,' *BMJ*, Nov. 6, 1909, 1372.
69 J.T.W. Leslie, 'An Address on Malaria in India: Delivered at the Opening of the Malaria Conference, Simla, October 1909,' *Lancet*, Nov. 20, 1909, 1483–1486.
70 Editorial, 'Engineering Works and Malaria,' *JTMH*, Jan. 1, 1910, 13, 8–10.
71 Editorial, 'The lesson of Mian Mir,' *JTMH*, May 16, 1910, 146–151.
72 W. King, 'The Prevention of Malaria,' *BMJ*, June 3, 1911, 1348.
73 *Memorandum by the Sanitary Commissioner with the Government of India regarding the Measures taken for the Suppression of Plague and Malaria,*' GOI Press, Department of Education, Sept. 22, 1911, reprinted in the *Lancet*, Oct. 28, 1911, 1127–1129.
74 'Suppression of Malaria and Plague in India,' *BMJ*, Oct. 28, 1911, 1127–1129.
75 'Suppression of Plague and Malaria in India,' *IMG*, Nov. 1911, 429–431, at 429.
76 'Suppression of Malaria and Plague in India,' Oct. 28, 1911, *BMJ*, Oct. 28, 1911, 1129.
77 See also, C.A. Gill, 'The Personal Factor in Sanitation,' *IMG*, Aug. 1911, 298–302.
78 C.P. Lukis, 'Presidential Address at the Second Meeting of General Malaria Committee at Bombay, 16th and 17th November 1911,' *Paludism*, 4, 1912, 1–9, at 5.
79 Lukis, 'Presidential Address,' 5–6.
80 *Proceedings of the Imperial Malaria Committee held in Bombay on 16th and 17th November 1911. Second Meeting of the General Malaria Committee,* reprinted in *Paludism*, 4, 1912, 1-129, at 75, 72–76 [hereafter Bombay Malaria Conf., 1911].
81 Bombay Malaria Conf., 1911, 127, 129.
82 'Antimosquito Measures in India,' *BMJ*, Jan. 6, 1912, 23–25.
83 As a delegate to the 1911 Malaria conference, the anti-mosquito enthusiasm of K.C. Bose was typical of many present: '[i]f . . . a crusade against mosquitoes is carried on there is every reason to hope that before long the country which is at present so beset with malaria will be freed. . . . [W]e all know that the anopheles are harmful and as such are to be annihilated'; 'Second Meeting of the General Malaria Committee,' 74.
84 Christophers refers to his Punjab report as already 'in the press' in a summary version that appears in the first 1911 issue of *Paludism*, well before the report was formally released; 'Epidemic Malaria of the Punjab,' 17–26, at 17.

85 'Tropical Medicine,' *BMJ*, Feb. 24, 1912, 432–433; Notes from India. 'Malaria in the Punjab,' *Lancet*, Nov. 18, 1911, 1439–1440; also, *Lancet*, Dec. 23, 1911, 1778.

86 'The present Position of Anti-malarial Methods in India,' *Lancet*, Jan. 13, 1912, 113. The *BMJ* went further, heralding the 'new sanitary era' in India in which anti-malaria measures were based 'on scientific knowledge, not upon empiricism. . . . There can be no doubt that the most effective way of dealing with malaria is by antimosquito measures . . . abolishing all collections of stagnant water, small or large, liable to be visited by mosquitoes.' In its public relations purpose, the Lukis Memorandum had clearly hit their target, the *BMJ* editorial concluding that India 'has at last awakened . . . to her responsibilities.'; 'Antimalarial Measures in India,' *British Medical Journal*, Jan. 13, 1912, 91–92. Bynum interestingly points out that 'British journals, such as the *Lancet* and *British Medical Journal*, ceased to contain much about Indian malaria after the [first world] war'; ' "Reasons for contentment",' 22.

87 'Malaria in the Duars' is listed, however, in J.A. Sinton's bibliography of malaria research in India under GOI publications; 'A Bibliography of Malaria in India,' *RMSI*, Oct. 1929, 1–200, at 112. In the introduction to his 1935–1936 series, 'What malaria costs India,' Sinton describes the 'frightful loss of life' in the Duars labour camps, yet cites as source an obscure lecture by Bentley, not 'Malaria in the Duars'; C.A. Bentley, *A Lecture on Malaria and an Appeal to the Dooars Planters* (Calcutta: Orphan Press, n.d.), 8 pp.; 'What Malaria Costs India, Nationally, Socially and Economically,' *RMSI*, 5, 3, Sept. 1935, 223–264, at 230.

88 S.R. Christophers, 'Sydney Price James,' *Obituary Notice of Fellows of the Royal Society*, 5 1945–1948, 507–523, 512; see also, Bynum, 'An Experiment that Failed,' 114.

89 R. Ross, *The Prevention of Malaria* (London: John Murray, 1911), 209.

90 *Indian Sanitary Policy. Being a Resolution issued by the Governor General in Council on the 23rd May 1914* (Calcutta: Superintendent Government Printing Office, 1914), 17–18.

91 With one exception. Slipped into the final text of the 1914 'Indian Sanitary Policy' statement was the decision to depute a malariologist and engineer to Italy 'to study methods of "bonification",' an add-on 'proposition' that perhaps reflected the recent appointment of W.W. Clemesha as GOI Sanitary Commissioner to replace J.C. Robertson; ibid., 18.

92 H. Evans, 'European Malaria Policy in the 1920s and 1930s: The Epidemiology of Minutiae,' *Isis*, 80, 1, Mar. 1989, 40–59, at 51.

93 R. Ross, 'A Memorandum on the Present Position of Malaria Prevention in India' [originally written in 1911], *Journal of Communicable Disease*, 29, 3, 1997, 187–200. For the circumstances and outcome of Ross's unpublished 1911 memorandum, see Bynum, 'An Experiment that Failed,' 117–119. Lukis similarly wrote of the 'tendency of malaria workers to divide up into two camps, namely, those who advocate anti-mosquito measures and those who pin their faith on quinine prophylaxis'; 'Proc. Imperial Malaria Committee [Bombay, Nov. 1911],' *Paludism*, 4, 1911, 1–9, at 4.

94 Watts, 'British development policies.' Interestingly, Christophers clearly recognised the criticism risk, nevertheless, concluding, 'It would not be right as searchers after truth to blur over what is . . . believed to be the truth, and this I have not attempted to do even *at the risk of being*

reactionary. Malaria prevention for plantations, industrial concerns, towns and cities . . . is one thing, a claim that rural malaria in India "is preventable" and therefore why not "prevented" is simply a quibble of ignorance'; in 'Note on Malaria Research and Prevention in India,' *Report of the Malaria Commission on its Study Tour of India* (Geneva: League of Nations, 1930), C.H./Malaria, 11–26, at 23, 25.

95 Ross, 'The Practice of Malaria Prevention,' 71.

96 Bentley, *Malaria in Bombay*; S.R. Christophers, J.A. Sinton, G. Covell, 'How to Take a Malaria Survey,' in *Health Bulletin* (Calcutta: GOI Press, 1928), 130.

97 Of concern for Leslie was 'insistence' by advocates of mosquito-extirpation 'on the universal value of their measure'; Leslie, 'Proposal for the Further Investigation of Malaria in India,' 90.

98 Bynum notes that in his 1910 *Prevention of Malaria* text the subject of India 'barely rated a mention . . . except as the site of Ross's own activities in the 1890s'; 'An Experiment that Failed,' 114. Subsequent 'vector sanitation' efforts of the Indian branch of the later Ross Institute would be directed to the tea plantation sectors.

99 In his 1910 private meeting with the Secretary of State for India, Ross 'plead[ed] my cause on behalf of the million people who are said to die of malaria in India'; *Memoirs: With a Full Account of The Great Malaria Problem and its Solution* (London: John Murray, 1923), 504.

100 Ross later argued that 'killing mosquito-grubs to prevent malaria may assist in giving to civilization the gift of another half a world – the tropics'; *Studies in Malaria* (London: John Murray, 1928), 58; as cited in Bynum, ' "Reasons for Contentment",' 20.

101 Ross for his part felt misrepresented by the term 'extirpationist'. It was not necessary, he insisted, to eradicate all anopheline mosquitoes in an area to achieve a reduction in malaria transmission. Yet, practically speaking, it was difficult to know where the distinction lay between sufficient 'reduction' and extirpation, and thus could hardly form the basis of a policy of general application, even aside from the recurring cost involved.

102 R. Ross, 'The Anti-malaria Experiment at Mian Mir,' *BMJ*, Sept. 17, 1904, 633.

103 He did, however, acknowledge, in passing, that '[f]amine, poverty and other diseases will reduce the recovery factor'; Ross, *The Prevention of Malaria*, 197.

104 R. Ross, 'Malaria and Feeding,' *JTMH*, May 1, 1929, 132.

105 Bynum highlights this 'optics' dilemma in ' "Reasons for Contentment," ' 25–26.

106 Christophers and Bentley, 'The Human Factor,' 83.

107 See, for example, Watts, 'British Development Policies.'

108 Christophers, 'What Disease Costs India: A Statement of the Problem Before Medical Research in India,' *IMG*, Apr. 1924, 196–200.

109 A. Hooton, Major IMS, Agency Surgeon. Kathiawar, letter to the *IMG*, dated Apr. 24, 1909, in *Trans. Bombay Med. Congress*, 93.

9   Post-Simla
Malaria control in practice

The practical outcome of the October 1909 Imperial Malaria Conference for malaria conditions in Punjab can be gauged in five policy areas: institutional framework, vector control work, access to treatment, flood control, and famine control. This chapter explores the extent to which the first four aspects, those raised directly in deliberations at Simla, would be acted upon in Punjab province over the ensuing years. Official action on the even larger issue of food (in)security is traced in the subsequent two chapters of the study. Here, however, by way of introduction to post-Simla policy shifts, we can discern at the outset a very different tone within the administration, with control of epidemic destitution front of mind for both malaria workers and public health officials.

The 'human factor' incorporated in malaria analysis

Behind the Lukis Memorandum's formal endorsement of malaria vector control in September 1911, the broader economic dimensions to 'exalted' malaria can be seen to have re-emerged in medical deliberations at a number of levels. At the second General Malaria Committee conference in Bombay two months later, the meeting's chairman raised the 'interesting point,' that 'economic stress may play an important part in deciding what effect malaria is going to have, whether there is likely to be a heavy mortality from it or not.'[1] In attendance at the November 1911 meeting, Christophers reminded delegates that mortality in Punjab epidemics was linked to severity of preceding harvest losses. '[T]here are two main crops in Punjab,' he elaborated,

> if one fails it does not matter very much. They can manage to tide over very well, but if both fail there comes a condition of stress, almost of famine, and the people are in a very bad way indeed and this seems to be one of the important causes of the epidemic.

Then turning to current conditions in the province, he noted the 'considerable failure of the monsoon' that year. 'I would like to know,' he asked, 'if an opinion has been formed regarding the possibility of another epidemic because if one finds that this is the case *we can prepare for it.*'[2] Senior officials in attendance clearly had anticipated the query '[R]egard[ing] the question of stress,' the Chair replied, 'I discussed it with Sir Louis Dane before I came here and he says that it does not exist this year,' adding that agricultural conditions for the previous two years had been 'very prosperous.' The Punjab Sanitary Commissioner, E. Wilkinson, in turn, confirmed that 'the late rains have been considerably in excess,' and concurred that 'there is no distress in the Punjab likely to attract an epidemic.'[3]

Attentiveness to prevailing economic conditions in assessing malaria risk extended beyond immediate harvest conditions. It was at the third meeting of the General Malaria Committee in November 1912 that Bentley first presented his broader analysis of the malaria problem in the 'dying river' tracts of lower Bengal as one lying squarely in the realm of agricultural decline.[4] Here, we briefly consider Bentley's investigations as further indication of the seriousness accorded the 'human factor' by the administration in shaping malaria policy during this period: confidence in Bentley's acumen would be reflected in his appointment as Bengal Sanitary Commissioner in 1915.[5]

'Burdwan fever' was an example of *endemically* 'pernicious' malaria induced by profound economic contraction. Beginning in the late 1840s, an intense form of malaria had begun to emerge in a number of formerly 'healthy' districts in the western Burdwan Division of the Bengal Presidency surrounding and to the north of Calcutta, soon eponymously referred to as 'Burdwan fever.'[6] Its appearance and trajectory coincided with construction of embankments along the western side of the Damodar river, a major tributary of the Ganges, as protection for rail lines and roads radiating from Calcutta. Highlighted in Christophers and Bentley's 1909 'Human Factor' paper[7] as triggered by associated 'aggregation of labour,' Bentley's subsequent investigation broadened that causal understanding of labour-camp destitution to include the hydrological consequences of embankment construction: generalised agricultural involution. As naturally occurring silt-bearing inundation flows were disrupted, immiseration and rising rates of fever mortality and depopulation followed. Previously, the Burdwan Division, Bentley asserted,

> was *the most prosperous and progressive Province in the whole of India*. But since 1860 conditions have greatly changed. . . . [O]wing to the confinement of the Damodar river . . . by marginal

embankments, the country has been deprived of needed moisture . . . [bringing] a progressive diminution in the net cropped area.[8]

Cropped area, Bentley estimated, was 'now a little more than half of what it was forty years ago. . . [with] only 5 per cent of this area twice sown because the supply of moisture is so small.' This compared with rates of 15 to 50 per cent in the eastern districts of Bengal. Meanwhile,

> year by year, enormous volumes of water flow through the Burdwan district unused, often causing immense flood damage in lower lying tracts which at present continually receive more water than they actually require. . . . [A]bandoned by the landowners and eventually even the more wealthy cultivators, . . . [t]he [fever] mortality among village beggars and the landless labourers is exceedingly heavy, because they are constantly *on the verge of starvation*.[9]

What Bentley was documenting in 1912 and in increasingly detailed subsequent reports could be termed endemic or 'slow' famine: a rural tract with a population already at bare subsistence level where food production and livelihood over the course of only a few years had been reduced virtually by half.[10] What the 'dying river' tracts needed, Bentley argued, was not 'drainage,' but *more* water, but of a particular kind: re-establishment of the naturally occurring inundation flows. In subsequent testimony at 1927 hearings of the Royal Commission on Agriculture in India, he estimated there were 'more than 6 million acres of cultivable land lying waste in Bengal' for lack of water and the naturally fertilising silt that could replenish it.[11] One half-century earlier, Arthur Cotton, a 19th century British engineer responsible for major irrigation works in the Madras Presidency, concluded that

> the first cause of this fatal [Burdwan] fever was the shocking state of the people in respect of even food, that they were so dreadfully underfed that they had no stamina, but succumbed at once to fever, that they might have otherwise thrown off with ease.[12]

The phenomenon of 'dead river' formation in lower Bengal was a naturally occurring process of shifting channels of the Ganges-Brahmaputra delta. What distinguished the 19th-century changes was their extent and speed,[13] a process of decline initially set in motion with the system of land tenure established under the 1793 Permanent Settlement between the East India Company and the region's large landlords (zamindars) that had led to multiple layers of tax-farming, absentee ownership, and neglect of local water and soil management. Decline was then markedly exacerbated from the mid-19th century in those areas where inundation waters were cut off by embankments constructed without adequate, or any, provision for the entry and egress of inundation flows.

'Burdwan fever' was a particularly stark example of the power of destitution to dramatically heighten the lethality burden of an 'ordinary,' endemic infection.[14] In his 1912 presentation, Bentley pointed to broader conceptual questions.

> The whole question of rural malaria in India, whether occurring as a mere infection or a disease manifestation, is bound up with the problem of agriculture. . . . The attempt to reduce malaria by such measures as drainage or the clearing of jungle unless accompanied by an extension of improvement in cultivation, is foredoomed to failure.[15]

Bentley's ongoing analysis of agricultural involution in lower Bengal continued during his tenure as Director of Public Health through the 1920s, as did his efforts to push for restoration of irrigation flows in the affected tracts.[16]

Bentley was not alone in his practical attention to conditions of human livelihood. In a 1917 memorandum on railway construction and malaria, W.W. Clemesha, recently appointed Sanitary Commission with the GOI, urged local Governments to place copies of the Christophers-Bentley paper on 'The Human Factor' 'into the hands of all large employers of labour.'[17] Describing the public health impacts of 'careless aggregation of labour' as 'far-reaching,' he stressed that 'everything should be done to maintain the whole of the employés, from the Chief Engineer down to the lowest paid coolie on the line, in a good and efficient state of health.' Recommending regular inspection of labour lines by Malaria Officers and provincial Sanitary Commissioners, Clemesha cited as a model the recent construction of the Lower Ganges bridge, urging that 'these excellent arrangements should be the rule and not the exception.'[18] Concern over the economic dimensions to malaria, in other words, was continuing to inform policy at the highest levels of the sanitary administration.

Post-World War I political and fiscal tensions, however, would bring the brief window of transparency in official deliberations largely to a close. The era of major malaria and sanitary conferences, with publicly distributed proceedings, came to an end with the 1914–1918 war.

Attention to economic factors in malaria, however, took other forms: in 1920s Punjab, expressed in efforts to predict malaria epidemics. As Chief Malaria Officer for the province, C.A. Gill established a system of annual epidemic forecasting that incorporated local July–August rainfall, June spleen rate, a district 'epidemic potential factor' (coefficient of variability of autumn fever death rate), and prevailing economic hardship (foodgrain price levels). District-level forecasts were prepared and issued in early September in anticipation of the local need for quinine, flood mitigation efforts, and economic relief.[19] In practice, however, forecasts devolved largely to rainfall and related flooding. By the mid-1920s, foodgrain prices generally failed to reflect local crop and employment conditions as price levels came increasingly to be determined by international conditions. And June spleen rates subsequently were determined to have little value in predicting autumn fever mortality.[20] Accuracy of the *thana*-level forecasts thus was limited, many areas either missed or inaccurately included in epidemic predictions,[21] and after 1924 their publication was abandoned.[22] Nonetheless, such efforts may well have reinforced the onus for 'timely' drought and flood relief measures, as will be discussed ahead.

Institutional organisation

The decision to establish a permanent all-India malaria organisation had already been taken as the delegates gathered at Simla in October 1909. Within weeks of the conference, a Central Malaria Bureau was founded at the Kasauli hill station near Simla, site of the Central Research Institute. Under the direction of Christophers, the Bureau functioned as a training centre, laboratory, and reference library for malaria work across the country. A Central Malaria Committee, headed by the GOI Sanitary Commissioner, advised on policy and control programs carried out by counterpart Provincial Malaria Officers. By 1914, 200 IMS officers and Assistant Surgeons had been trained in mosquito identification techniques and malaria survey methods.[23] A General Malaria Committee that included provincial delegates met annually to discuss and disseminate ongoing research and control experience, with proceedings published in *Paludism*, the first medical journal in India dedicated solely to malaria, edited by S.P. James.[24] In 1911, a second edition of a text on Indian anopheline mosquitoes by James and W.G. Liston was published,[25] and by the mid-1920s, a map of malaria transmission levels and principal vectors was completed for the entire subcontinent.[26] In Punjab, C.A. Gill as Chief Malaria

Officer, conducted malaria surveys of a number of major towns in 1914–1915, and annual rural spleen surveys were initiated amongst school children under the age of 10, survey work that continued through to the 1940s.[27]

By late 1911, malaria research now came under a sub-committee of the newly established Indian Research Fund Association (IRFA), with Ronald Ross as advisory member. In 1913, the *Indian Journal of Medical Research*, co-edited by the Director General of the Indian Medical Service and Christophers, replaced *Paludism* and the earlier ad hoc *Scientific Memoirs* series, Lukis urging contributors to 'show the world what the medical profession in India is doing for the benefit of humanity.' In the first year of the IRFA, Rs 5,00,000 (£33,333) was directed to research, a large proportion for urban anti-malaria measures as trial operations, and a further Rs 82 lakhs (£548,866) to district (rural) boards in some provinces for rural sanitation.[28]

These activities, however, would soon be curbed at the onset of World War I, with most medical officers called up for military duty. At the war's outbreak, Harrison notes, there were 748 IMS officers in India, but only 56 remained for its duration.[29] With the British invasion of what would become Iraq, Christophers had been appointed as Malaria Officer to the Mesopotamian Expeditionary Force in 1916 and put in charge of the Central Laboratory in Basra, later describing the war period as having had 'a disastrous effect' on the organisation of malaria work in India when 'officers of the calibre and status previously available could no longer be spared for antimalaria work.'[30] In Punjab, the post of Chief Malaria Officer was eliminated in 1918 and remaining activities assigned to the Inspector-General of Hospitals.[31]

Fiscal retrenchment

War-time retrenchment of special provincial malaria officers would not be reversed after 1918. The earlier organisational commitment to malaria research and control efforts would never fully be resumed in a post-war period characterised by marked fiscal stringency. Under the 1919 Montagu-Chelmsford constitutional reforms, many administrative powers and portfolios, including sanitation (in 1921 renamed 'public health'), were transferred to local (provincial) jurisdictions, with funding now largely the responsibility of provincial governments. Waning prominence accorded public health was reflected in a dramatic reduction in the content of the annual provincial public health reports. As well, pre-war All-India malaria and sanitary conferences were not re-instated, the decision perhaps as much a political one as fiscally prompted, an anonymous contributor to the *Indian Medical Gazette* noting that 'some of the resolutions of previous conferences had proved distinctly embarrassing to the Government of India.'[32] They were replaced by much smaller annual meetings beginning in 1923 limited to medical researchers,[33] with proceedings no longer circulated to outside institutions. Although the annual provincial public health reports continued to be prefaced with foodgrain price, wage level, rainfall, and harvest data, the brief period of transparency had come to a close.

In 1923, further cutbacks in all spheres, including medical research, were mandated by the Inchcape Commission.[34] In the ensuing reorganisation, the mandate of the Malaria Bureau was broadened to encompass other epidemic and endemic infectious diseases, thereby 'weakening the efforts towards the study of malaria.'[35] Christophers, now Director of the Central Research Institute in Kasauli, added his own voice of concern regarding the state of medical research, in an open letter in the *Indian Medical Gazette* in 1924, stressing the price 'a country pays for a bad sanitary reputation.'[36]

Christophers's uncharacteristic public admonishment appears to have had some impact. At the Medical Research Workers' Conference of 1925, his proposals for the re-establishment of an efficient central malaria organisation received unanimous approval and led in 1927 to the formation of the Malaria Survey of India under the Directorship of J.A. Sinton (1927–1936), replacing the earlier Central Malaria Bureau. Financed through the IRFA and private contributions,[37] it included commitment to a new journal dedicated solely to malaria, *Records of the Malaria Survey of India*, and to a permanent rural research field station at Amritsar, later moved to Karnal district as the Ross Experimental Station for Malaria. In 1938, an enlarged Malaria Survey of India was moved to New Delhi now under the name of the Malaria Institute of India.[38] Valuable research on malaria transmission continued in Karnal district and on the malariogenic effects of irrigation in Sind, the lower tract of the Indus river system as well as on malaria chemotherapy. But in Punjab province, only in 1937 would district-level anti-malarial investigation teams be sanctioned, plans that once again would be undermined with the outbreak of war in 1939.[39]

Vector control

Following the 1911 Lukis Memorandum, considerable effort was directed to vector control in selected urban centres. In Bombay city, anti-larval work was carried out involving supervision of public and private cisterns and wells, the chief sites of *A. stephensi* breeding, as determined by Bentley in 1909. The municipal Malaria Department, however, was disbanded in 1918 and malaria would reappear episodically in Bombay thereafter.[40] The Malaria Commission of the League of Nations remarked in 1929 that 'much still remain[ed] to be done' in Delhi as well.[41] The most ambitious urban anti-mosquito operations were undertaken in Saharanpur, a town of 60,000 in the western United Provinces where high levels of endemic malaria prevailed. Anti-larval operations begun in 1912 included stone-lining of drainage ditches and urban streams, and canal irrigation was prohibited within a one-mile radius of the town. '[G]reat improvement' in 'malariousness' eventually was achieved, with the spleen rate falling from 78.8 to 7.3 per cent between 1910 and 1923.[42]

Malaria control efforts through the 1920s on several industrial plantations also met with initial success: in the Cachar plantations in southern Assam, the spleen rate fell to 10 per cent.[43] At the Ennur casuarina plantation on the Madras coast, vector extirpation met with some success, but, as in the case of Bombay, was not maintained.[44] It was in industrial labour camps where malaria control operations brought the most demonstrable benefits, such as completion of the Nagpur-Bengal railway line, previously abandoned due to intense malaria. But other facets beyond anti-larval operations appear to have played a major role. In a 1928 study, R. Senior White acknowledged that railway company managers were 'accustomed to use up their coolies as they do their tools,' noting the prevailing catchphrase ' "a death a sleeper" '[railway tie].[45] His malaria recommendations included systematic quinine treatment of seasonal malarial fever, removal of local populations from construction sites and, in the case of the Bengal-Nagpur railway, a second replacement labour force to alternate with those labourers sick and recuperating from malarial fever.[46] In other words, rather than discarding workers, economic pragmatism had led to keeping them on the workforce by nourishing them back to health.

Such shifts in labour conditions were by no means universal. Successes in controlling vector transmission, moreover, were almost all in 'enclave' projects, with Hehir concluding in 1927 that '[u]p to the present, malaria in India has only been toyed with, and that perfunctorily.'[47] Two years later, the League of Nation Malaria Commission (LNMC) highlighted a further irony: that most of the *anti-mosquito* malaria control efforts across the country had been directed to urban centres, where malaria 'in fact is not a problem at all. . . . It occurs in patches. . . [and] is extremely local.'[48] Muraleedharan has described anti-mosquito efforts in the Madras Presidency in similar terms, '*ad hoc* investigations,' amounting to 'tinkering with the problem.'[49]

Saharanpur as 'model'?

Even where urban trials of vector control had achieved success, important questions remained. In the case of Saharanpur town, the cost (six annas per person annually) exceeded the entire annual per capita health budget for the province,[50] and when Government of India funding was ended, the program was not taken over by the municipality.[51] The project appears to have triggered deep debate about larger economic costs as well. The prohibition on irrigation ultimately would be overturned in 1922, to the dismay of the lead investigator of the trial, J.A.S. Phillips. 'The whole of this question,' he acknowledged, 'raised problems which economists might delight to argue about; "should prosperity be considered before health." To the sanitarian there is only one answer to the question and it is a firm negative.'[52]

Phillips's reaction exemplifies the epistemic consequences of a narrowed sanitationist framework of public health: compartmentalised attention to germ-transmission infection in isolation from the human host and its subsistence. But the Saharanpur trial raised an equally important practical question. In his brief to the LNMC India study tour, Christophers noted that despite the apparent reduction in malaria transmission in Saharanpur, *overall* mortality figures for the town were 'not greatly affected.' The crude death rate was 50.3 per mille in 1921, a level as high or higher than in the preceding decade.[53] This suggests that as malaria deaths declined, other endemic infections took malaria's place, an observation that raised the much larger question of competing risk of death.[54]

By the mid-1920s, another troubling question for public health policy in relation to malaria transmission control had begun to be openly discussed: the possible consequences of declining levels of acquired immunity, should control programs falter. '[S]hort of some very complete degree of improvement,' Christophers questioned whether 'a diminished child immunity might be a serious change to introduce.'[55] The issue would preoccupy malaria workers three decades later with respect to holoendemic regions in Africa in relation to post-World War II global eradication policy. Certainly, the question was raised at the Third General Meeting of the LNMC, its 1933 report ultimately recommending 'acquisition of a "relative immunity" through a non radical treatment of the infected people living in highly endemic areas.'[56] The issue may have acted as a further brake, beyond fiscal stringency, to aggressive efforts at control of malaria transmission.

What was not in question was the unfeasibility of anti-mosquito operations for the general (rural) population of India. The League of Nations Malaria Commission in 1929 would readily acknowledge what the 'Indian School of Malaria' had recognised long before, that the rural population was, practically speaking, unreachable with methods then available.[57] This was a conclusion even Rockefeller Foundation consultant, Paul Russell, appears to have initially acknowledged, suggesting in 1936 that 'for rural India' efforts must be directed to 'cheap, automatic, naturalistic methods . . . as primarily improve agricultural yields.'[58] As to experimental vector control work, there was a quiet shifting of government effort to Rockefeller Foundation malaria workers through the 1930s.[59]

Post-1920 vector control policy can be seen, then, to have been in a holding pattern. Limited enclave work had brought growing awareness of the technical difficulties involved in controlling malaria transmission, and raised larger questions, fiscal and immunological. Unofficially, government malaria control policy was one of awaiting rising living standards and possibly new synthetic drugs, while in the background addressing the worst forms of epidemic and endemic starvation. The Malaria Survey of India would reinstitute a modest level of ongoing epidemiological research at the Punjab research station at Karnal, in Sind province, and in Bengal. But the major part of research activities was now directed to therapeutics: investigation of effective forms of quinine, treatment regimes, and distribution methods. The British Raj was content at this point to let the Rockefeller Foundation take over much of the face-saving anti-mosquito task of 'doing something about malaria transmission,' experimenting with Paris green and in the later years of the decade, pyrethrum and 'natural' systems of vector control. Instead, the meagre resources allotted to malaria would be channelled to the two key issues emphasised in Christophers's 1911 report: flood control – strictly speaking, the responsibility of the Irrigation and Public Works departments – and quinine access.

Flood control

In his 1911 call for flood control as *'the first step in the sanitation of a rural tract*,'[60] Christophers was only echoing long-standing calls for amelioration of obstructed surface water drainage in Punjab province. Though standing waters likely enhanced levels of malaria transmission, flood water was a malaria mortality problem most importantly for its economic effects: both in its immediate paralysis of the agricultural economy and its longer-term consequences for soil productivity. Certainly, the latter was reflected in the Baker-Dempster Commission's recommendation for Karnal district realignment of the Western Jumna canal. By the 1880s, local sanitary officials had recognised these serious consequences, arguing that the health benefits from surface drainage works would far outweigh those from 'village sanitation' (conservancy and water supply).[61] A Provincial Sanitary Board was established in 1890, mandated to initiate a detailed survey, by district, of areas where natural surface drainage was intercepted by rail, canal, or other embankments, in addition to reporting conditions of water supply and conservancy. But by the mid-1890 reporting of 'rural circle' drainage, conditions had dwindled to a brief appendix.[62]

The issue, however, would hardly fade away. In the wake of the 1908 epidemic associated with severe flooding, the need for concerted remedial action on flood control could no longer be ignored, despite the enormous practical challenges. In 1919, a separate Drainage Board was created to take the place of the Sanitary Board in rural areas, with a dedicated Engineer appointed,[63] and one decade later, an Irrigation Research Institute was established.[64] Through the 1920s, considerable progress was made on the construction of seepage drains in the water-logged tracts of the Upper Chenab and Upper Jhelum Canal, along with 'extensive remodelling of the distribution channels' where the canal network was causing obstruction of natural drainage lines.[65] In eastern Punjab, work was undertaken in Gurgaon district to repair 35 bunds – low, earthen embankments designed to capture inundation flows and surface rainwater for irrigation purposes – that had fallen into disrepair in earlier years of British rule.[66] In neighbouring Rohtak district, storm water drains were remodelled, and in the sub-montane districts of Hoshiarpur and Karnal, desilting of stream beds undertaken and several major drainage channels constructed.[67] Such measures amounted, in effect, to rural 'bonification' for the localities involved, though how much of the rural population was reached by these efforts is difficult to gauge from published reports.

At the same time, however, canal construction continued apace. The area canal-irrigated nearly doubled from 6.04 million acres in 1907–1908 to 11.16 million two decades later, out of a total cultivated area in the province of 30 million acres.[68] Ecological effects inevitably mounted. By the late 1920s, the administration was turning much of its attention to a problem more threatening to its agriculture revenues than episodic flooding: the spread of alkaline salts across the canal-irrigated tracts. Upward evaporation of irrigation waters was drawing up the salts of sub-surface water and depositing them on the surface soil, a phenomenon that was rapidly extending into the southwest even where water tables were low.[69] The cost to government revenues associated with acute (short-term) flooding was now a small fraction of the cost of the portion of land permanently going out of cultivation due to salinization.[70] Bald fiscal calculus would prevail: official attention swung to alkalisation – and with it, funding and research.[71] With further fiscal retrenchment, the issue of seasonal flood control receded even further down in the administration's list of priorities. By the mid-1930s, proposed surface drainage schemes languished for lack of sanctioning, and those projects approved often faced delays.[72]

Compounding the flooding problem, larger projects that attempted to mitigate underlying causes, such as reforestation of the submontane hills, generally also met a similar fate. Initial land revenue (tax) 'settlements' in the 19th century had included the forests of the Siwalik hills in the northeast of the province, tracts formerly village commons. Hundreds of thousands of acres of hill forests soon were destroyed to feed the appetite for railway ties, locomotive fuel, and domestic uses, a process which 'upset the whole agricultural economy' of the region.[73] From the earliest decades of the colonial period, the disastrous effects of soil erosion in the submontane hill catchment areas were evident.[74] By 1900, the hills in Hoshiarpur district were 'stripped almost bare.'[75] Tree felling and grazing restrictions were easily evaded, and only 'spasmodic' efforts were made at reforestation.[76] The result was predictable. In northeastern Hoshiarpur district alone, 'the soil of hundreds of thousands of fertile fields ha[d] been washed away or buried under sand,' a senior official in the Forestry Service, reported in 1944.[77] These effects, Sir Harold Glover emphasised, extended across the breadth of the northern submontane districts of the province, leading to silting up of the canals and rising river beds in the plains, compounding the problem of flooding.[78]

Assessing trends in incidence and severity of flooding across the province is difficult for lack of specific year-to-year data. An indirect gauge, however, is seen in figures on land revenue (tax) remissions grantly on account of flooding. Beginning in 1908, these records indicate acreage in each canal zone for which irrigation charges were remitted due to crop damage related to flooding and to 'bad soil,' the latter a heading which included waterlogging and salinization (Table 9.1). There are limitations to these data. Available only from 1908, no comparison with the pre-1908 period is possible.[79] As well, they appear to apply mainly to the canal-irrigated tracts of the province. Nonetheless, they suggest little decline in the extent of severe flooding across the post-1908

Table 9.1 Area (hectares) irrigation charges remitted for flooding and 'bad soil,' Punjab, 1908–1937, 1945

Year	Flooded area (hectares)	Total irrigated area	% flooded	Oct.–Dec. fever death rate	'Bad soil'
	1	2	3	4	5
1908	140,767	7,353,146	1.9	18.0	29,444
1909	36,640				55,697
1910	20,132				62,132
1911	4,139				125,476
1912	8,236				71,385
1913	15,208				37,061
1914	56,145				86,315
1915	1,111				73,852
1916	33,662				120,501
1917	302,707	9,063,541	3.5	14.4	100,085
1918	1,737				82,785
1919	24,195				142,521
1920	2,836				150,360
1921	32,930				172,846
1922	12,757				227,020
1923	22,229				186,685
1924	55,834				161,593
1925	29,729				136,225
1926	24,171				229,895
1927	3,603				168,247
1928	3,635				174,958
1929	226,692	12,475,305	1.8	7.6	223,948
1930	16,109				290,927
1931	25,416				362,244
1932	22,032				359,560
1933	182,631	12,017,455	1.5	8.4	259,684
1934	11,575				181,274
1935	10,121				230,999
1936	21,510				104,885
1937	3,164				317,342
..					
..					
1945	15,817				478,193

Source: Punjab. Annual Report, Public Works Dept., Irrigation Branch; *Annual Report of the Sanitary Commissioner*, Punjab; after 1921, *Report on the Public Health Administration of the Punjab*, various years.

period, either in terms of absolute area flooded (Table 9.1, col. 1) or as a percentage of total irrigated area (Table 9.1, col. 3).

Narrative accounts of flooding in the annual administrative reports also suggest little decline through the 1920s and 1930s. In 1933, flooding destroyed 580,000 acres of crops and over 132,000 houses in southeastern Punjab.[80] In 1947, severe flooding caused much 'hardship to the stranded [Partition] refugees.' Three years later, 'catastrophic' floods destroyed 850,000 acres of crops and 200,000 houses in (East) Punjab State. Food had to be air-dropped to large numbers of villages completely isolated, and again in 1955 when floods deluged 7,000 (East) Punjab villages.[81] Thus, although local rural tracts undoubtedly benefitted from improved drainage, the previous accounts suggest little decline in frequency or severity of flooding in Punjab province, if any at all, across the final decades of the colonial period.

What did change after 1908 was the imperial government's *response* to flooding: in taxes remitted for flood-related harvest losses (Table 9.1), and in provision of direct food relief. The nature and timing of changes in flood- and drought relief after 1908, and their likely impact on starvation vulnerability, will be explored in chapters 10 and 11. But first, we turn to consider post-1908 changes at the medical level in terms of access to treatment (quinine), the second of the major recommendations coming out of the Simla conference.

Quinine availability

Three full days devoted to quinine deliberation at Simla had revealed, and left unresolved, myriad problems both in popularising the drug and in distributing it in the absence of any effective rural health infrastructure. Along with an array of competing interests within the imperial body politic, these difficulties would continue to bedevil quinine policy for the remainder of the colonial period – despite the undisputed value of the drug itself against uncomplicated malaria infection.

The anti-malarial properties of the Peruvian cinchona bark, from which quinine and related alkaloids were extracted, had long been recognised and exploited by Europeans in their imperial possessions. Cultivation of cinchona in South Asia began in 1860.[82] Within two decades, 1 million pounds of cinchona bark were being produced annually in India for military and administrative use, a figure that reached 16 million pounds in Ceylon by 1887.[83] Dutch planters in Java, however, were expanding production even more rapidly, leading to a glut of bark on the international market by the 1880s and 1890s, and to plummeting prices. In response, planters in India and Ceylon shifted to more remunerative tea and coffee cultivation.

The cinchona species most suited to climatic conditions in the subcontinent was *C. subbrarubra*, rather than the 'less hardy' yellow bark species, *C. ledgerianna*, which flourished in Java and produced a higher content of quinine.[84] In the early years of cultivation, 'cinchona febrifuge,' a mixture of quinine and quinine-related alkaloids, was still the standard form of the drug. By the mid-19th century, however, techniques of extraction and pharmaceutical promotion had made the pure form of quinine (quinine sulphate) preferred by medical practitioners in Europe, a preference that rapidly extended to India despite 1860s trials suggesting similar anti-malarial effectiveness of the febrifuge. Quinine ascendancy over febrifuge was further entrenched with the 1874 Bengal government decision to encourage private planters to switch from cultivation of the red bark *(C. subbrarubra)* to *C. ledgerianna*.[85] Under provincial government proprietorship, limited quinine cultivation continued in Bengal and Madras, sufficient to guarantee official requirements. But private sales, which made up three-quarters of all quinine consumed in India at the turn of the 20th century, depended largely on imports manufactured from Java bark.[86]

As price levels continued to fall, increasing amounts of quinine began to be made available to the civilian population in India. Between 1887 and 1894, the annual quantity distributed free by 'medical depots, hospitals and charitable dispensaries' amounted to 3,720 pounds, sufficient to provide symptomatic treatment (45 grains) for 600,000 of the estimated 100 million malaria cases a year.[87] In an effort to extend access beyond the largely urban institutions, a 'pice packet' scheme was initiated in 1890 in Bengal and gradually taken up in other provinces, where single 7-grain doses of quinine powders were sold through local post offices for one pice, 'the smallest coin in general daily use among the people.' Post office sales, however, remained generally low, by 1910 amounting to less than 8,000 pounds per year for India as a whole (Table 9.2).[88] To reduce adulteration risk, quinine increasingly was distributed in 5-grain tablet form, a packet of three tablets costing in 1911 half an anna,[89] or one-quarter of the prevailing maximum adult male labourer daily wage.

By 1909, quinine prices had fallen to Rs 7–14–0 per pound from Rs 15 four years earlier[90] and consumption doubled to 165,976 pounds over levels in 1900, sufficient for symptomatic treatment of 24 million malaria cases.[91] Yet cost and inaccessibility continued to exclude most of the population, an issue that dominated Simla conference deliberations that October. Moreover, within four years of the 1909 malaria conference, any prospect of further price decline was extinguished. Dutch producers, with 97 per cent of world production of cinchona bark now coming from Java, had combined to set a 'floor' on market prices.[92] The Kina Agreement set the international price of quinine at Rs 18 per pound, a level maintained through to the final decades of the colonial period. Following severe World War I shortages of the drug

Table 9.2 Quinine consumption (lbs), Punjab and British India, 1895–1910

	Pice-packet quinine sold (lbs)		Total quinine (lbs), Br. India
	Punjab	Br. India	
1895	6	2,470	n.a.
1900	22	3,954	85,104
1902	16	5,027	85,196
1904	28	6,968	100,361
1906	106	7,404	105,565
1908	156	7,549	128,373
1909	88	7,701	165,976

Source: S.P. James, 'A Note on Some of the Measures that have been taken to make quinine available to the poor in India,' *Paludism*, 3, 1911, 10–14.

and soaring prices triggered by European military demands,[93] the GOI in 1921 signed on to the Kina Agreement,[94] guaranteeing supplies – but not access for the large majority of South Asians. At 160,000 pounds in 1922, annual consumption increased to 211,000 pounds by 1930–1931, a level which remained 'remarkably steady' through the 1930s,[95] the internal private market for quinine being saturated long before most of the population had access.[96]

Quinine access in Punjab

In Punjab, sporadic efforts had been made from the 1880s to distribute quinine during local epidemics, often through charitable organisations, and in the case of the 1881 Amritsar epidemic, through municipal authorities.[97] The first systematic attempt to distribute quinine free to rural communities during epidemics began in 1890 in the southeastern Delhi division of the province through district Boards, with provincial assistance. Regular use of quinine in all the jails of the province followed in 1893. One year later, the pice packet scheme was introduced in Punjab province on an experimental basis again in the southeast and extended provincially in 1902. The scheme was unpopular, however, with annual sales amounting to 88 pounds by the end of the decade,[98] prompting major changes in distribution policy in January 1908. School teachers, native druggists, and other minor officials were enlisted as selling agents, and the commission for postmasters selling pice packets was increased. As well, the policy of providing quinine free during epidemics was regularised, with 'district boards and municipalities to supply the dispensaries under their control and to zaildars and others for distribution to those who are unable to purchase it for themselves.' During the malaria epidemic that followed eight months later, 6,000 pounds of quinine would be distributed free through this expanded network with eight 'itinerant hospitals' sanctioned for rural distribution.[99]

With post-World War I expansion in public medical facilities, malaria cases treated annually at the 398 hospitals and locally funded dispensaries in the province had risen three-fold to 2 million by the 1930s, increasing to 3 million in epidemic years,[100] potentially reaching between 7 and 15 per cent of the population in particular years (Table 9.3). Thus, the timing of the increase in general quinine availability and medical treatment corresponds closely to the period of epidemic malaria decline in Punjab. Yet a significant role for quinine in that decline hinges on the degree to which available supplies reached those most vulnerable to dying from the infection, raising questions of both geographic and economic access. Quinine provided largely free in the province through public health facilities, remained low, at 0.9 grains *per capita* (0.8 quinine, 0.1 cinchona febrifuge), below even the all-India mean (Table 9.4).[101]

The issue of rural access was one that preoccupied provincial public health administrators from the earliest years of quinine distribution. Establishment of rural clinics in the 1920s was an effort to ensure at least one medical facility per 100 square miles. In 1929, a further scheme of 4,174 quinine depots and sub-depots was set up, with schoolmasters as local distribution agents provided with supplies of

Table 9.3 Malaria cases (in- and out-patient) and deaths, govt hospitals and dispensaries, by year, Punjab Province, 1921–1940

	Cases	*Deaths*		*Cases*	*Deaths*
1921	658,568	58	1931	2,133,153	84
1922	645,640	43	1932	1,876,293	74
1923	561,112	72	1933	3,062,837	103
1924	1,315,664	90	1934	2,174,764	101
1925	1,236,688	120	1935	1,846,147	68
1926	1,518,961	94	1936	1,994,392	80
1927	1,339,754	120	1937	1,568,000	50
1928	1,194,323	102	1938	1,494,267	49
1929	2,105,174	97	1939	1,673,530	32
1930	2,192,986	134	1940	2,736,899	60

Source: Dial Das, *Vital Statistics of the Punjab, 1901–1940* Board of Economic Inquiry, Punjab, No. 80, 1942, Appendix 1, 97, 45.

Table 9.4 Quinine and cinchona febrifuge (lbs, grains* per capita), issued by public health, medical, and other departments, by province, India, 1937

	Quinine		Cinchona febrifuge		Total (grains p.c.)
	lbs	Grains p.c.	lbs	Grains p.c.	
British India	33,793	1.1	8,667	0.3	1.4
Punjab	3,070	0.8	496	0.1	0.9
United Provinces	4,741	0.6	4,075	0.5	1
Bihar	2,166	0.4	75	0.02	0.4
Orissa	1,506	1.5	472	0.5	2
Central Provinces	3,687	1.6	850	0.4	2
Bombay	6,105	2.2	402	0.1	2.3
Madras	5,305	0.8	738	0.1	0.9
Bengal**	12,849	1.5	12,100	1.4	3

*one grain = 65 mg. **data for 1940. *Note*: Bengal figures may include additional quinine distributed through local Co-operative Anti-Malaria Societies.
Source: *Ann. Rpt. Public Health Commission*, GOI, 1938, p. 285; 1940–1944, Statistical *Appendices*, pp. 110–117.

quinine, the intent to make malaria treatment available at a distance of no more than five miles from any village.[102] Through the 1930s, quinine and/or cinchona febrifuge distributed through the depots and sub-depots averaged 1,500 pounds a year (Table 9.5). In practical terms, however, quantities remained limited, amounting to less than one-half pound of quinine per depot per year, sufficient for minimal symptomatic treatment (30 grains) for 60 cases of malaria in a rural area comprising 10 villages. Even assuming the non-medical distribution agents could accurately distinguish malaria from other fevers and that most of the allotted quinine went to actual malarial patients, the proportion of all malaria cases treated each year through the depot scheme would have been marginal: in epidemic years, most of the 60 treatments likely going to fever cases within the agent's own village, and insufficient at that.

Alternative schemes, variously employing travelling dispensaries and part-time medical practitioners, also met with little apparent success: in 1938, the Punjab Public Health Commissioner decried 'the haphazard giving of quinine to anyone who comes asking for it' as 'utterly futile,' that left '[t]he really ill people in villages, who are unable to

Table 9.5 Annual quinine and cinchona febrifuge distribution (lbs) by public
health, medical, and other departments, Punjab, 1929–1940

	Depots/sub-depots (lbs)	Hospitals, dispensaries	Total
1929	3,374	n.a.	n.a.
1930	1,887	n.a.	n.a.
1931	1,702	n.a.	n.a.
1932	1,469	n.a.	n.a.
1933	4,132	n.a.	n.a.
1934	1,096	n.a.	n.a.
1935	1,659	n.a.	n.a.
1936	1,699	2,048	3,747
1937	1,799	1,767	3,566
1938	n.a.	n.a.	n.a.
1939	n.a.	2,727	3,931
1940	1,963	2,881	4,844

Source: *Ann. Rpt. Public Health Administration*, Punjab, various years.

leave their beds . . . notoriously neglected.'[103] By the early post-Independence period, the number of malaria cases treated at in- and out-
door health facilities in East Punjab in 1949 remained at early 1930s
levels: 697,962 cases recorded in East Punjab compared with 1.4 million cases in double the population of pre-Partition Punjab province.[104]

In an effort to overcome the dismally low aggregate figures for quinine availability, targeted distribution on the basis of malaria forecasts
was attempted from the early 1920s. The year 1933, as we have seen,
was marked by destructive flooding, rainfall exceeding 1908 levels.
Efforts, for the first time, were made to provide a four-day course
of quinine (30 grains) to fever cases, and 378,379 such treatments
were distributed to 'known malaria patients' in 3,023 villages in worst
affected districts such as Rohtak and Karnal. Here, per capita availability reached 3 and 6 grains per capita respectively (Table 9.6),[105] a
level that may well have saved many lives: autumn fever death rates
were one-quarter the level seen in earlier epidemics such as 1908, as
discussed in chapter 6 (Table 6.2). Still, the question remains whether
quinine targeting could account for lower overall fever mortality in
1933. Malaria infection rates were high in many districts in the autumn
months of 1933, the number of hospital/dispensary cases almost doubling provincially (Table 9.3) and spleen rate levels rose in most districts, particularly in the northern and western districts.[106] Most malaria
cases in the province, in other words, would have gone untreated.

Table 9.6 Quinine/cinchona febrifuge availability (grains* per capita), July–Sept. rain (% normal), Oct.–Dec. fever death rate (per 1,000), and spleen rate, 23 plains districts, Punjab, 1933

District	Quinine + cinchona febrifuge, grains p.c.	July–Sept. rain (% normal)	Oct.–Dec. FDR (per 1,000)	Spleen rate (Nov.)	
				1932	1933
Southeast:					
Hissar	1	191	7.7	9.3	10.8
Rohtak	6	300	9.4	7.4	13.8
Gurgaon	3	163	9.3	10.2	13.6
Karnal	2	157	9.5	13.1	19.8
Amballa	2	200	6.8	11.3	13.2
Central:					
Hoshiarpur	1	158	6.2	9.0	12.4
Jullundur	1	182	5.4	3.6	5.1
Ludhiana	1	147	4.2	4.1	10.0
Ferozepur	1	162	6.6	7.6	6.4
Lahore	1	145	3.2	14.1	12.1
Amritsar	1	199	5.4	5.4	6.9
North:					
Gurdaspur	1	165	7.4	22.9	17.4
Sialkot	1	152	10.0	8.9	38.0
Gujrat	1	202	12.3	8.3	28.9
Gujranwala	2	209	17.8	9.3	32.3
Jhelum	1	155	9.5	9.5	23.9
West/ Southwest:					
Shahpur	1	220	11.1	4.4	22.4
Jhang	1	119	5.9	11.6	17.4
Montgomery	2	261	6.9	13.1	29.8
Multan	1	145	10.6	8.4	35.2
Dhera Ismail Khan	1	163	10.1	34.5	25.1
Muzaffargarh	1	108	11.8	25.3	55.1
Dhera Ghazi Khan	1	224	9.9	16.4	21.1

* one grain = 65mg.
Source: See Table 4.1; GOI-PHC 1933, 335; M. Yacob, S. Swaroop, 'Malaria and spleen rate in the Punjab,' *Ind. J. Malariology*, 1, 4, Dec. 1947, 469–487.

The inescapable problem in Punjab, as for the rest of British India, remained insufficient gratuitous supply. Indeed, total quinine distributed (depot plus hospital/dispensary distribution) in 1933 appears to have been considerably less than the 6,000 pounds distributed in 1908.[107] And in Bengal where per capita quinine figures were considerably higher, supplies were still considered 'hopelessly inadequate.'[108] Through to the final years of the colonial period, senior public health officials continued to lament that supplies were sufficient to treat at most one-seventh of the malaria cases occurring annually in the country, and that treatment for the estimated 100 million malaria cases in 1930s India would require almost the entire world production of quinine.[109]

Reluctance to expand cinchona cultivation in India went beyond the long-term investment lead times required for cinchona cultivation (eight to 15 years for maximum production).[110] It no doubt also lay in growing prospects for the development of synthetic quinine or quinine substitutes. Plasmochin was introduced in 1926 by the German Bayer Company, and three years later, Atebrin. Neither were serious rivals for reasons of cost, side effects, and effectiveness against falciparum malaria, but they clearly signalled that '[t]he days of quinine [were] numbered.'[111]

At another level, many IMS officials were concerned over potential side effects of the quinidine alkaloid contained in the febrifuge mixture, in particular, quinidine's cardiac depressant effects. Yet this hardly applied to the low and episodic doses provided at public-sector health facilities.[112] Moreover, the solution was development of a standardised form of the mixture that limited quinidine content, a task taken up by the League of Nations Malaria Commission in the wake of its 1929 study tour of India: the resulting mixture termed 'totaquina.'[113] Yet, as of 1937, the amount of totaquina distributed through the government health facilities remained marginal (3,642 pounds).[114]

Most immediate constraints were imperial fiscal priorities. Post-war, the Inchcape Committee had called for 'drastic . . . economy' in all spheres of government,[115] cutbacks already marked in other areas of public health. The four-anna cost of a single treatment (45 grains) of quinine, for example, exceeded the entire per capita annual public-sector health budget in 1920 British India, the latter amounting to scarcely three annas for all expenditures, personnel, and supplies, in addition to drugs.[116] Even malaria patients treated in government hospitals frequently received amounts of quinine well below that required for minimal symptomatic treatment.[117] Expanded access would have entailed not just the febrifuge cost, but of a rural health infrastructure capable of distributing it. In the context of Inchcape retrenchment, aversion to either was reinforced by the provinces' repeated refusal to assume responsibility for greater quinine costs. Post-war devolution of constitutional powers had shifted fiscal as well as administrative responsibilities to local (provincial) governments, including medical and public health services. The main source of revenue granted the provinces in the Government of India Act, 1919 was land revenue. But unlike other forms of revenue retained by the central government such as customs and income tax, land revenue at this point was a largely inelastic income source for provincial treasuries.[118]

Disinclination to fund greater subsidisation of quinine/febrifuge was fuelled as well by concerns that patients treated at public clinics often did not represent that subgroup most at risk. A recurring complaint was that 'cheap quinine is purchased not by the poor, but by others who can well afford to pay the market rate.'[119] Already in 1908–1909, the Punjab administration, in recognising 'the popularity of the institutions maintained by local bodies,' was asking 'how to exclude from their benefit well-to-do persons able to pay a private practitioner.'[120] Moreover, it was argued – not without reason – that lowering the price of quinine in India would only lead to supplies being bought up privately and exported for sale at international prices.[121] At the same time, as a prized commodity there was little prospect of avoiding 'profiteering,' adulteration undermining, in turn, public confidence in quinine as an anti-malarial.[122]

Nevertheless, through the 1920s and early 1930s, access to quinine did increase as hospital and municipal dispensary services gradually expanded. In 1937, 42,460 pounds of quinine and cinchona febrifuge, or approximately one-fifth of total supply, were distributed through government facilities (Table 9.4), with much of this amount, it appears, supplied free or at subsidised rates (Table 9.7).[123] By the late 1930s, over 12 million cases of malaria, approximating 5 per cent of the population of British India, were being treated at public-sector facilities annually. Still, overall per capita quinine/cinchona febrifuge availability through public facilities remained low, ranging between 1.5 and 2 grains annually, levels that were acknowledged as 'totally inadequate to meet existing needs.'[124] In Punjab, 3,566 pounds were distributed free of charge in 1937; a level, however, that still amounted to only 0.9 grains per capita (Table 9.4). Under such supply constraints, it seems unlikely that rural access to quinine after 1908 could have shifted substantially to the most at risk.

Questions of efficacy

In attempting to gauge the contribution of quinine to epidemic decline in Punjab, a further question arises regarding efficacy of the drug itself. Practical difficulties of quinine treatment had long been recognised

Table 9.7 Quinine and cinchona febrifuge distributed free, or sold (lbs) by public health, medical, and other departments, in selected provinces, British India, 1940

	Rural		Urban		Total	
	Free	*Sold*	*Free*	*Sold*	*Free*	*Sold*
Punjab	3,838	17	1,006	nil	4,844	17
United provinces	3,793	697	1,748	nil	5,541	6,972
Bengal	22,475	27,830	2,583	6,549	25,058	34,379
Central provinces	1,103	632	862	721	1,965	153
Madras	5,878	1,773	2,449	94	8,327	1,867
British India	47,661	33,255	16,155	11,279	63,816	44,534

Source: *Ann. Rpt. Public Health Commission*, GOI, 1940–1944, *Statistical Appendices*, 110–119.

by public health officials related to the drug's bitter taste[125] and side effects of nausea, vomiting, and diarrhoea. The latter, already prominent among malnourished children, would only enhance parents' concerns.[126] In his major text, *Malaria in India*, Hehir acknowledged that in a young child who 'has already a little diarrhea which the quinine aggravates, very little quinine is being absorbed.'[127] Gastrointestinal symptoms were particularly prominent amongst severe cases of malaria. Thus, therapeutic response to the drug amongst the most at risk was often limited – and a common observation. During the Bengal famine of 1943, medical witnesses reported that 'destitutes attacked by malaria often failed to respond to appropriate treatment and succumbed readily to the disease, while healthy people attacked by malaria in the same area recovered after treatment in the usual way.'[128] Well before, malaria workers had concluded that 'starved and overworked people with chronic malaria require something more than quinine to cure them.'

> Cases of chronic malaria on quinine and attending the out-patient dispensary or hospital for months without any effect on the disease, if admitted into hospital, put to bed, properly fed, and given quinine under supervision, lose their paroxysms and, maybe, are permanently cured.[129]

These serious limitations to efficacy do not mean quinine did not save lives among the millions with public-sector access to it over the final decades of colonial rule. The question is not whether quinine could be a useful anti-malarial, but rather under what conditions. Ultimately, assessment of quinine's role in the decline in malaria mortality after 1908 requires placing the numbers of lives saved through timely access to the drug within the context of the total malaria mortality regularly occurring in epidemic years. What is clear is that among those groups most at risk of dying from malaria infection, young children and the undernourished and famished, quinine was not only least accessible but also least effective.

We turn, then, in the final portion of the study, to examine in closer detail the fifth area of malaria control policy coming out of the 1909 Simla conference, if not apparent in its published proceedings: changes in government relief policies to address 'scarcity' as the central determinant of epidemic malaria mortality.

Notes

1 *Proceedings of the Imperial Malaria Committee Held in Bombay on 16th and 17th November 1911* (Simla: Government Central Branch Press, 1912), reprinted in *Paludism*, 4, 1911, 1–129, at 85 [hereafter Bombay Malaria Conf., 1911].
2 Ibid., 82 [emphasis added].
3 Ibid., 82–83.
4 C.A. Bentley, 'Some Problems Presented by Malaria in Bengal,' in *Proceedings of the Third Meeting of the General Malaria Committee Held at Madras, November 18–20, 1912* (Simla: Government Central Branch Press, 1913), 71–84.
5 Obituary: C.A. Bentley, *British Medical Journal*, Dec. 3, 1949, 1299.
6 B. Chaudhuri, 'Agricultural production in Bengal, 1850–1900,' *Bengal Past and Present*, 88, 2, 1969, 152–206, at 158. 'An ague . . . becom[ing] pernicious' with economic hardship, Fayrer noted, was a well-recognised phenomenon, citing numerous instances designated by the locality's name, such as Terai fever, Peshawar fever, Moultan fever, Scinde fever, Deccan fever, all 'merely . . . local varieties with no fundamental differences'; Sir Joseph Fayrer, *On the Climate and Fevers of India* (London: J&A Churchill, 1882), 61.
7 S.R. Christophers, C.A. Bentley, 'The Human Factor,' in W.E. Jennings, ed., *Transactions of the Bombay Medical Congress, 1909* (Bombay: Bennett, Coleman & Co., 1910), 78–83.
8 *Report of the Royal Commission on Agriculture in India* (London: HMSO, 1928) Vol. 4, 'Bengal,' 241–246 [hereafter *RCAI*], [emphasis in original].
9 *RCAI*, v. 4, 242 [emphasis in original]; Bentley, 'Some Problems Presented,' 62–64, 78.
10 For a concise overview, see C.A. Bentley, 'Some Economic Aspects of Bengal Malaria,' *IMG*, Sept. 1922, 321–326. See also S.N. Sur, *Malaria Problem in Bengal* (Calcutta: Bengal Public Health Department, 1929); C.A. Bentley, 'A New Conception Regarding Malaria,' 3rd Meeting of the General Malaria Committee, Nov. 18–20, 1912, held at Madras (Simla:

Government Central Branch Press, 1913), 61–84; __, *Report on Malaria in Bengal: The Past and Present Distribution of Malaria in Bengal and its Influence Upon the Population* (Calcutta: Bengal Government Press, 1916); __, '*Malaria and Agriculture in Bengal: How to Reduce Malaria in Bengal by Irrigation* (Calcutta, Bengal Government Press, 1925), 188. For subsequent analysis, see R. Mukherjee, *Changing Face of Bengal: A Study in Riverine Economy* (Calcutta: University of Calcutta, 1938); A. Biswas, 'The Decay of Irrigation and Cropping in West Bengal, 1850–1925,' in B. Chattopadhyay, P. Spitz, eds., *Food Systems and Society in Eastern India* (Geneva: United Nations Research Institute for Social Development, 1987), 85–131.

11 *RCAI*, v. 4, 245.

12 Sir Arthur Cotton, *The Madras Famine* (London: Simpkin, Marshall & Co., 1877) Appendix B (letter to Editor of *Illustrated News*, June 29, 1877).

13 W. Schüffner, 'Notes on the Indian Tour of the Malaria Commission of the League of Nations,' *Records of the Malaria Survey of India*, 11, 3, Sept. 1931, 337–347, at 340 [hereafter *RMSI*].

14 By the later 1930s, lower subsoil water and silt content levels resulting from reduced irrigation flows were found to enhance breeding of the main anopheline vector, *An. philippinensis*; M.O.T, Iyengar, 'Studies on Malaria in the Deltaic Regions of Bengal,' *Journal of the Malaria Institute of India*, Dec. 1942, 435–446 [hereafter *JMII*]. Yet, as discussed in ch. 12, malaria mortality in the 'healthy' high water-table tracts of eastern Bengal would soar during the 1943 famine to heights similar to those in the dead-river regions, with no change in subsoil water tables or climate, suggesting the primacy of economic factors over entomological.

15 Bentley, 'Some Problems Presented,' 77–78.

16 Schüffner, 'Notes on the Indian Tour of the Malaria Commission,' 341. Mukerjee describes colonial efforts to re-establish flow irrigation in the Bengal 'dead-river' tracts; *The Changing Face of Bengal*, 91–109. In discussing anti-malaria agricultural 'bonificazione', Christophers later noted 'the magnificent work of Bentley . . . on control measures connected with the great deltaic area of decaying rivers in Bengal north of Calcutta'; 'Measures for the Control of Malaria in India,' *Journal of the Royal Society of the Arts*, Apr. 30, 1943, 285–295, at 289.

17 W.W. Clemesha, 'Note on the Influence of Railway Construction on Malaria,' in 'Collected Memoranda on the Subject of Malaria,' *RMSI*, 1, 2, Mar. 1930, 163–170.

18 Ibid.

19 C.A. Gill, 'The Forecasting of Malaria Epidemics with Special Reference to the Malarial Forecast for the Year 1926,' *Indian Journal of Medical Research*, 15, 1, July 1927, 265–276, at 272 [hereafter *IJMR*]; __, 'The Prediction of Malaria Epidemics,' *IJMR*, 10, 4, 1923, 1136–1143.

20 M. Yacob, S. Swaroop, 'Malaria and Spleen Rate in the Punjab,' *Indian Journal of Malariology*, 1, 4, Dec. 1947, 469–489.

21 Gill, 'The forecasting of malaria epidemics,' 273, 275; M. Yacob, S. Swaroop, 'The Forecasting of Epidemic Malaria in the Punjab,' *JMII*, 5, 3, June 1944, 319–335, Table VI.

22 C.A. Gill, *The Genesis of Epidemics and Natural History of Disease* (London: Bailliere, Tindall & Cox, 1928), 191.

23 G. Covell, 'The Malaria Survey of India, 1927–1937,' *JMII*, 1, 1, Mar. 1938, 1–17, at 3.

24 For accounts of the 1910 and 1911 meetings of the General Malaria Committee, see *Paludism* 1911, 2, 1–16; and 1912, 4, 1–129.

25 S.P. James, W.G. Liston, *The Anopheline Mosquitoes of India*, 2nd ed. (Calcutta: Thacker, Spink & Co., 1911).

26 S.R. Christophers, J.A. Sinton, 'A malaria map of India,' *IJMR*, 14, 1, 1926, 173–178.

27 Spleen surveys in Punjab towns in 1914 and 1915 showed 45 to be highly endemic (25–50 per cent) and a further 14, hyper-endemic with a spleen index above 50 per cent; Punjab Malaria Bureau, *Report on Malaria in the Punjab* (Lahore: Government Press, 1915), 3–4.

28 *Proc. Third All-India Sanitary Conference, held at Lucknow*, Jan. 1914 (Calcutta: Thacker, Spink, 1914), 113, Appended Resolution, 2.

29 M. Harrison, *Public Health in British India: Anglo-Indian Preventive Medicine 1859–1914* (Cambridge: Cambridge University Press, 1994), 233.

30 S.R. Christophers, 'Note on Malaria Research and Prevention in India,' in *Report of the Malaria Commission on its Study Tour of India* (Geneva: League of Nations, 1930), 11–26. [hereafter, LNMC, India Tour]; __, 'Policy in Relation to Malaria Control,' *Indian Journal of Malariology*, Dec. 1955, 297–303, at 302 [hereafter *IJM*].

31 GoP, *Report on Malaria in the Punjab* (Lahore, 1918), 4.

32 Special Article, 'The Need for a Public Health Policy for India,' *IMG*, Oct. 1927, 575–582, at 580.

33 *Sanitary Conference, Lucknow*, Appended GOI Resolution, 1.

34 *GOI-PHC*, 1924, 102; 'Public Health and Medical Research in India,' *British Medical Journal*, Apr. 14, 1923, 640; A. Balfour, H.H. Scott, *Health Problems of the Empire* (London: W. Collins Sons & Co., 1924), 134.

35 D.R. Mehta 'Malaria control in Punjab,' *IJM*, 9, 4, Dec. 1955, 334.

36 S.R. Christophers, 'What Disease Costs India: Being a Statement of the Problem Before Medical Research in India,' *Presidential address at the Medical Research Section of the Fifth Indian Science Congress, IMG*, 1924, Apr. 1924, 196–200, at 200.

37 In 1926, the IRFA received its first public contribution of Rs 1 lakh from the Maharaja of Parlakimedi.

38 The journal *Records of the Malaria Survey of India* was replaced in 1938 by the *Journal of the Malaria Institute of India*, which, in turn became the *Indian Journal of Malariology* in 1947. For an overview of the Malaria Survey of India and Indian Research Fund Association, see S.R. Christophers, 'John Alexander Sinton, 1884–1956,' *Biographical Memoirs of Fellows of the Royal Society*, 2, 269–281; __, *History of Malaria Research in India* LNMC, India Tour, 12–15. See also W.F. Bynum, 'Malaria in Inter-War British India,' *Parassitologia*, 42, 25–31, 2000.

39 *Report of the Health Survey and Development Committee*, Vol. I (New Delhi: GOI Press, 1946), 93–94.

40 G. Covell, 'Developments in Malaria Control Methods During the Past Forty Years,' *IJM*, Dec. 1955, 305–312, at 306. See also, T. Ramachandra

Rao, *The Anophelines of India,* 1st ed., (New Delhi: Malaria Research Centre, ICMR, 1984), 137–150.

41 LNMC, India Tour, 60–61.

42 J.A.S. Phillips, 'On the Results of Anti-Malaria Measures in Five Towns in the United Provinces,' *IMG,* May 1924, 221–228; LNMC, India Tour, 16, 61.

43 Despite energetic mosquito control operations on the Meenglas estate in the Duars, the LNMC noted spleen rates remained high in 1929; LNMC, India Tour, 53–54.

44 LNMC, India Tour, 63–64.

45 R. Senior White, *Studies in Malaria as It Affects Indian Railways,* IRFA, Technical Paper, 258 (Calcutta: Central Publications Branch, 1928), 7, 1.

46 LNMC, India Tour, 16, 54–56, 58–59; Senior White, *Malaria as it Affects Indian Railways.*

47 P. Hehir, *Malaria in India* (London: Humphrey Milford, 1927), 428.

48 LNMC, India Tour, 36, 62, 66.

49 V.R. Muraleedharan, 'Malady in Madras: The Colonial Government's Response to Malaria in the Early Twentieth Century,' in D. Kumar, ed., *Science and Empire: Essays in Indian Context (1700–1947)* (New Delhi: Anamika Prakasshanin, 1991), 101–112; V.R. Muraleedharan, D. Veeraraghavan, 'Anti-Malaria Policy in the Madras Presidency: An Overview of the Early Decades of the Twentieth Century,' *Medical History,* 36, 1992, 290–305, at 291, 300.

50 LNMC, India Tour, 61, 30.

51 Ibid., 61.

52 Phillips, 'Anti-Malaria Measures in Five Towns,' 225.

53 LNMC, India Tour, 16. 'Anti-Malaria Policy in the Madras Presidency,' 290–305.

54 For further discussion, see ch. 12, 384.

55 Christophers, 'Note on Malaria Research and Prevention,' in LNMC, India Tour, 23.

56 M.J. Dobson, M. Malowany, R.W. Snow, 'Malaria control in East Africa: The Kampala Conference and Pare-Taveta Scheme: A Meeting of Common and High Ground,' *Parassitologia,* 42, 2000, 149–166; G. Corbellini, 'Acquired Immunity Against Malaria as a Tool for the Control of the Disease: The Strategy Proposed by the Malaria Commission of the League of Nations,' *Parassitologia,* 40, 1998, 109–115; J.L.A. Webb, *The Long Struggle Against Malaria in Tropical Africa* (New York: Cambridge University Press, 2014).

57 LNMC, India Tour, 50.

58 P.F. Russell, 'Malaria in India: Impressions from a Tour,' *American Journal of Tropical Medicine,* 16, 6, 1936, 653–664.

59 S. Zurbrigg, *Uncoupling Disease and Destitution: The Case of Malaria,* in preparation.

60 S.R. Christophers, 'Malaria in the Punjab,' *Scientific Memoirs by Officers of the Medical and Sanitary Departments of the Government of India* (New Series), 46 (Calcutta: Superintendent Government Printing Office, 1911), 132 [emphasis in original].

61 *PSCR* 1891, 3.

62 J.C. Hume, 'Colonialism and Sanitary Medicine: The Development of Preventive Health Policy in the Punjab, 1860 to 1900,' *Modern Asian Studies*, 20, 4, 1986, 703–724, at 722.

63 Punjab, *Annual Report, Public Works Department, Irrigation Branch*, 1920–1921, para. 30 [hereafter *PPWIB*]; *PLRA* 1920–1921, 2; Gill, *Genesis of Epidemics*, 214.

64 By the later 1920s, hydrological research had identified an underground rock ridge running across the Punjab at right angles to the direction of the flow of the rivers, a factor thought to be contributing to waterlogging propensity upstream of the ridge in the northern two-thirds of the province; E. McKenzie Taylor, M.L. Mehta, 'Some Irrigation Problems in the Punjab,' *The Indian Journal of Agricultural Science*, 11, 2, 137–169, at 138, 141–144. See also, Indu Agnihotri, 'Ecology, Land Use and Colonisation: The Canal Colonies of Punjab,' *IESHR*, 33, 1, 1996, 37–58, at 51.

65 *PPWIB* 1919–1920, 9; *PPWIB* 1921–1922, 9; *PPWIB* 1922–1923, 7; *PPWIB*, 1925–1926, 8.

66 H.K. Trevaskis, *The Punjab of Today* (Lahore: Civil and Military Gazette Press, 1931), 232.

67 *PPWIB* 1929–1930, Drainage Circle report, 9; *PPWIB* 1931–1932, 6; *PPWIB* 1927–1928, 42.

68 As the sanitary and medical establishment sat deliberating at Simla, three more major irrigation canals were nearing completion, composing the Triple Canal system: the Upper Chenab (1912), Lower Bari Doab (1913), and Upper Jhelum (1915) canals.

69 *PPWIB* 1926–1927, 8. By the 1940s, over 250,000 acres in Gujranwala district had gone out of cultivation due to soil salinzation compared with 4,636 acres due to waterlogging; in Montgomery district, 120,000 acres were alkali affected though waterlogging acreage was negligible; K.B. Yacob, S. Swaroop, 'Preliminary Forecasts of the Incidence of Malaria in the Punjab,' *IJM*, 1, 4, 1947, 497–499.

70 In six northern districts, uncultivated 'alkali' land had reached 249,188 acres by 1928–1929 compared with 28,587 waterlogged acres; *PPWIB* 1926–1927, 8; *PPWIB* 1929–1930, 9.

71 *PPWIB* 1931–1932, Report of the Rural Sanitary and Waterlogging Circle, 9. By 1945–1946 report, salinization was estimated to be affecting 16.43 lakh acres, compared with 4.19 lakh acres in 1937–1938, much of the increase accounted for in terms of earlier under-reporting; McKenzie Taylor and Mehta, 'Some Irrigation Problems in the Punjab,' 164; *PPWIB* 1945–1946, ix. A 1967 study found that '44% of irrigation water was lost to seepage in unlined canals before reaching intended fields, with a further 27% field loss to subsoil water'; Interim Report, National Committee on the Use of Plastics in Agriculture, 1982, cited in A. Agarwal. *India's Environment – 1984–1985: The Second Citizen's Report* (New Delhi: Centre for Science and Environment, 1986), 111.

72 *PPWIB* 1937–1938, 64. By 1950, it was estimated that one in four acres of land irrigated by canal water had been lost, most to salinity; *Agricultural Statistics of the Punjab, Pakistan 1901–1902 to 1946–1947*. Board of Economic Industry, Punjab, Pakistan, Publication No. 97, 1950, 13–15; cited in A.K. Dasgupta, 'Agricultural Growth Rates in the Punjab, 1906–1942,' *IESHR*, 18, 3–4, 1981, 327–348, at 346.

73 H.K. Trevaskis, *Land of the Five Rivers* (London: Oxford University Press, 1928), 225, 244–245; H. Banerjee, *Agrarian Society of the Punjab, 1849–1901* (New Delhi: Manohar, 1982), 40.

74 '[W]herever the Forest Department have not the power of control, the wood is being cleared away remorselessly'; *PLRA* 1876–1877, Exts. from the Dep. Cmr. rpts., 14.

75 Sir Harold Glover, *Erosion in the Punjab* (Lahore: Civil and Military Gazette, 1944), 113–114.

76 Trevaskis, *The Punjab of Today*, 384.

77 Glover, *Erosion in the Punjab*, 17–20.

78 Ibid.

79 *PPWBR* 1924–1925, 7; *PLRA* 1924–1925, 2.

80 In 1933, in Gurgaon district 78 per cent of crops were lost, in Rohtak district, 57 per cent; *PLRA* 1933–1934, 2.

81 C. Ramaswamy, *Meteorological Aspects of Severe Floods in India, 1923–1979* (New Delhi: India Meteorological Department, Hydrology Monograph No. 10, 1987), 13, 42, 92, 106, 142–144; C. Ramaswamy, *Review of Floods in India during the Past 75 Years* (New Delhi: Indian National Science Academy, 1985), 17, 32, 63.

82 Historical accounts of cinchona cultivation in India include A.J.H. Russell, 'Quinine Supplies in India,' *RMSI*, 7, 4, Dec. 1937, 233–244; S.P. James, 'A Note on Some of the Measures that Have Been Taken to Make Quinine Available to the Poor in India,' *Paludism*, 3, 1911, 10–14; Editorial, 'The Need for a Cheap and Efficient Anti-Malarial Drug in India,' *IMG*, Apr. 1941, 225–229. For recent accounts, see V.R. Muraleedharan, 'Quinine (cinchona) and the Incurable Malaria,' *Parassitologia*, 42, 2000, 91–100; __, 'Cinchona' Policy in British India: The Critical Early Years,' in A.K. Bagchi, K. Soman, eds., *Maladies, Preventives and Curatives: Debates in Public Health in India* (New Delhi: Tulika Books, 2005), 32–43; A. Kumar, 'The Indian Drug Industry under the Raj, 1860–1920,' in B. Pati, M. Harrison, eds., *Health, Medicine and Empire: Perspectives on Colonial India* (Hyderabad: Orient Longman, 2001).

83 Editorial, 'The Need for a Cheap Anti-Malarial,' 225.

84 Editorial, 'Cinchona Policy,' *IMG*, Oct. 1935, 567–571. *C. ledgeriana* cultivation trials in 1920s Burma encountered repeated setbacks.

85 Editorial, 'The Need for a Cheap Anti-Malarial,' 225.

86 James, 'Note on Some of the Measures,' 13.

87 Ibid., 11.

88 Ibid., 1; Simla Conf., 88.

89 Bombay Malaria Conf., 1911, 110–111.

90 Simla Conf., 68.

91 James, 'Note on Some of the Measures,' 13.

92 *GOI-PHC* 1936, 55.

93 Editorial, 'Quinine Supplies in India,' *IMG*, Sept. 1918, 343–344; *GOI-SCR* 1920.

94 Muraleedharan, 'Quinine and Incurable Malaria,'*Parassitologia*, 42, 2000, 92; Simla Conf., 88.

95 *GOI-PHC* 1922, 103; *GOI-PHC*1936, 58–59.

96 Muraleedharan, 'Quinine and Incurable Malaria,' 97.

97 *PSCR* 1881, ii; __, 1882, 20; __, 1892, 18; *PLRA* 1884–1885, 35.

98 C.A. Gill, 'Summary of Anti-malarial Measures'; Simla Conf., 64–67.

99 Ibid.
100 *GOI-PHC* 1937, 46; Dial Das, *Vital Statistics of the Punjab, 1901–1940*, Board of Economic Inquiry, Punjab, 80, 1942, Appendix 1, 97, 45.
101 *GOI-PHC* 1936, 308. A comparative figure for Italy was 15 grains; ibid., 58.
102 *PPHA* 1929, 17.
103 'Memorandum on anti-malaria measures in the Punjab,' Mar. 18, 1937; reprinted in League of Nations, Malaria Commission, C.H./Malaria/258, Geneva, May 28, 1938. See also, F.H.G. Hutchinson, 'Remarks on the Notes of Sir Leonard Rogers and Dr. C.A. Bentley on the Forecasting of Malaria Epidemics and the Popularization of the Use of Quinine,' reprinted in *RMSI*, Mar. 1930, 190–192.
104 GOI, *Statistical Abstract, 1951–1952* (New Delhi: Government Printing Office, 1953), 56. Synthetic antimalarials in India in 1949 included 980,000 paludrine tablets and 531,000 mepacrine tablets; *Report for the Quadrennium, 1949–1952*. Directorate General of Health Services, Ministry of Health, 51.
105 *GOI-PHC* 1933, 335, Table M.
106 Yacob and Swaroop, 'Malaria and Spleen Rate in the Punjab.'
107 For a detailed account of rural quinine distribution efforts in 1908, see *PSCR* 1908, 18–19.
108 *GOI-PHC* 1930, 58; Simla Conf., 11.
109 Hehir, *Malaria in India*, 427; *GOI-PHC* 1922, 103.
110 *GOI-PHC* 1936, 61.
111 Muraleedharan, 'Quinine and Incurable Malaria,' 97. Quinine was synthesised in 1944. See also, *Malaria in India*, 299; and for German production of synthetic antimalarials, Leo B. Slater, *War and Disease, Biomedical Research on Malaria in the Twentieth Century* (New Brunswick, NJ: Rutgers University Press, 2009).
112 Editorial, 'Cinchona Policy,' 570; Editorial, 'The Romance of Cinchona,' *IMG*, Apr. 1931, 211–214. Yet febrifuge quinidine content (16 to 75 mg. per 5-grain tablet) was, in fact, a small fraction of thrice-daily 300 mg doses used to control heart arrhythmias; J.A. Sinton, 'The Relative Values of the Cinchona Alkaloids in the Treatment of Malarial Fevers,' *RMSI*, 1, 4, 1930, 451–472.
113 Russell, 'Quinine Supplies in India,' 243.
114 Editorial, 'Cinchone Policy,' 570; *GOI-PHC* 1936, 59; *GOI-PHC* 1937, 47. The 1935 *IMG* editorial cautiously directed their critique of 'monopolist' practices to Java, suggesting the 'introduction of totaquina is definitely against the interest of the Dutch monopolists'; Editorial, 'Quinine Policy,' 569.
115 Russell, 'Quinine supplies in India,' 236–237.
116 Roger Jeffery has estimated public-sector health expenditures increased from 0.15 rupees per capita in 1900 to 0. 34 in 1930; *The Politics of Health in India* (Berkeley: University of California Press, 1988), 73.
117 *GOI-PHC* 1922, 103. In Bengal, treatment was 15 grains, not infrequently adulterated to half-strength, with many patients given only a single day's quinine dose. 'It is not reasonable,' A.H. Procter commented, 'to expect a malaria patient to walk several miles daily to obtain 15 grains of quinine'; 'The Dispensary Treatment of Malaria in India,' *IMG*, Jan. 1927, 36–38.

118 The proportion of government revenues contributed by land revenue (taxation) fell from 53 per cent in 1900–1901 to 23 per cent three decades later; D. Kumar, 'The Fiscal System,' in *Cambridge Economic History of India*, Vol. 2 (Cambridge: Cambridge University Press, 1983), 905–944, at 929.

119 F.H.G. Hutchinson, 'Note on the Supply of Quinine as an Anti-Malarial Measure,' [1920], reprinted in *RMSI*, 1, 2, 1930, 193–195, at 194.

120 *PLRA* 1908–1909, 1.

121 Muraleedharan, 'Cinchona' Policy in British India,' 40. Overriding all, perhaps, were geo-political concerns. Cinchona expansion in India directly threatened assured quinine supplies under the Kina Agreement; G. Covell, 'A Brief Review of the History and Development of the More Important Antimalarial Drugs,' *IJM*, 1, 2, June 1947, 231–241 at 234. Competition with the German pharmaceutical industry was intense and bore major implications for global military supremacy, as already witnessed during the 1914–1918 war when European armies regularly battled malarial debility in their respective colonial theatres of war.

122 Adulteration jeopardised even hospital supplies; Editorial, 'The Quinine Fraud,' *IMG*, Oct. 1939, 623–624.; R.N. Chopra, 'Present Position of Anti-Malarial Drug Therapy in India,' *IMG*, July 1938, 418–423.

123 *GOI-PHC* 1937, 47. These figures rely on incidental data appearing in provincial and GOI annual reports where meanings of key terms such as 'sold' and 'free' are at times unclear, or inconsistent. Substantial year-to-year fluctuation in reported quantities possibly reflect variation in local government requisition of supplies more than actual distribution or use. In the case of Bengal, figures may include additional quinine/febrifuge bought by and distributed through the non-governmental Co-operative Anti-Malaria Societies.

124 *GOI-PHC* 1936, 308, 54.

125 Simla Conf., 68.

126 '[L]east cooperation has obtained in the case of babies under two years of age'; H.G. Timbres, 'Studies on Malaria in Villages in Western Bengal,' *RMSI*, 5, 4, Dec. 1935, 366.

127 Hehir, *Malaria in India*, 281.

128 Famine Inquiry Commission, *Report on Bengal* (New Delhi: Government of India Press, 1945), 121. This has been documented more recently among Rwandan refugees; D. Wolday, T. Kibreab, R. Hodes, 'Sensitivity of *P. Falciparum* in Vivo to Chloroquine and Pyrmethamine-Sulfadoxine in Rwandan Patients in a Refugee Camp in Zaire,' *Transactions of the Royal Society of Tropical Medicine and Hygiene*, 89, 1995, 654–656, as cited in P. Bloland, H. Williams, *Malaria Control During Mass Population Movements and Natural Disasters* (Washington, DC: The National Academies Press, 2003), 21.

129 Hehir, *Malaria in India*, 281.

Part III

Shifts in food security, 1868–1947

10 Relief of 'established' famine, 1880–1900

With harvest failure 'two thirds of the ordinary supply of agricultural labor is cast loose on a market where it is absolutely without value.'
– Col. R. Baird-Smith. *Report on the Famine of 1860–1861* [1861], Pt. I, 3.

In Punjab '[t]he people clamoured for village works such as the Government has through all the famine operations deprecated and discouraged.'
– *Punjab Land Revenue Administration* 1877–1878, Ext., 4.

This portion of the study attempts to trace in general terms the timing of, and factors underlying, the decline in epidemic destitution in the early decades of 20th-century Punjab. How close was the temporal association between the escape from famine in Punjab and malaria mortality decline? Certainly, any causal relationship between the emergence of a formal system of famine relief and epidemic malaria decline in the province at first glance appears implausible. Fulminant malaria epidemics continued unabated a full quarter century following the institutionalisation of famine relief under the 1883 provisional Indian Famine Code. Indeed, though the famine of 1899–1900 is considered to be the last 'great' famine in British India, severe malaria epidemics continued in Punjab, in 1908 and again in 1917.

Official declarations of famine, of course, are unreliable guides to epidemic starvation. What constitutes 'famine' was, and remains, influenced by political considerations and imperatives. Definitional issues aside, it is clear that the famines which formerly swept away millions of lives across the Indian subcontinent in the 19th century receded quite abruptly in the early years of the 20th century. The escape from famine was bound up inevitably with broader shifts in the economy associated with developments in transportation and communications; however, much of this infrastructure was in place before the 'great' famines at the turn of the century. More closely related temporally to the decline in famine and epidemic malaria after 1920 were a series of changes in the character of Indian famine relief in the early decades of the 20th century. From palliative relief of 'established' famine as set out in the 1880 Famine Commission Report,[1] famine relief policy from 1901 increasingly was directed to early, pre-emptive support of the agricultural economy *before* frank famine had declared itself.

Though these early 20th century changes held major implications for starvation vulnerability, limited analysis to date has been directed to their nature or impact. In part this reflects the relative invisibility of such policy shifts, enacted, as they were, largely unheralded by the colonial administration. But it relates also to the changing character of relief itself. As famine relief increasingly took the form of pre-emptive measures to prevent periodic drought from developing into famine, and as these measures became a routine aspect of local land revenue administration, special accounts of such activities in the form of massive famine inquiry reports disappear from the archival records, as do also the humanly compelling images characteristic of overt famine. Increasingly termed 'drought relief' or 'scarcity relief,' only sparse details appear in the interstices of regular administrative reports and unpublished *Famine Proceedings*, and thus these measures have generally been less evident to modern researchers.

One consequence of their relative invisibility is that South Asian famine historiography has tended to focus upon the earlier 'unprevented' famines. Bhatia and Srivastava's classic studies of the administrative practices, and flaws, of relief operations through the major famines of the later 19th century have offered invaluable entry points into the often-daunting primary-source famine literature.[2] But the focus remains the great famines. Srivastava's 1968 account importantly extends to 1918 and identifies a number of key policy changes post-1901, but with little analysis of their implications.[3] Renewed attention by historical demographers has also focused on the major 19th-century famines, and understandably post-Independence famine relief administration.[4] But this has left the early 20th century relief policy shifts still overshadowed, and the question of the early 20th century escape from famine – with the exception of the 1943–1944 Bengal famine – largely unexamined. Effective famine *prevention*, in turn, has come to be seen as awaiting the post-Independence period and systematic public intervention in national food supply, with explanations of famine decline in the early 20th century gravitating to economic 'modernisation' and favourable climatic patterns.[5] The latter are, of course, valid areas of investigation, but in the absence of analysis of pre-emptive famine prevention measures, their relative contribution remains difficult to assess and this crucial period still poorly understood.

An important exception to the post-1901 hiatus in famine control analysis can be seen in the work of Arup Maharatna. In his study of famine relief during the 1907–1908 famine in the United Provinces, Maharatna identifies a clear shift to more 'liberal and rational' relief measures and links these changes to a much lower mortality toll.[6] The 1907–1908 famine, however, marked only the first stage in the transformation of official famine policy from that initially articulated in the famine inquiry report of 1880.[7] From reluctant, minimalist (if highly costly) relief of 'established' famine, as formalised in the provisional Indian Famine Code of 1883,[8] emphasis shifted in the decades following the last 'great' famine in 1900 to activist famine *pre-emption*. After 1908, 'drought relief' in Punjab increasingly became a policy of routine application during times of *local* harvest shortfall, in contrast to 1880 policy that limited government intervention to years of widespread and catastrophic harvest failure.[9] From 1920 onward, relief measures also began to be sanctioned for other causes of mass subsistence dis-'entitlement': in particular, for flooding and, following the 'disastrous' experience of World War I hyper-inflation, on the basis of famine-level ('scarcity') foodgrain prices alone without famine ever being declared. The cumulative effect was to make relief available both earlier and more frequently: in effect, catching starvation with a finer – or, perhaps more accurately, less coarse – net. The timing of these later policy changes clearly was compelled by considerations beyond the humanitarian, as seen in the growing notoriety of malaria epidemics in this period. Nonetheless – or perhaps *because of* the larger political imperatives involved – their impact on food security was real.

Here, then, we turn to explore when and in what ways post-1901 policy changes affected relief efforts in Punjab, and their likely impact on vulnerability to starvation in the context of the larger economic shifts taking place. What follows is not a detailed account of famine relief measures across the colonial period. The focus instead is on the *general* framework of relief, beginning with the provisional Indian Famine Code of 1883, tracking how such efforts, and later policy changes, potentially limited, undermined, or ultimately supported, continuity in access to food through periods of acute food crisis, and to what extent these changes correspond in their timing to epidemic malaria decline in Punjab. Inevitably, such an account becomes also an exploration of the massive shifts in attitudes towards destitution and economic theory that underlay these changes, a subject lying at the core of the region's broader economic and health history.

Hailed as a milestone in political conduct and colonial administration in many accounts of British colonial rule, the Indian Famine Code of 1883 was the first systematic attempt to predict and 'mitigate' famine across the vast territory of the South Asian subcontinent. Based upon recommendations of a Commission of enquiry set up in the wake of the disastrous 1876–1878 South Indian famine, the provisional Code of 1883 established standard criteria for defining famine and a set of early warning signs of impending distress. In doing so, it reduced the ad hoc nature of famine relief and lifted much of the onerous responsibility for the decision to embark on public relief from individual lower officials to the provincial administration. By regularising monthly reporting of crop conditions by district officials, and requiring public relief works plans to be drawn up in advance of actual famine, famine 'preparedness' was institutionalised.

In systematising relief procedure, the Code undoubtedly helped to reduce starvation mortality in the final decades of the 19th century in comparison to levels in earlier famines. As horrifying as descriptions of mass starvation were in the famines of 1896–1897 and 1899–1900, in no region did depopulation occur on the regional scale experienced in the 1833 Guntur famine, for example, or in Orissa in the 1860s, where one-quarter of the population perished.[10] But enormous gaps in continuity of relief remained, along with relief rations often bordering semi-starvation levels. That the practical effectiveness of the Famine Code remained limited was dramatically demonstrated in the very high death rates across the closing decade of the 19th century. At the time, the administration argued that the late 19th-century famines were triggered by unprecedented drought and crop failure. Undoubtedly, some of the 1900 famine death toll can be attributed to the proximity of this famine to that three years earlier, but it is difficult to see the drought leading up to the 1896–1897 famine as unique in severity. Crop losses across India, though large, were similar to those experienced in 1891–1892, and again in 1907–1908 (Table 10.1).[11]

So the question remains: why, despite a formally instituted system of famine relief and far greater capacity for movement of foodgrain by rail into deficit regions, did starvation continue to claim so many millions of lives? And conversely, how can the disappearance of major famine only after 1920 be explained? Ultimately, success in preventing mass starvation, it is argued, was an achievement involving more than efficient transportation capabilities, administrative protocols,

Table 10.1 Annual foodgrain availability, output plus net trade flow (100,000 tons), British India, 1891–1947

	Foodgrain output	Net trade flow	Gross availability		Foodgrain output	Net trade flow	Gross availability
1891–1892	38.6	-2.1	36.5	1919–1920	55.3	1.8	57.1
1892–1893	45.4	-1.2	44.2	1920–1921	43.1	0.5	43.6
1893–1894	47.3	-0.8	46.5	1921–1922	55.8	1.1	56.9
1894–1895	50.3	-0.7	49.6	1922–1923	55.8	0.0	55.7
1895–1896	45.9	-1.0	44.9	1923–1924	49.0	-1.0	48.0
1896–1897	36.5	0.2	36.8	1924–1925	49.2	-1.8	47.6
1897–1898	54.3	0.0	54.3	1925–1926	48.2	0.3	48.5
1898–1899	54.3	-1.5	52.8	1926–1927	47.9	0.1	48.1
1899–1900	43.9	-0.4	43.6	1927–1928	45.2	0.4	45.6
1900–1901	48.1	0.5	48.6	1928–1929	49.1	1.3	50.4
1901–1902	48.1	-0.2	47.9	1929–1930	51.4	1.1	52.5
1902–1903	54.3	-1.3	53.0	1930–1931	51.0	0.6	51.6
1903–1904	52.3	-2.0	50.4	1931–1932	51.4	1.0	52.4
1904–1905	47.6	-2.8	44.8	1932–1933	49.0	0.8	49.8
1905–1906	45.5	-1.3	44.2	1933–1934	48.3	1.6	50.0
1906–1907	50.3	-0.6	49.7	1934–1935	48.5	2.3	50.8
1907–1908	39.7	-0.6	39.1	1935–1936	45.9	1.8	47.6
1908–1909	46.6	0.6	47.2	1936–1937	50.4	1.2	51.7
1909–1910	59.3	-0.7	58.6	1937–1938	48.9	0.5	49.3
1910–1911	59.1	-1.5	57.6	1938–1939	44.6	0.9	45.4
1911–1912	54.5	-2.9	51.5	1939–1940	48.1	2.0	50.1
1912–1913	52.0	-3.3	48.7	1940–1941	44.7	0.9	45.6
1913–1914	47.4	-1.4	46.0	1941–1942	46.9	0.4	47.2

(Continued)

Table 10.1 (Continued)

	Foodgrain output	Net trade flow	Gross availability		Foodgrain output	Net trade flow	Gross availability
1914–1915	51.9	-0.1	51.8	1942–1943	48.8	-0.3	48.4
1915–1916	56.7	-0.7	55.9	1943–1944	53.0	-0.1	52.9
1916–1917	58.3	-0.6	57.7	1944–1945	51.3	0.3	51.6
1917–1918	57.8	-2.4	*58.4	1945–1946	47.3	0.3	47.6
1918–1919	39.4	-0.5	38.8	1946–1947	47.3	0.9	48.2

* The gross availability figure for 1917–1918 appears incorrect, possibly a typographical error for 55.4.
Source: G. Blyn, *Agricultural Trends in India, 1891–1947* (University of Pennsylvania Press, 1966), p. 334.

and formal guidelines. It entailed, as well, a shift in attitude towards hunger and markets, and in the relationship of the colonial state to the people over which it ruled, changes that did not occur immediately with publication of the 1880 Famine Commission Report.

Pre-1880 famine relief

The notion of government obligation to provide relief during periods of famine did not originate with the 1880 Famine Commission Report. Pre-British native rulers often assumed responsibility for granting agricultural loans *(takavi)* and remission of agricultural taxes ('land revenue') during periods of harvest failure, and made some effort to control grain hoarding, profiteering, and market speculation.[12] Nevertheless, there is little evidence of systematic methods of famine prevention or relief to the extent organised, for example, by the Qing dynasty in 18th-century China.[13] Costs of transporting large quantities of grain overland were prohibitive, and preoccupation with military concerns often took precedence – indeed, war and political instability were recurring triggers of famine, as elsewhere historically.[14]

Under the East India Company, famine relief efforts through the later 18th century were even more limited. Ten million people perished in the famine of 1770, one-third of the population of Bengal.[15] Only in the 1837–1838 northern India famine did British officials acknowledge an obligation to provide employment 'for all those willing to labour' during severe harvest failures. [16] Shaped by the tenets of political economy and Malthusian views of 'surplus' population,[17] however, relief measures were harsh and extremely limited, and major famines continued.

The sheer scale of the suffering in the 1866 Orissa famine left many minds 'seared by the horrors witnessed.'[18] Moreover, rapid extension of modern communications and railway transportation through the 1860s and 1870s had brought growing recognition that mass starvation was unnecessary technically, and thus increasingly untenable politically. The first major shift towards effective relief came in 1873, under the district administration of A.P. MacDonnell. Response to the failure of the winter crops in Bihar and Orissa included extensive relief works, generous gratuitous relief administered for the first time through local village relief organisations, and the import on public account of almost half a million tons of grain into the drought-stricken areas of northern Bihar and Bengal where transportation was as yet poorly developed.[19] With a change in the reins of viceregal power, however, the pendulum of official relief sentiment quickly swung back to 'strict economy' and assiduous non-interference in the grain markets. When famine struck again in 1876–1877 in southern India, relief measures under the new viceroy, Lord Lytton, and Finance minister in Council, Sir John Strachey, were harsh, disorganised and delayed, reflecting intense disagreement between provincial officials and a central government demanding greater 'stringency.' Despite an expenditure of over 80 million rupees (£6 million), more than 3 million people perished in the Madras Presidency alone.[20]

Relief in the South Indian famine of 1876–1877 was not only an expensive disaster in human and financial terms, but also for the first time under British rule it was clearly documented as such. Employing the mortality returns from the recently instituted system of vital registration, W.R. Cornish, the Madras Sanitary Commissioner, produced a stark portrait of the intimate relationship between foodgrain prices and death rates over the course of the 1876–1877 famine period, an account that would form the backdrop to the Famine Commission Report of 1880.[21]

But the 1876–1878 famine was historic also in being the first where foodgrains continued to be exported out of the subcontinent throughout the crisis, triggering famine-level prices and starvation far beyond the regions affected by drought. Harvests in northern India had not been affected in 1876, but foodgrain prices rose to famine level virtually simultaneously with those in the south. In the event, the northwest experienced severe drought and crop failure a year later, in 1877. Grain exports continued, however, and prices remained at famine level for a third year into 1879, despite the return of good rains and harvests in the south in 1877 and in the north in 1878.

Such transcontinental price behaviour was unprecedented. What the 1876–1879 famine starkly demonstrated was that with South Asian grain prices half those of European levels, international demand for Indian grain could occur even with local prices at famine levels. Grain riots during famines had already posed a major problem through the early 19th century. Though studiously omitted from later published famine reports, over 400 grain riots occurred in 1877–1878 eastern Punjab alone.[22] Considered crucial to the balance of payments of the British Raj,[23] subsidised grain exports, nevertheless, would proceed apace, the consequences of which were played out in the 1887 and 1890 malaria epidemics in Punjab, as we have seen in chapter 5.

Beyond grain exports, opposition to agricultural taxation policy was also rapidly growing, the leading source of revenue for the GOI. Particularly resented was the rigidity of tax (land revenue) collection, set at half the level of average net returns, irrespective of harvest conditions.[24] Throughout the 1876–1879 famine, the colonial government had continued to collect agricultural taxes across the famine tracts, a policy that increasingly was seen to contribute to rural indebtedness and enhanced liability to famine.[25] Criticism from leading English-language newspapers,[26] and increasingly from prominent figures in Britain,[27] made more effective famine relief a minimum political prerequisite for reassertion of *laissez-faire* economic theory, and more immediately, for law and order.

The GOI under Lytton, however, was determined to limit the cost at a time of growing fiscal pressures. The recent devaluation of silver had increased administrative costs and, in particular, the value of remissions back to London. Alongside soaring military costs in Afghanistan, Bhutan, Burma, and Abyssinia, campaigns financed from Indian revenues, and pressure from British manufacturing interests, had recently led to the repealing of cotton import duties, a further loss of Indian revenue. Appointment of the Indian Famine Commission in 1878 was above all, then, an exercise in containment, an administrative reining in of those provincial governments whose beginning leniency in famine relief was seen as attracting more than the absolutely destitute. This quest for 'economy' reflected Sir John Strachey's commitment to 'to keep famine relief as cheap as possible, so as to avoid raising new taxes,'[28] and helps to explain the serious constraints the Famine Commission's 1880 report imposed on actual famine prevention.

The 1880 Famine Commission Report

Three 'main principles' of famine relief framed the 1880 Famine Commission Report and the ensuing provisional Famine Code of 1883: provision of 'employment to those deprived of work,' gratuitous relief for those too ill or aged to work, and support of agricultural production through loans to landowners and an easing of inelastic land revenue (tax) collection.[29] Employment was to be made available to all who sought relief, with extremely low wages functioning as a 'self-acting' test of need. The Code clearly recognised that the immediate trigger of mass starvation lay in collapse in employment (livelihood) and purchasing power via soaring grain prices: in Amartya Sen's terms, loss of 'entitlement' to food.[30] After 1883, vast public works projects provided employment for literally millions of people in a manner better organised than virtually all prior relief efforts, save those in 1874 Bengal.[31] The question remains, then, why famine mortality continued to run also in the millions until well after the turn of the 20th century.

This failure to avert famine has often been attributed to inexperience. But this ignores the administrative success of Bengal famine relief in 1873–1874. A more persuasive explanation lies with two additional principles framing relief under the 1883 Famine Code: the first, aversion to interference in the rural economy; and second, the goal one of mitigating 'established' famine rather than famine prevention. These two desiderata dictated the timing of relief, its location, and its deterrent character, aspects that often undermined its ultimate effectiveness in terms of saving lives. Overruling advice from the Agriculture and Revenue Department, non-intervention in the economy ordained that employment generation was to be provided primarily on large public works, geographically and economically separate from village agriculture.[32] As late as 1899–1900, the Government of India insisted that 'in no other way can . . . enforcement of the labor test . . . be secured [except through] the discipline and incommodities of large works.'[33] The 1880 Famine Commission Report has at times been interpreted as rejecting the 'distance test,' perhaps because of the ambiguity in the language employed.[34] Yet only in the subsequent 1898 Famine Commission Report would a specific guideline appear, with 'excessive distance' defined as more than 15 miles.[35] With wage rates at bare subsistence levels, daily travel back and forth to the distant work camps was physiologically impossible, making residence on the famine works largely unavoidable -- Klein aptly describing the policy as 'put[ting] distance and work between the famine-stricken and a bowl of grain.' In practice, applicants from neighbouring villages routinely were directed to more distant relief works.[36]

Famine relief thus was premised upon a 'self-acting' distance test, policy that changed unambiguously only after 1901. Officially termed a 'labour test' of need, it was, in fact, a test of frank destitution. Residence on the large relief works entailed highly hazardous living conditions, with families physically exposed to intense crowding, summer heat, crude water and sanitation facilities, and for women and children, additionally, exploitation and sexual abuse. Only for the 'respectable' cultivating classes did the 1880 Famine Commission Report recommend village-level works, a directive left vague, and little implemented.

Further contradictions

In taking on provision of 'employment to all,' the administration in 1878 faced an inherent dilemma. For even in non-famine years, substantial sections of the population regularly faced seasonal unemployment and acute hunger during agriculturally slack periods ('hunger seasons'). It was impossible under such circumstances to devise a 'labour test' capable of distinguishing between ordinary unemployment and famine unemployment, for all would seek such livelihood. Moreover, the policy of waiting for 'established famine' meant resort to relief works was that much greater still. Thus, a third principle implicitly flowed from the first and second: deterrence, meaning in practice setting wages at bare survival levels.

Deterrence began with the method of testing for 'established famine': initial trial relief works to gauge severity of rural employment collapse. The procedural trigger for initiating the test was scarcity foodgrain prices: levels 40 per cent or more above normal. If increasing numbers of people were willing to submit to test work conditions, 'famine' was officially declared and such 'test works' were expanded into regular famine relief works. The definition of 'famine,' then, was an operational one: increasing resort to 'test work' relief – the bar set by conditions on the works. In theory, wage levels were similar to those on regular famine relief works, well below half the normal rate for unskilled labour – at times, even lower.[37] Unlike on regular famine relief works, however, wages were based on output, with no minimum for incapacity, no rest-day wage, and no allowance for dependents. As such, they were of questionable adequacy for the labourer himself or herself given the heavy labour involved such as stone breaking, and left nothing for other family members unable to labour. The test thus obliged the abandoning of 'unproductive' family members, including young children. Rather than a 'labour' test, it was a measure in effect of the classic marker of established famine, social breakdown.

Relief wage levels

Wage levels recommended in the 1880 Famine Commission Report on relief works were themselves kept to 'no more than strictly required.'[38] The maximum wage for men, intended for 'seasoned' labourers performing heavy labour was one and a half pounds of the cheapest foodgrain available, providing between 2,200 and 2,500 calories per day. For 'light work,' 1.25 pounds. Women were to be paid 'a little less' than men; working children between 7 and 12 years, half the male rate (1,100–1,250 calories); and children under 7 years, half as much again (625 calories).[39] A 'minimum' rate was set at 18 ounces, and a 'penal' wage was 15 ounces.[40]

As such, 1880 relief wages were slightly lower even than prevailing jail rations which themselves were set to provide only minimally adequate consumption.[41] They fell far below what in modern terms is considered recommended calorie allowance for manual labour,[42] with the gap especially large for children. No doubt many famine victims were physically small (stunted), with somewhat lower calorie requirements. But this would have been offset by the added energy demands entailed in stone breaking, digging earthworks, and carrying heavy loads, work that could increase calorie requirements as much as 50 per cent or more. Wages 'sufficient for the purpose of maintenance' was understood, it seems, as maintenance in the short term only, enough to keep many, not necessarily all, workers alive while on the relief works. Moreover, workers routinely faced wage deductions, official and non-official. Ineffective supervision on the large works and corruption of lower functionaries was endemic, inherent to the enormous and hastily organised work sites. Often, wages were paid on a weekly basis rather than daily, which forced workers to borrow from local moneylenders at exorbitant interest rates. As well, across-the-board wage reductions were at times decreed in an effort to limit the often-overwhelming numbers coming onto relief.[43]

But the logic of deterrence also led to critical *gaps* in relief. The question of timing of relief work closure was addressed only fleetingly in the 1880 Famine Commission Report, though there were few aspects more important. In a single seemingly offhand remark, the Commission suggested that 'the effects of famine may be expected to wear off a month or two before the crops are actually cut.'[44] In practice, this meant that closure of relief works in the two great famines of the 1890s generally began with the arrival of the monsoon rains. Forcing people off relief works often involved reducing already insufficient wages. With little or no valedictory dole, or savings, many faced several months of negligible access to food until the harvesting of subsequent crops, or as agricultural labourers, with real wages a fraction of normal (bare subsistence) levels. Two months of semi- or frank starvation was, of course, better than 10, in the absence of employment on relief works altogether. But the end result in many instances may have been simply to shift much mortality to a later stage of the famine, judging from characteristic post-monsoon malaria lethality in famine years.

Rationalising 'stringency'

The 1880 Famine Commission Report openly acknowledged that keeping relief at razor-edge levels of adequacy involved risks, but these risks were argued as necessary to the larger purpose of avoiding 'demoralization' of those accepting public relief. Any breakdown in the 'habits of frugality and foresight . . . would be an incalculable misfortune,' the 1880 report had warned.[45] Yet did 'all experience' confirm such fears? The official report of the 1874 Bengal famine had concluded that those on relief had 'no willingness to continue to be treated as paupers, but . . . [went] back to their fields and ordinary occupations as soon as the first harvest was ripe.'[46] Moreover, the minimalist stance of the 1880 Famine Commission Report extended well beyond the labouring 'surplus' poor. Relief to the landowning classes was subject to similar constraints. Agricultural loans should not be given, the report cautioned, 'unless the applicant is able to show he is in serious need,' and even then, only in cases 'without serious risk of ultimate loss.'[47] Thus, instead of a general policy aimed at supporting the agrarian economy, the policy of *takavi* loans was reduced to sporadic aid to more 'secure' larger landowners, and thus its wider potential lost.

A similar excessive caution coloured tax relief policy as well. '[N]obody should be forced . . . to borrow in order to pay the land revenue,' the report initially suggested; yet elsewhere it specified that suspensions (temporary deferment of tax payments) be allowed only in 'extraordinary drought. . . [where] *the great majority* will not have sufficient means both to pay the revenue and to provide for their own support.'[48] This qualification limited suspensions to widespread crop failure so severe that even larger landowners were forced to borrow. Even then, individual case by case approval was required, making delays unavoidable, as subsequent experience was to prove. No provision whatever was made in the 1883 Code for remission (cancellation) of land revenue demand in years of harvest failure.[49]

Thus, while on the one hand, accepting responsibility for systematic relief, the 1880 Famine Commission Report conveyed, on the other, often paralysing ambivalence for just such relief: a reflection of continuing ideological aversion to 'State intervention' in the economy. The resulting ambiguity could not help but kindle hesitancy and confusion when the Famine Code was applied to actual famine conditions by local officials in the ensuing decades. As late as the 1899–1900 famine, for example, village-level employment projects in Punjab required individual 'special' approval at the highest provincial level.[50]

Ironically, the decision to make large and distant public works the central 'pillar of relief' meant famine relief would be costly no matter how meagre and deterrent the wages offered. Public works entailed large administrative costs and in the end were often of questionable utility, but the indirect costs were greater still. Reliance on distant public works for employment generation prescribed a recurring drain of labour and capital out of the agricultural economy precisely at a time of peak need for both. In other words, 1880 relief policies compounded the problem of drought-triggered capital depletion, leaving rural communities increasingly vulnerable to subsequent 'vicissitudes of climate.' To no small extent, the cumulative drain over the preceding decades may help explain the increasing 'ready resort' to relief works in the final 'great' famine of the 19th century. Caught in this vicious circle, the only response of the Government of India in the course of the 1899–1900 famine was to exhort even greater strictness to stem the flood of applicants onto relief works.

Agricultural commercialisation and foodgrain supply

In the aftermath of the 1876–1878 famine, the question of adequacy of foodgrain supply was perhaps the most problematic issue the colonial government faced. With grain exports crucial to the balance of payments of the British Raj, there were pressing fiscal reasons for arriving at a sanguine assessment of foodgrain supplies. In the end, the Commission optimistically estimated a surplus of 5 million tons out of a total 'normal' annual output of 51.5 million tons.[51] It also assumed continuing availability of village stores of grain.[52] Both assumptions were highly questionable. The 51 million ton figure was closer to bumper harvest levels than average (Table 10.1), and credible testimony to this effect was presented by two dissenting members of the Commission.[53] Inter-regional railway grain trade was *replacing* rather than supplementing traditional village storage practices, a predictable outcome already evident in 1880.[54] Traditionally, such stores had been used by larger landowners during times of drought to pay agricultural labourers in preparation for the hoped for return of the rains, their decline thus accentuating vulnerability to both 'work famines' and price-induced starvation.[55] Even where local supplies were adequate, the prospect of famine-level prices meant local traders were reluctant to sell grain, awaiting even higher prices.[56] Compounding subsistence vulnerability still further, scarcity grain prices increasingly were failing to return to pre-famine levels[57] in the final decades of the 19th century, but with little corresponding increase in wage levels (Figures 3.4a-b).[58]

The effects of this general price-wage squeeze were further compounded by increasing sensitivity of foodgrain markets to harvest fluctuations. In the past, famine usually only followed upon two or more consecutive years of drought. By the early 1890s, a single year, or indeed a single season, of poor harvests was enough to trigger famine-level grain prices. Moreover, these changes were taking place against a backdrop of a rapid decline of village textile industries. Between 1850 and 1880, millions of weaving and spinning jobs were lost, a sector estimated to have given full-time employment to 1 to 2 per cent of the population and many more engaged in such work on a seasonal basis.[59] The subsistence significance of hand spinning to many rural households lay not in overall income contribution but in the role such work played in filling seasonal gaps in employment and earnings. The loss of such income further undermined traditional village survival strategies.

The decline in local grain stores and rising foodgrain prices were inevitable effects of the growth in modern transportation and commercialisation of agriculture taking place across the second half of the 19th century. The point here is not that these effects could have been completely avoided, once set in train. But, rather, that in its 1880 Famine Commission Report the colonial administration chose to minimise and largely ignore them in devising famine relief policies across this period.[60] By a narrow three to two vote,[61] the majority opinion prevailed, the Commission categorically rejected both relief for 'scarcity' prices, or any intervention in the grain markets. Within the decade, grain exports would rise to over 2 million tons annually. Thus, the British Indian government entered the final years of the 19th century with a famine policy capable of reducing some of the mortality impact of 'work famines,' but ideologically unprepared to acknowledge either the new behaviour of prices as a trigger of mass starvation, or the cumulative capital drain out of the agricultural economy induced by inflexible tax demand and a relief framework based on distant relief works.

The first 'great' famine: 1896–1897

The first major test of the 1883 Famine Code came in 1896–1897. Although drought and harvest failure in 1896 was widespread, crop losses across the subcontinent were not substantially worse than in 1891–1892. What distinguished the 1896–1897 period as a 'great famine' was the rapidity with which foodgrain prices rose throughout India.[62] Relief was provided on an enormous scale, peaking at 3.3 million persons, at a cost of Rs 72 million. In the Madras Presidency, mortality levels rose only 4 per cent, and in Bengal, relief operations appear to have actually reduced the death rate from that prevailing before 1896.[63] Elsewhere, however, relief was often harshly administered, delayed, or prematurely terminated.[64] In the Central Provinces and Berar, the crude death rate in 1897 more than doubled.[65]

In the wake of an official death toll of well over 1 million,[66] another commission of inquiry was established. The 1898 Famine Commission recommended several important policy changes, including special measures for tribal populations and the weaver communities, somewhat increased wage levels, and an additional allowance for nursing women.[67] But final recommendations amounted in effect to fine-tuning of the framework set out in 1880, with large public works remaining the 'backbone' of relief, and 'stringency' deemed essential to containing costs.[68]

Yet in the final pages of the 371-page 1898 report, hints of shifting attitudes foreshadowed more fundamental policy changes to take place after 1901: above all, a new concern for the timing of relief. Here, the report identified return of the rains as the peak period of famine risk requiring intensification of efforts in the form of expansion of village works, gratuitous relief and loans for purchase of seed.[69] Indeed, the very basis of 'self-acting' tests upon which the entire system of Famine Code relief was premised was openly questioned, revealing plummeting confidence in the underlying principles framing the 1883 Code as well as in the tenets of *laissez-faire*.

These key insights, however, failed to be translated into unambiguous recommendations. The issue of inflexible land taxation, for example, identified as the 'most questionable feature' of 1896–1897 relief in Bombay Presidency, was ignored entirely.[70] As in 1880, it was as if two quite separate voices were speaking, with the voice of leniency repeatedly overridden by that of stringency. Huge questions had been raised in the concluding paragraphs of the 1898 report, but they were for the most part left unanswered, leaving provincial governments, in turn, quite unprepared to respond to another severe drought. Yet within months of its publication, the north-central and northwestern region of India was well along the path to yet another 'great' famine, that of 1899–1900.

Notes

1 *Report of the Indian Famine Commission* (London: HMSO, 1880), [hereafter *FCR* 1880].
2 B.M. Bhatia, *Famines in India* (Bombay: Asia Publishers House, 1963); H.S. Srivastava, *The History of Indian Famines, 1858–1918* (Agra: Sri Ram Mehra, 1968).
3 Srivastava, *History of Indian Famines*, 285–324.
4 T. Dyson, 'On the Demography of South Asian Famines,' *Population Studies*, 45, 1991, Parts 1 & 2, 5–25; 279–297; J. Drèze, 'Famine Prevention in India,' in J. Drèze, A. Sen, eds., *The Political Economy of Hunger*, Vol. 2 (Oxford: Clarendon Press, 1990), 13–122.

5 M. McAlpin, *Subject to Famine: Food Crises and Economic Change in Western India, 1860–1920* (Princeton, NJ: Princeton University Press, 1983); S. Guha, 'Mortality Decline in Early Twentieth Century India: A Preliminary Enquiry,' in S. Guha, ed., *Health and Population in South Asia: From Earliest Times to the Present* (London: Hurst, 2001), 86.

6 A. Maharatna, 'Regional Variation in Demographic Consequences of Famines in Late Nineteenth and Early Twentieth Century India,' *Economic and Political Weekly*, June 4, 1994, 1399–1410 [hereafter *EPW*]; __, *The Demography of Famines: An Indian Historical Perspective* (New Delhi: Oxford University Press, 1996). See also A.R. Vasavi, 'The Millet Drought': Oral Narratives and the Cultural Grounding of Famine-Relief in Bijapur,' *South Indian Studies*, 2, July–Dec. 1996, 205–233 at 218–220.

7 *FCR 1880*.

8 Revenue and Agriculture Department *Famine Proceedings*, 49, June 1883. The provincial Governments framed their individual codes upon the 1883 Provisional Famine Code, the GOI 'reserv[ing] the power of correcting errors . . . and giv[ing] final sanction to the Codes'; Srivastava, *History of Indian Famines*, 169.

9 The exception were famines during both World Wars when the Famine Code was not invoked in some affected provinces.

10 *FCR 1880*, Part III, *Famine Histories* (London: HMSO, 1885), 21, 45 [hereafter, *Famine Histories*].

11 G. Blyn, *Agricultural Trends in India, 1891–1947* (Philadelphia: University of Pennsylvania Press, 1966), 334; S. Guha, 'Introduction,' in S. Guha, ed., *Growth, Stagnation or Decline? Agricultural Productivity in British India* (New Delhi: Oxford University Press, 1992), 1–48.

12 M.A. Kaw, 'Famines in Kashmir, 1586–1819: The Policy of the Mughal and Afghan Rulers,' *IESHR*, 33, 1, 1966, 59–71; A. Loveday, *The History of Indian Famines* (London: G. Bell & Sons, 1914); D. Curley, 'Fair Grain Markets and Mughal Famine Policy in Late Eighteenth-Century Bengal,' *The Calcutta Historical Journal*, 7, 1, 1977, 1–27; David Hardiman, 'Usury, Dearth and Famine in Western India,' *Past and Present*, 152, Aug. 1996, 113–156. Jos Mooji, *Food Policy and the Indian State: The Public Distribution System in South India* (New Delhi: Oxford University Press, 1999), 64.

13 P. Will, R. Bin Wong, *Nourish the People: The State Granary System in China, 1650–1850* (Ann Arbor: University of Michigan, 1991).

14 For analysis of internecine warfare and food insecurity in South Asian history, see Deepak Lal, *Cultural Stability and Economic Stagnation, India c. 1500 BC – AD 1980* (Oxford: Clarendon Press, 1988), 47–48.

15 W.W. Hunter, *Annals in Rural Bengal* (London: Smith, Elder, 1868), 402; cited in Loveday, *History of Indian Famines*, 33.

16 'Famine Histories,' 22 [emphasis added]. For a detailed account of the 1837–1838 famine and its significance as 'the first when relief on "modern principles" was begun by the provision of "works of public utility",' see S. Sharma, *Famine, Philanthropy and the Colonial State* (New Delhi: Oxford University Press, 2001), ix.

17 S. Ambirajan, 'Malthusian Population Theory and Indian Famine Policy in the Nineteenth Century,' *Population Studies*, 30, 1, Mar. 1976, 5–14; __, *Classical Political Economy and British Rule in India* (Cambridge:

Cambridge University Press, 1978), ch. 3; __, 'Political Economy and Indian Famines,' *South Asia: Journal of South Asian Studies*, 1, 1, Aug. 1971, 20–27, at 22; L. Brennan, 'The Development of the Indian Famine Codes: Personalities, Politics and Policies,' in B. Currey, G. Hugo, eds., *Famine as a Geographic Phenomenon* (Dordrecht: D. Reidel Publishers, 1984), 91–111; P. Bandopadhyay, *Indian Famine and Agrarian Problems: A Study on the Administration of Lord George Hamilton, Secretary of State for India 1895–1903* (Calcutta: Star Publishers, 1987); M. Alamgir, *Famine in South Asia: Political Economy of Mass Starvation* (Cambridge, MA: Oelgeschlager, Gunn and Hain, 1980); A. Rangasami, 'Systems of Limited Intervention: An Evaluation of the Principles and Practice of Relief Administration in India,' in J. Floud, A. Rangasami, eds., *Famine and Society* (New Delhi: Indian Law Institute, 1993), 185–198; K. Currie, 'British Colonial Policy and Famines: Some Aspects and Implications of 'Free Trade' in the Bombay, Bengal and Madras Presidencies, 1860–1900,' *South Asia*, 14, 2, 1991, 23–56.

18 FCR 1880, 43; I. Klein, 'When the Rains Failed: Famine, Relief, and Mortality in British India,' *Indian Economic and Social History Review*, 21, 2, 1984, 185–214, at 192 [hereafter *IESHR*]; B. Mohanty, 'Orissa Famine of 1866: Demographic and Economic Consequences,' *EPW*, 28, 2–9, Jan. 1993, 55–66.

19 'Famine Histories,' 111–113, 125. Excess mortality across the 1873–1874 famine period was negligible, 'an illustration,' Klein observes, 'of the art of the possible'; 'When the Rains Failed,' 193.

20 Brennan, 'Development of the Indian Famine Codes,' 97; M. Davis, *Late Victorian Holocausts: El Niño, Famines and the Making of the Third World* (London: Verso, 2001). Maharatna estimates 1876–1878 famine 'excess' mortality as 8.2 million; *Demography of Famines*, 15.

21 *Report of the Sanitary Commissioner, Madras* 1877, 1878 [hereafter *MSCR*]; FCR 1880, Part II, 'Measures of Protection and Prevention,' 107.

22 N. Singh, *Starvation and Colonialism: A Study of Famines in the Nineteenth Century British Punjab 1858–1901* (New Delhi: National Book Organisation, 1996), 66, 204. See also D. Arnold, 'Famine in Peasant Consciousness and Peasant Action: Madras 1876–1878'; in R. Guha, ed., *Subaltern Studies III: Writings on South Asian History and Society* (New Delhi: Oxford University Press, 1984), 62–115; Hardiman, 'Usury, Dearth and Famine'; Sharma, *Famine, Philanthropy*), 79–134.

23 Prasannan Parthasarathi suggests cheaper subsistence labour costs in India had long been seen to undercut British textile exports and interests. Agricultural grain yields in India were more than double those in England in the 18th century, accounting in part for lower foodgrain prices and wages. Importing cheaper Indian wheat would lower British wage rates and manufacturing costs, leading to increased competitiveness with a previously dominant Indian textile industry. The export of Indian foodgrains also increased prices internally in South Asia, likewise helping reduce British:Indian wage differentials; 'Rethinking Wages and Competitiveness in the Eighteenth Century: Britain and South Asia,' *Past and Present*, 158, Feb. 1998, 79–109.

24 E. Stokes, *English Utilitarians and India* (Oxford: Clarendon Press, 1959), 134.

25 A. Cotton, *The Madras Famine* (London: Simpkin, Marshall, 1878), reprinted in A. Cotton, *Famine in India* (New York: Arno Press, 1976); Brennan, 'Development of the Indian Famine Codes,' 98.

26 In 'Sir George Couper and the Famine in the North Western Provinces,' a booklet published by *The Statesman*, containing the letters of Rev. T.J. Scott and its own editorials critical of famine relief; Bhatia, *Famines in India*, 99–100. See also, J.W. Furrell, 'Famines in India and the Duty of Government,' *The Calcutta Review*, LVIII, 5, 1874, 153–156, cited in Ambirajan, 'Malthusian Population Theory,' 87.

27 J. Gourlay, *Florence Nightingale and the Health of the Raj* (Aldershot, Hants: Ashgate, 2003); FCR 1880, 26.

28 J. Strachey to R. Strachey, Sept. 19, 1877; in Brenner, 'Development of the Indian Famine Codes,' 92. C.A. Elliott, Secretary to the Famine Commission argued, like Strachey, the inevitability of famine mortality: 'The campaign against famine, like other wars, if properly conducted must have its butcher's bill'; FCR 1880, Appendix II, 'Miscellaneous Papers bearing upon The Condition of the Country and People of India,' 110.

29 *Report of the Indian Famine Commission, 1898* (Simla: Government Central Printing Office, 1898), 255–256 [hereafter FCR 1898]. The Punjab government issued a Famine Code in 1888, prepared on the combined model of the Bombay Code Draft code and the 1883 Provisional Code, and was first used in 1891; Singh, *Starvation and Colonialism*, 184.

30 A. Sen, *Poverty and Famines: An Essay on Entitlement and Deprivation* (Oxford: Clarendon Press, 1981).

31 Klein estimates peak numbers on relief works as 3.5 million during the 1896–1897 famine and 2.7 million in 1899–1900, compared with 877,000 in 1876–1878; 'When the Rains Failed,' 190.

32 FCR 1898, 239; Brenner, 'Development of the Indian Famine Codes,' 106–107. See also, P. Gray, 'Famine and land in Ireland and India, 1845–1880: James Caird and the Political Economy of Hunger,' *The Historical Journal*, 49, 1, 2006, 193–215. Two of the five members of the 1880 Commission also dissented, J. Caird and H.E. Sullivan; FCR, 1880, 86–92.

33 *Circular*, 2 Famine, dated Dec. 27, 1899, from GOI Press, Revenue & Agriculture Department to Government Punjab; in Punjab Revenue Department, *The Punjab Famine of 1899–1900*, Vol. 2, Lahore, 1901, 103–106 [hereafter FCR (Punjab), 1900–01].

34 Dreze, 'Famine Prevention in India,' 29.

35 Klein, 'When the Rains Failed,' 197; FCR 1880, 57; FCR 1898, 246.

36 FCR (Punjab) 1900, Vol. 1, 25.

37 The 1898 Famine Commission acknowledged that test work wages had often fallen to the minimum Code wage 'in recent years'; FCR 1898, 243. The maximum (digger) wage was two annas; providing 2,200 calories with grain prices at 20 seers per rupee; D. Kumar, *Land and caste in South India: Agricultural Labour in the Madras Presidency during the Nineteenth Century* (Cambridge: Cambridge University Press, 1965), 146.

38 FCR 1880, 57.

39 FCR 1880, 80–81. By comparison, 1962 Maharashtra famine relief wage rates were 18 *chhataks* or 36 ounces; 16 ounces for non-working dependants; Government of Maharashtra, *The Bombay Scarcity Manual* (draft) (Bombay: Revenue Department, 1962), 46–52.

40 FCR 1898, 256. Some gratuitous relief was provided at village level to the elderly and infirm incapable of labouring on the distant works. But young dependants of those on relief works were required to reside on the works to qualify for this relief.

41 W. Digby, *The Famine Campaign in Southern India 1876–1878*, Vol. 2 (London: Longmans Green, 1878), 254.

42 Modern recommended caloric intake for children 4–6 years of age is 1,690; 7–9 years, 1950; adult females (moderate work), 2,225; adult males, 2,875; adult males (heavy work), 3,800, levels that include a safety margin of up to two standard deviations; C. Gopalan, B.V. Ramasastri, S.C. Balasubramanian, *Nutritive Value of Indian Foods* (Hyderabad: National Institute of Nutrition, 1995).

43 Half the workers on a large relief work in Bombay Presidency in 1896–1897 were reported to be receiving the penal wage of 15 ounces; and the remaining, the minimum wage; V. Nash, *The Great Famine* (London: Longmans Green, 1901), 32; as cited in *Famines in India*, 256.

44 FCR 1880, 36.

45 Ibid., 48–49.

46 'Famine Histories,' 146.

47 FCR 1880, 76, 75.

48 Ibid., 75, 74 [emphasis added].

49 Ibid., 74; *Famines in India*, 121.

50 FCR (Punjab), 1900–01, 103.

51 The Commission also assumed the 1876–1877 crop shortfall of 6 million tons as the worst harvest shortfall to be expected; FCR 1880, 68–69. Yet harvest losses in 1918 would reach almost 18 million tons (Table 10.1).

52 FCR 1880, 73.

53 Ibid., 88–91.

54 MSCR 1877, 8–9; A.P. Macdonnell, *Report on the Food-Grain Supply and Famine Relief in Behar and Bengal, 1873–1874* (Calcutta: Bengal Secretariat Press, 1876), 8. The practice of storing *ragi* in underground pits was reported as declining in Mysore state by the 1870s under pressure of the emerging grain trade and 'the more rigorous system of collecting the land tax'; A.K. Connell, 'Indian Railways and Indian Wheat,' *Royal Statistical Society*, 48, June 1885, 248–249.

55 Connell, 'Indian Railways,' 249; FCR (Punjab) 1898, Exts., v. W.R. Cornish detailed the storage of *cholum* and *ragi* in Southern India in 'underground pits . . . excavated to a depth of 10 or 12 feet. . . [and] usually made to hold about 10,000 seers of grain each; MSCR 1876, 12; FCR 1901, Appendix, Vol. 5, 'Evidence of Witnesses, Madras, Bengal, NWPs, Punjab and Ajmer,' 3–4.

56 PLRA 1891–1892, Exts., 18–19.

57 S.E. O'Conor, *Prices and Wages in India* (Calcutta: GOI Department Finance and Commerce, 1886), 14–19.

58 N. Bhattacharya, 'Agricultural Labour and Production: Central and South-east Punjab,' in K.N. Raj et al., eds., *Essays on the Commercialization of Indian Agriculture* (New Delhi: Oxford University Press, 1985), 105–162, Figs. II (b), III. See also, H. Banerjee, *Agrarian Society of the Punjab (1849–1901)* (New Delhi: Manohar, 1982), 191; C. Bates, 'Review of *Subject to Famine*,' *Modern Asian Studies*, 19, 1985, 868.

59 M. Twomey, 'Employment in nineteenth Century Indian Textiles,' *Explorations in Economic History*, 20, 1983, 52, cited in B.R. Tomlinson, 'The Economy of Modern India, 1860–1970,' in *The New Cambridge Economic History of India*, Vol. 3 (Cambridge: Cambridge University Press, 1993), 102.

60 Three years earlier, with the subcontinent in the throes of severe famine, Sir John Strachey, described 'high prices. . . [as] the salvation of a country, [since] consumption not essential is sternly checked, and the reduction of stocks is lessened'; *The Indian Famine of 1877*. Statement made in the Legislative Council of the Governor-General of Calcutta, on December 27, 1877 (London: Kegan Paul, 1878), 34–35.

61 'Dissent on certain points,' *FCR* 1880, 89–90.

62 *FCR* 1898, 176.

63 *FCR* 1901, 4; L. Brennan, L. Leathcote, A. Lucas, 'The Causation of Famine: A Comparative Analysis of Lombok and Bengal 1891–1974,' *South Asia*, 7, 1, 1984, 1–26. Criticised by the 1898 Commission as 'unduly lenient,' the Madras provincial administration was unrepentant, defending its decision to raise wage rates to 48 ounces in Mar. 1897 by pointing to lower mortality rates and arguing the higher expenditure was sound economic investment because 'the famine will leave few permanent traces behind it'; *FCR* 1898, 270, 180–181; Bhatia, *Famines in India*, 248–249.

64 *FCR* 1898, 175.

65 The crude death rate reached 69.3 per 1,000 in the Central Provinces in 1897 and 52.6 in Berar compared with 25.4 per 1,000 in Madras; *Statistical Abstract relating to British India* (London: HMSO, 1840–1920).

66 The 1901 Census estimated famine mortality across the 1891–1900 decade as 5 million; *General Report of the Census of India, 1901* (London: HMSO, 1904), 84. Kingsley Davis estimated 6 million 'excess' deaths in the two famine years of 1897 and 1900; *The Population of India and Pakistan* (New York: Princeton University Press, 1951), 36, 39.

67 *FCR* 1898, 260, 271–273.

68 Ibid., 220.

69 Ibid., 208.

70 Ibid., 318, 186, 354.

11 The shift to famine prevention

The folly of collecting revenue from people, who by reason of severe drought have no food in their houses, and whose credit with the grain-dealer is well nigh exhausted, seems obvious, but in this matter routine has sometimes proved strong enough to overpower common sense.
  – H.K. Trevaskis, *The Punjab of Today* (Lahore: 'Civil and Military Gazette' Press, 1931), 161.

The 1901 Famine Commission Report

It would be the 1901 Famine Commission, under the chairmanship of A.P. MacDonnell (1844–1925), that succeeded in turning around the ideological ship of state from mitigation of 'established famine' to one of famine prevention. Considered 'by far the most capable administrator' in India,[1] the larger significance of the MacDonnell appointment lay in his role three decades earlier as district Collector in the successful famine relief program in northwestern Bihar, then part of the Bengal Presidency. In the wake of the 'great' famine of 1899–1900, no longer was the 1873–1874 Bengal famine cited as an example of profuse and unnecessary famine relief expenditure, but rather as one in which 'a great principle was finally asserted; and methods of relief administration were devised.'[2]

That 'great principle' was the preventability of famine mortality, and of 'famine' itself. Up to this point, the administration had consciously set limits to the responsibility it was willing to assume for famine-related deaths. Deaths due to epidemic disease in the course of a famine, the 1880 Famine Commission had argued, were inherently beyond the means of the State to control. Citing the 1879 'severe outbreak of malarial fever' in the northwest (Punjab and the Northwest Provinces), it contended that 'no scarcity whatever existed' to explain the high mortality; thus, it concluded, 'the hope that any human endeavours will altogether prevent an increase of mortality during a severe famine is untenable.'[3]

MacDonnell emphatically rejected this 'fatalistic view.' In 11 pages of detailed analysis of 1899–1900 famine mortality, the 1901 report pointed out that deaths were due largely to ordinary (endemic) infectious diseases simply rendered more lethal by starvation. Singling out the enormous autumn mortality at the close of the 1900 famine, he insisted that '[o]f fevers, it can only be said that they often are *in origin* climatic, but their *fatality* is, owing to the reduced power of the people to resist them, largely due to famine.'[4] Government, in other words, could not be absolved from responsibility for such deaths.

Gone was the rote optimism about the 'recuperative powers of the peasantry' that so characterised the 1880 report. Instead, 1901 Census figures were cited, showing population decline in many provincial jurisdictions, the entire decade ending with the 1899–1900 famine one of general 'misfortune and distress.'[5] Gone as well were lingering Malthusian assumptions that relief was only postponing the day of reckoning for the 'surplus' poor. In their place now was a sense of urgency to 'get it right,' in no small measure impelled by growing recognition of the profound consequences of recurrent famine on the agricultural economy.[6] Criticism of past errors and 'misconceptions' was unequivocal, at times scathing. Test works in Bombay in 1899 had been 'unduly prolonged' which led to 'disastrous' delays in initiating any form of relief. The strict conditions imposed on requests for agricultural loans came in for special criticism, along with 'the desire of the subordinate officials to avoid all risk.' Even those loans granted often came too late and so lost 'a great deal of their value.'[7]

While criticising specific administrative failures, the 1901 report also targeted inadequacies in the Famine Code itself. Long delays in establishing gratuitous relief was 'one cause of the great mortality,' an issue that 'was touched, but only lightly, by the Commission of 1898; it was scarcely even considered by the previous [1880] Commission.' Likewise, 'village works were heavily discounted . . . by the universal absence of a programme,'[8] again a problem directly attributable to the framework of relief set forth by the 1880 Famine Commission.

Shift to village-level employment generation

Beyond critiquing past failures, the 1901 Commission's central task was articulation of a fundamentally different framework for state intervention in times of harvest failure. The general principles were similar to those of the 1883 Famine Code – an early warning system, preparedness, and employment generation. But the approach to the latter differed radically. Up to this point, village-level relief had been limited mainly to gratuitous (free) relief for the infirm and aged. What was proposed in 1901 was making support for village agriculture the primary locus for employment generation. Village works were

> more economical, more useful, less exposed to outbreaks of cholera and epidemic disease, less open to . . . interference with the labour market, neglect of agricultural dwellings and stock. . . [and] less likely to loosen moral and domestic ties.[9]

Success hinged above all on public confidence in official support from the earliest stages of distress. Officials were exhorted to 'give heart to the people' in a 'moral strategy' to pre-empt constriction of local credit and agricultural operations. 'It is scarcely possible to overstate the tonic effect upon the people, of *early* preparation, of an *early* enlistment of non-official agency, of liberal advances in the *earliest* stages, and of *early* action in regard to suspensions of revenue.' In contrast to previous 'wait and see' policy, this required publication early on of a comprehensive plan to demonstrate clarity of purpose and method as well as devolution of control to the rural communities themselves.[10]

The new strategy thus marked a fundamental change in the timing of relief. Under the 1883 Code, no action was taken until sufficient resort to test works signalled a formal declaration of famine. Under the 1901 proposals, 'relief' was initiated *before* there was any certainty or official declaration of famine, to include 'liberal advances' for the repair and construction of wells, and purchase of seed for the coming *rabi* season. Adequate preparation, the Commission acknowledged, meant accepting financial risk. '[M]oney spent in preparation may, indeed, be wasted, but the loss is trifling in comparison with the expenditure which want of preparation entails'[11] – a stance starkly at odds with Sir John Strachey's 1878 admonition to 'choose to err on the side of too little rather than too much.'[12] Loans were to be made not on an individual basis but as a general policy so as to be available immediately to convince agriculturalists of the state's support. This required devolution of spending authority to allow lower level officials on tour to distribute agricultural loans 'on the spot.' Lists also were to be drawn up for suspensions and remissions of the land tax and for gratuitous relief,[13] to be available immediately in the event that drought proceeded to formal declaration of famine. Liberal and early expenditure was the key to ultimate cost-effectiveness. '[E]conomy' ultimately lay instead in assuring subsequent harvests and hastening recovery from drought. Pragmatism, in other words, was replacing punitiveness, deterrence, and ideology as the central informing principle.

Large public works might still be required, the Commission acknowledged, but they would no longer be the 'backbone' of relief.[14] Wherever possible, they were to be located nearby, thus enabling cultivators as well as agricultural labourers to attend to their animal stocks and prepare for resumption of agricultural activities. Moreover, the distance test was categorically rejected, the 1901 Commission 'condemn[ing]' earlier compulsory residency requirements.[15] It also recommended abolishing the 'penal wage,' arguing that regular resort to fining in Bombay in the 1899–1900 famine had been as much the result of administrative failure to provide sufficient employment at public works sites as reluctance of relief workers to work. To avoid the problem of 'contumacy,' work requirements 'must be carefully matched to capability.' Weaker persons were now to be placed in separate gangs to ensure reduced and 'sufficiently elastic' task loads[16] rather than being penalised by a reduced wage, one inadequate to bring them back to a state of health. Here, the Commission was challenging the central 'moral' principle of the 1883 Code that based payment (food rations) on work output rather than need.

Filling in the gaps

The report then turned to address gaps in relief access. Prompt admission and initial relief of new comers onto large relief works was essential: past delays had 'occasioned much suffering.' It condemned 'the evils of deferred [weekly] payment,' recognising this involved considerable reduction of the wage by forcing the workers to live upon credit with local moneylenders or the headman of the work gang, entailing onerous interest rates. It condemned, as well, the practice of across-the-board wage reductions, pointing out the obvious, that this 'affect(s) the weak and the needy far more than those who do not require relief.' For those who still 'cling to the works' after other employment is available, this should be done, it advised, only through raising tasks rather than reducing wages, and even at that, only for the able-bodied. Even here, they added, 'To be on the safe side, it. . . [should] require the sanction of the Commissioner.'[17] Here, again, the basic framework of relief administration was being turned upside down: now it was punitive measures, rather than lenient, that required special sanction.

This attention to relief continuity culminated with four and a half pages devoted to 'Rains Policy.' Like the 1898 report, the 1901 commissioners recognised the final stage of famine as the most hazardous. But unlike earlier reports, the 1901 report provided explicit procedures.

> *[B]efore* the rains break, and in time for the prudent use of the money, advances for cattle and seed should be given [to] . . . set free the capital of the country for agricultural effort. . . . [A]s the hot weather draws to its close, [those] people, if employed on large works, should be dispersed over small public works near their homes and village works.[18]

Here, however, they cautioned that a 'few [large] works should always be kept open, to meet any unexpected contraction in the labour market.' Above all, the 1901 Commission stressed the much greater need for gratuitous relief during the rains which should continue until the ripening of the first crops. Even at this point, those still in receipt of relief were to receive a two-week 'valedictory dole.'[19]

This attention to relief continuity distinguishes the 1901 report from all previous official famine policy. It was as if the authors had finally placed themselves in the 'shoes,' or bare-feet, of the starvation-vulnerable, thinking through the question 'How do they eat?' each step of the way from initial failed rains to re-establishment of regular village agricultural economic activity. It was a strategy based on pragmatic understanding that a single interval of starvation, if only a few weeks' duration, could render all previous effort and expenditure ineffective in terms of 'the ultimate test of lives saved.'[20]

Granted, the amount eaten was carefully calculated – one could argue, with the same exquisite attention – to be not an ounce more than bare subsistence, and in individual cases perhaps not even that. Indeed, maximum wage rates recommended in the report for famine relief works were marginally lower than those recommended by the 1898 Famine Commission, 36 ounces rather than 40. Upward revisions were made, however, for children: 20 ounces for those over 10 years; for young children, the daily allowance was doubled to eight ounces; and the recommended age of working children raised from 7 years to 10.[21]

It was the 1901 Famine Commission Report as well that categorically rejected use of relief 'kitchens' as a general measure of relief for those unable to work. Aside from being 'more costly than the dole [gratuitous relief],' the 'ill-cooked food materially affect[ed] the health of people.' Revulsion to cooked food relief, they pointed out, was acknowledged in earlier reports but never acted upon. Used in effect 'as a test of distress' in 1899–1900, relief kitchens had been resorted to in unprecedented numbers, and in the Bombay Presidency the policy 'was carried out with a certain want of intelligence,' with people in one district expected to travel to a kitchen if they lived within eight miles of it.[22]

Dry, practical, in no sense could these changes be considered lenient. But together, they reduced gaps in food access, allowing those facing imminent starvation to survive the period of acute famine. Their impact no doubt was wider still: increasing levels of resistance to disease when return of the monsoon rains brought famine to a close but renewed malaria transmission as well.

The broader diagnosis

The 'pre-emptive' task also involved reducing underlying vulnerability to harvest-fluctuations, the larger agenda for Macdonnell's 1901 Famine Commission report. Citing 1901 Census figures confirming population decline in large regions of British India between 1891 and 1901, the final portion of the report thus turned to broader agricultural policy questions.[23] Land revenue policy, 'protective' irrigation, and rural credit and debt were extraordinarily sensitive subjects, all of them lying at the heart of the anti-imperialist critique. Among them, agriculture taxation was the most politically contentious, producing revenues upon which the fiscal and ideological foundation of the imperial project rested.

It has often been assumed that under the 19th-century land revenue system of the British Raj, remissions were granted in years of poor harvests.[24] Yet remissions were intended solely for 'unforeseen accidents': *localised* hailstorms, crop pests, or very unusual flood conditions. Drought-induced losses, by contrast, were considered a predictable calamity 'arising from the normal vicissitudes of the season,' and qualified only for temporary deferment ('suspension') of land revenue demand – and, even here, generally only when harvest failure was both severe and widespread.[25] Such recurring losses, it was argued, were 'anticipated by the Settlement officer in framing his [tax] assessments.'[26]

In practice, the term 'suspension' was largely a euphemism for land revenue that local officials were unable to collect.[27] During the severe drought of 1878–1879, for example, 95 per cent of land revenue was collected in the worst affected tracts of Punjab. Even where granted, official sanction for suspensions generally came late in the course of a famine in an effort to discourage others from applying for relief.[28] If uncollected for three years despite a battery of coercive legal measures, the 'suspension' was ultimately recorded as a 'remission.' These rules continued to apply under the 1883 Famine Code: during the 'great' famine years of the late 19th-century, remissions granted were negligible (Table 11.1, col. 3).[29]

It has been assumed also that land revenue demand by the turn of the century was so low 'that the economic impact of post-1900 taxation changes could not have been large.'[30] Yet while not excessive by earlier historical standards, the impact of inflexible tax collection on smallholders most certainly was oppressive.[31] The assumption that cultivators would have surplus in normal years to save for payments in years of drought may have applied to larger landowners, but it ignored the position of subsistence cultivators, many of whom resorted to wage labour even in good years to fill in seasonal consumption (hunger) gaps. Forty per cent of cultivators 'in the Delhi area' in the 1930s, for example, had no surplus to sell even in normal harvest years and another 33 per cent 'had to part with all of their surplus to pay their debts.' Only 27 per cent of cultivators were in a position 'to market their surplus for profit.'[32] The standard tax rate in Punjab from the 1860s was one-half 'net assets,' after deducting cultivation costs including that of labour.[33] This demand amounted to 12 per cent of a 'normal' harvest. For subsistence households, a 50 per cent harvest loss – not infrequent – meant hunger even before taxation. But the fixed tax levy reduced this further, leaving 38 per cent of an average harvest, an amount that could not begin to cover costs of production and subsistence needs.

Aside from the highly regressive character of the policy, the smallholder was at a further disadvantage. In requiring immediate payment in cash rather than in kind, those households without grain reserves were forced to sell their crops when prices were at their lowest level, and then to purchase grains at the end of the agricultural year for household consumption when prices were highest. Coercive methods, not surprisingly, were routinely required to collect the land revenue. All but the larger ('surplus') landowners were forced to borrow to pay in years of crop failure, often under 'great oppression.'[34] Tax demands in such years came at a critical point of acute depletion of assets. For tenants, landowners demanded payment well in advance of the government collection, itself demanded before the marketing of the harvested crops.[35] Inelastic taxation also applied to harvest failure caused by flooding, an issue of particular economic significance for Punjab.

Even where suspensions were granted, as in the two 'great' famines of the late 1890s, cultivators were required to pay back the suspended amount at the first good harvest in addition to the current year's demand, when all possible resources were needed instead to make up famine-induced losses of seed and cattle and to repay debts. Thus, despite notional adoption of suspensions as a form of indirect famine relief within the 1883 Famine Code, in practice, the rigid land revenue system remained largely intact through to 1900, despite vocal concerns by experienced local officials over increasing rural indebtedness. S.S. Thorburn, former Commissioner of Rawalpindi Division, calculated that over the final three decades of the 19th century, a period of 'several prolonged fodder famines and quite a dozen poor harvests' in Sialkot district, suspensions had totalled a mere Rs 6,450 and remissions Rs 1,694 on account of hail.[36]

During the 1896–1897 and 1899–1990 famines, larger sums were ultimately suspended, in Punjab amounting to Rs 2 million and 4.3 million respectively out of a total tax demand of Rs 26 million.[37] In effect, individual peasant cultivators could hope for temporary tax deferment only when they shared their ruinous conditions with literally millions of others. Remissions granted, however, during these 'great' famine years were negligible amounting to 13,128 rupees in 1896–1897, and in 1899–1900, 4,838 rupees.[38] Singling out the Punjab administration, the 1901 Famine Commission pointed to the province's 1897 reluctance to grant remissions as another 'great evil,' and attributed failure of economic recovery leading up to the 1899–1900 famine to rigid tax collection.[39] It was not until 1901–1902, after the tabling of the 1901 Famine Commission Report, that the backlog of suspensions from these two major famine years was finally remitted (Table 11.1, col. 4).

As a policy to impoverish and force subsistence producers to mortgage their land, the inelastic land revenue system could hardly have been more effective. In theory, government agricultural loans *(takavi)* were intended to offset such capital drain. In practice, this rarely was the case. Despite the Agriculturist (loan) Acts of 1883 and 1884, the 1885–1895 decade that encompassed several years of severe harvest losses in Punjab saw an average of 50,000 rupees *takavi* loans granted per year: a minute fraction of the land revenue collected annually from the province.[40] The 1894–1895 Punjab Land Revenue Administration report explained the 'unpopularity' of these loans as due to 'the adoption of stringent measures by the Revenue authorities for recovery.'[41] Loans did increase substantially during the major famines of 1896–1897 and 1899–1900 to Rs 1.6 million and 2.8 million respectively in Punjab. Yet much of the potential benefit was lost due to zealously cautious administration[42] and bureaucratic delays accompanying individual assessment.[43]

Table 11.1 Annual suspensions and remissions of land tax (in 100,000 Rs), Punjab, 1888–1939

	Suspensions during year	Amount under suspension remitted during the year	Remissions due to current year calamities	Total remissions during current year*
	1	2	3	4
1888–1889	n.a.	n.a.	0.1	1.4
1889–1890	n.a.	n.a.	<0.1	0.2
1890–1891	2.0	0.7	1.3	2.1
1891–1892	3.5	0.3	0.1	0.9
1892–1893	0.6	0.4	0.2	1.1
1893–1894	0.3	0.4	0.3	0.9
1894–1895	0.5	0.3	0.7	1.2
1895–1896	4.8	0.3	0.3	0.7
1896–1897	20.0	0.3	0.2	0.7
1897–1898	1.6	0.2	0.1	0.4
1898–1899	10.2	0.5	0.3	1.1
1899–1900	43.1	3.1	<0.1	6.4
1900–1901	2.5	3.4	0.1	6.2
1901–1902	25.6	42.5	8.4	80.8
1902–1903	12.2	1.1	0.1	2.3
1903–1904	3.8	0.0	0.1	0.1
1904–1905	4.5	3.4	0.2	4.2
1905–1906	22.8	4.6	0.6	9.7
1906–1907	3.7	5.2	1.0	10.4
1907–1908	40.8	1.7	0.4	3.3
1908–1909	4.8	2.1	0.5	3.1
1909–1910	1.0	7.5	0.2	8.0
1910–1911	0.7	0.8	0.2	1.5
1911–1912	13.7	0.5	0.2	1.0
1912–1913	4.6	0.2	0.2	0.7
1913–1914	7.6	0.7	<0.1	0.8
1914–1915	1.4	0.5	n.a.	n.a.
1915–1916	12.8	0.3	0.3	0.6
1916–1917	0.6	0.2	0.2	0.4
1917–1918	3.8	1.3	0.5	1.8
1918–1919	22.4	0.4	<0.1	0.5
1919–1920	2.7	0.9	0.3	1.0
1920–1921	30.0	0.8	<0.1	0.8
1921–1922	8.3	2.1	0.7	2.8
1922–1923	1.0	0.8	0.1	1.0
1923–1924	1.8	0.7	0.2	2.6
1924–1925	2.1	0.5	2.9	1.5
1925–1926	5.2	1.2	0.9	n.a.
1926–1927	2.9	0.8	0.3	n.a.

	Suspensions during year	Amount under suspension remitted during the year	Remissions due to current year calamities	Total remissions during current year*
1927–1928	n.a.	n.a.	n.a.	n.a.
1928–1929	20.2	1.9	0.8	4.1
1929–1930	22.9	1.6	4.7	8.3
1930–1931	16.2	13.9	<0.1	14.5
1931–1932	9.3	16.4	0.1	17.5
1932–1933	19.6	19.2	0.3	20.3
1933–1934	3.6	5.9	15.2	23.1
1934–1935	13.0	7.9	0.6	10.7
1935–1936	8.5	3.3	0.5	6.4
1936–1937	7.8	8.3	0.6	16.5
1937–1938	18.8	6.9	1.0	14.4
1938–1939	35.3	7.6	2.0	15.9

Source: J. Lindauer, Sarjit Singh, *Land Taxation and Indian Economic Development*, Delhi: Kalyani Publ., 1979.

*includes 'remissions due to former year calamities'

Remarkably, the 1901 Famine Commission Report presented the problem of taxation-induced indebtedness as indisputable, one no longer worthy of debate. It harkened back to 1831 recommendations that had urged 'elasticity in the collection of the land tax,' opinions intentionally ignored in the belief that it was important 'to get land out of the hands of the cultivators unable to pay their way and to transfer it to cultivators with more capital.'[44] The view that land should be transferred to larger holders in the interests of agricultural development reflected three centuries of ideological argument in support of enclosure in England and Ireland.[45] Transposed to India, the utilitarian thesis, buttressed by Malthusian 'overpopulation' theory, informed colonial economic thought and taxation policy through much of 19th century British rule.[46] Here, the frankness of Macdonnell's accusation signalled a frontal challenge to prevailing economic orthodoxy, one that possibly could only be levelled with such credibility by an Irish nationalist chairman deeply conversant with its famine consequences in Ireland a half-century earlier.[47]

The 1901 Famine Commission land revenue recommendations were unequivocal: suspension of revenue demand must be pre-emptive, extensive, and expeditiously granted, and not restricted to years of disastrous crop failure. They were followed by a further five and a half pages devoted to the subject of agricultural development and the urgent need for 'popular institutions for organized credit . . . at the very doors of the cultivator,' in effect, a blueprint for at least partial redirection of government funds from rail and canal construction to village-level 'minor' irrigation works such as wells and tanks.[48]

Famine relief after 1901

The question remains to what extent the 1901 Famine Commission's recommendations were acted upon. Many have argued that the Government of India remained far more receptive to spending on famine relief measures – acute crisis management – than on broader-based agricultural development,[49] and this appears to have been largely the case. A special commission was appointed within months of the 1901 Famine Commission Report's submission, charged with inquiring into expansion of irrigation across rural British India. Pointing to the 'scandal' of famine, the Irrigation Commission's 1903 report decried the extent to which small-scale village irrigation systems had been allowed to fall into 'disrepair so serious as to diminish largely, and in some case, even destroy altogether, their efficiency.' It called for reinvestment in 'protective' village irrigation works, and for such 'small works' to form the 'backbone' of famine relief rather than large canal projects,[50] as articulated in the 1901 Famine Commission Report.[51] Yet these recommendations failed to be fully embraced.[52] In the case of Punjab, irrigation investment continued to be directed mainly to massive canal irrigation projects. By 1940, well irrigation had increased by only 25 per cent to 4.9 million acres, whereas canal irrigation reached 11.7 million.[53]

Nonetheless, fundamental changes in the nature of acute crisis relief did take place, with the 1901 Famine Commission Report now 'the standard authority on famine prevention and relief' over the final decades of colonial rule.[54]

1907–1908 famine in the United Provinces

The decade following the 1900 famine was marked, like the decade before it, by a number of poor harvest years. The 1907–1908 drought across north-central India was the most severe, by any account qualifying in turn-of-the-century terminology as a 'great famine,' with British India foodgrain output at 39.7 million tons considerably below even 1899–1990 levels. Hardest hit were the United Provinces to the east of Punjab, where crop failure was estimated at well over 7 million tons out of a normal harvest of 12 million, losses following upon two previous drought years. 'Such figures,' the subsequent Famine Commission Report observed, 'are too great to be easily grasped; there is probably no other country in the world except China where calamities on this scale are possible.'[55]

Provincial response was immediate. Along with early suspension of land revenue demand, Rs 12.8 million in loans and advances were distributed in October–November 1907 in an effort to counter contraction in credit and ensure the following winter *(rabi)* harvest. It was strategy lifted virtually verbatim from the 1901 Famine Commission Report: to 'encourage the people to continue to work in the fields and to sow as large an area as possible of spring crops instead of crowding on to relief works.' So great was the demand for labour that wage rates rose in some districts, rather than dropping as was typical in times of drought. Sown areas 'doubled or even tripled with the aid of advances' in many districts, and in spite of late and inadequate winter rains, a 1908 *rabi* harvest 60 per cent of normal was eventually harvested.[56]

By the final days of 1907, additional employment generation, however, was required in many tracts. In December, famine was officially declared and large public works were set up in five districts, increasing to 19 districts by March 1908. In a major departure from even 1901 recommendations, normal market wage rates were offered to relief workers in some areas in the later stages of the famine. Gratuitous relief was given to dependents of relief workers, ultimately amounting to 54 per cent of the total persons relieved, a level above even that recommended by the 1901 Famine Commission. Among those newly qualifying for gratuitous relief were children 7 to 10 years, no longer required to labour on relief works.[57]

Numbers on relief peaked in March 1908 at 1.4 million, and with the approach of summer rains many were shifted to village-level relief, with corresponding expansion of village-aided works and gratuitous relief. Closure of the larger works was carried out to ensure continuity of relief at village level. Lists of dependents, arranged by villages, were sent to local circle officers. 'To obviate all risks, all dependents, or their guardians, were given an advance of [one and two weeks'] allowance . . . to enable them to subsist until . . . registered for gratuitous relief.'[58] At the same time, additional loans were advanced for the summer sowing and gratuitous relief was further expanded, peaking at 550,000 persons by early August. All those still on large works were discharged with a one-month food dole.[59]

This attention to continuity of relief was unprecedented. Arup Maharatna's demographic study of the 1907–1908 U.P. famine confirms that mortality rose only marginally during the actual famine period, despite the severity and geographic extent of preceding harvest losses.[60] This contrasts with earlier famines, he points out, where mortality generally rose *in spite of* rising numbers on relief works.[61] Interestingly, he further shows that the 1907–1908 famine was the only major colonial period famine where correlation between severity of district crop failure and mortality was low, and attributed this to 'liberal and rational' relief in the famine-designated districts.[62]

Death rates for U.P. as a whole, however, did rise sharply by 34.6 per cent in the final months of 1908. Much of this increase however occurred in the western-most districts of the province, those districts bordering Punjab that had not been officially designated as famine-affected and which had received very limited, or no, relief over the course of the famine (Table 11.2). Here, autumnal malaria was

Table 11.2 Crude death rate (per 1,000), by district, United Provinces, 1908

District	CDR (per 1,000)	District	CDR (per 1,000)
Bareilly	81.2	Mainpuri	53.4
Budaun	78.8	Fatepur	52.1
Muttra	77.9	Muzaffargarh	50.6
Hardoi	75.2	**Sultanpur**	50.5
Agra	72.7	**Banda**	48.7
Moradabad	72.6	Saranpur	48.0
Farrukhabad	72.6	**Gonda**	48.0
Shahjahanpur	71.3	**Hamirpur**	47.0
Pilibhit	70.0	Partabgarh	46.2
Bijnor	69.1	**Mirzapur**	45.1
Aligarh	66.6	Benares	45.1
Etah	66.6	**Jaunpur**	45.1
Bulandshahr	66.6	**Fyzabad**	44.7
Cawnpore	62.6	Allahabad	44.1
Jalaun	62.0	**Jhansi**	42.7
Kheri	60.7	**Basti**	40.9
Lucknow	60.4	Almora	39.7
Etahwah	59.8	Garhwal	39.6
Sitapur	59.4	Azaragarh	38.1
Unao	56.7	Nainital	35.2
Rae Bareili	56.5	Ghazipur	33.3
Meerut	55.3	Gorakpur	31.5
Bahraich	55.1	Dehra Dun	29.7
Bara Banki	53.6	Bhallia	27.4

Note: 'Famine'-declared districts in bold.

Source: *Annual Report, Sanitary Commissioner*, U.P. (1908).

visited upon on a population stressed by poor crops and famine-level foodgrain prices, hardship compounded by severe floods bordering the Jumna river, and Punjab.[63] By contrast, among the 19 'famine' districts, only four experienced Sept.–Dec. fever death rates substantially above the provincial mean of 23.9 in 1908, and two of these were bordering Punjab (Table 11.3).

The relative success of 1907–1908 relief in the famine districts of the United Provinces has been attributed by some to increased opportunities for emigration out of the famine-affected tracts.[64] But the official provincial famine report suggests that famine migration in 1907–1908 was not marked, observing that 'there was no organized movement of the population from the distressed areas in search of work . . . and in fact no noticeable wandering at all.'[65] Even assuming optimistically that all those who did emigrate were successful in finding employment,

Table 11.3 Sept.–Dec. fever death rate (per 1,000), by district, United Provinces, 1908

'Famine' districts		'Scarcity' districts		'Normal' districts	
Muttra	52.8	Budaun	48.9	Bulandshahr	43.8
Agra	42.0	Bareilly	46.2	**Aligarh**	41.1
Hardoi	40.7	**Moradabad**	39.3	**Meerut**	30.7
Etawah	29.6	**Farrukhabad**	36.5	**Muzaffarnagar**	30.0
Jalaun	27.6	**Etah**	36.2	Saharanpur	24.5
Sitapur	24.2	Pilibhit	35.5	Partagarh	16.6
Bara Banki	21.1	**Bijnor**	34.2	Naini Tal	14.6
Kheri	20.1	Shahjahanpur	33.5	Gorakhpur	6.9
Sultanpur	20.1	**Mainpuri**	30.4		
Banda	17.2	Unao	28.8		
Hamirpur	17.2	Lucknow	27.4		
Fyzabad	15.3	Rae Bareli	26.2		
Jhansi	15.2	Cawnpore	24.9		
Bahraich	15.0	Fatehpur	19.2		
Allahabad	14.6	Azamgarh	12.8		
Gonda	13.9	Ghazipur	12.3		
Jaunpur	12.3	Benares	10.6		
Mirzapur	12.1	Dehra Dun	9.7		
Basti	10.5	Ballia	9.2		
		Almore	9.2		
		Garhwal	9.2		

Note: Western Jumna-Ganges doab districts are in bold.

Source: J. Chaytor White, 'Report on the outbreak of malarial fever in the United Provinces during the period September to December 1908,' *Records of the Malaria Survey of India*, 1, 2, Mar. 1930, 114–130.

it seems unlikely their numbers were comparable to the 1.4 million persons on relief in early 1908, in addition, that is, to those directly engaged in village agriculture by virtue of *takavi* advances. What also distinguished relief during the 1907–1908 famine was the large increase in indirect forms of relief, loans and advances totalling over 27 million rupees, whereas direct relief (public works and gratuitous relief), as substantial as it was, reached 16.8 million rupees. By comparison, total loans and advances across all six provinces in the 1896–1897 famine amounted to 18.4 million rupees.[66]

The experience of famine relief in 1907–1908 thus suggests marked movement away from the earlier restricted and punitive character of relief – beyond even those recommendations embraced by the 1901 Famine Commission. This shift reflected growing recognition that famine prevention was not simply imperative politically but was in the economic interests of government as well. 'The rapidity with which the country resumed its normal conditions was extraordinary,' the 1908 U.P. famine report remarked, 'and is in itself a splendid justification of the liberality with which gratuitous relief was given earlier in the year.' Twenty-five thousand permanent wells and many more temporary wells had been constructed during the course of the famine, and the fact was 'clearly established that given adequate . . . wells, cattle and seed . . . a district can at least feed itself from April to September, after a drought as severe as that of 1907.'[67]

The 1907–1908 famine has merited only passing reference in many accounts of South Asian famine history, an omission that can hardly be explained by lack of primary documents. The inattention appears to be a function of how uncharacteristic this famine was in relation to those only a few years earlier. Official relief efforts virtually eliminated the classic markers of famine: social breakdown and mass wandering. Relief measures appear also to have limited famine-related mortality in over half the famine districts. That 1907–1908 has not been seen as a 'great famine' year, at the time, or subsequently by historians, itself hints at the change in effectiveness of relief.[68]

'Scarcity' relief, post-1908

But the 1907–1908 famine also dramatically highlighted continuing limitations of the Famine Code. Throughout the 1907–1908 famine, the provincial administration had been concerned about the impact of high foodgrain prices upon 'the poorer classes' elsewhere in the province where test works had failed to attract sufficient labourers to qualify as 'famine' districts. In the event, the U.P. government chose to depart from previous policy by distributing gratuitous relief in an additional 24 districts, subsequently declaring them to be 'scarcity districts . . . in order to satisfy account requirements.'[69] *Per capita* expenditure, however, was only a tiny fraction of that in the famine districts and was limited primarily to urban centres.[70] The 1907–1908 famine, then, also demonstrated the continuing failure of the Indian Famine Code to address that privation not qualifying for relief under the test work definition of need, nor that starvation caused directly by foodgrain prices. Moreover, the very substantial autumn 1908 fever mortality surge occurred after virtually all relief had been terminated, suggesting that lingering debility was still taking an unnecessary toll.

The impact of high foodgrain prices ('scarcity') was an issue the Government of India had assiduously avoided up to this point. Foodgrain price levels were a signal to begin 'testing' for famine. But 'scarcity' itself had never been acknowledged in itself to be a direct cause of starvation. It is in this context that the 1908 granting of gratuitous relief in non-famine tracts of the United Provinces, token as it was, takes on greater significance. For it is here that famine policy history intersects crucially with epidemic malaria history.

The need for 'scarcity' relief in 1908 was amplified further by 'fulminant' malaria in neighbouring Punjab province in the autumn months of the year. Punjab had also been affected by severe drought in 1907, if less prolonged than that in U.P. As we have seen, large quantities of foodgrains, nevertheless, were exported eastward out of Punjab to the famine tracts of the United Provinces in response to prices there, and by late 1907, Punjab grain prices had reached historic levels as well.[71] Test works in drought-affected Punjab districts, however, attracted insufficient workers to trigger declaration of famine.[72] In concluding that 'scarcity' was a central factor underlying the 'disastrous' malaria epidemics in Punjab, it is inconceivable that Christophers was unaware of the larger significance of the term.[73] His deputation to the Punjab malaria inquiry was arguably a transparent effort from within the administration to provide scientific justification for this most political of conclusions: acknowledgement of 'price famine' as both a problem, and one qualifying for public intervention. *Malaria in the Punjab* thus publicly sounded beginning retreat from a most basic tenet of classical *laissez-faire* doctrine.

Drought and flood relief, post-1908

The practical significance of the decision to relieve starvation induced by grain prices was profound. It made relief available not only earlier in the course of a drought, but also available more frequently since it was no longer restricted solely to years of catastrophic crop failure. In his history of Indian famines, Srivastava astutely noticed the shift, pointing to five years of 'famine relief' between 1909 and 1917 in which gratuitous relief, agricultural loans and village-aided works were instituted not on the basis of mass resort to test works, but simply high prices and localised crop failure. Interestingly, this was a period of almost continuous good to excellent harvests in India as a whole – in only one of these nine years had all-India foodgrain output dipped below 50 million tons.[74] In 1915, the concept of 'scarcity district' was formally distinguished from that of 'famine district' as warranting official relief.[75]

These episodes of famine (or scarcity) relief also saw increasing instances where ordinary wages rates were offered on relief works. As well, earlier in 1903, a provision was added to the Famine Code for special fodder operations during drought to preserve draught cattle.[76] But of even greater significance for Punjab province perhaps was the inclusion of flood-induced crop failure as qualifying for relief, a policy that first appeared in the Bengal code in 1908 but was extended more broadly in 1920.[77] It was during these years also that the government began to permit direct intervention in the foodgrain market, with local government advancing loans to grain merchants to import foodgrains, a measure strictly prohibited in the past.[78]

With this quiet transformation in post-1908 relief came new administrative terms such as provincial 'Scarcity Departments' and 'drought relief,' rather than, or in addition to, famine relief. Relief measures were still open to criticism as Srivastava has noted.[79] Yet the policy changes witnessed in this period demonstrably broke the stranglehold of a non-interventionist relief system restricted to periods of exceptionally severe harvest failure. By the early 1920s, the shift in locus and timing to pre-emptive village-level employment generation had become routine, and its impact on agriculture recovery from drought, in turn, apparent to local officials.[80]

The timing of formal incorporation of these changes into provincial Famine Codes varied from region to region. In the case of Punjab, official adoption of price ('scarcity') relief did not occur until the 1930 revision of the provincial Famine Code.[81] But well before this, there is evidence of an increasingly inclusive definition of agricultural distress qualifying for sanctioned gratuitous relief and village-aided works. Starting from the 1920s, the annual Land Revenue Administration reports for Punjab began to include accounts of flood damage and details of emergency distribution of free food to flooded villages along with *takavi* advances. In 1923–1924, Rs 37,731 worth of food and blankets was reported distributed in flood-affected tracts of Mianwali and Muzaffargarh districts along with 480,000 rupees in *takavi* loans.[82] Floods along the Jumna river the following year occasioned 2.9 million rupees in *takavi* loans and Rs 150,000 distributed as gratuitous relief as well as provision of high-grade (dry) wheat seed to flooded tracts where crucial supplies were likely lost.[83] In 1928–1929, the first account appears in the provincial administrative reports of the army being called in to distribute food and agricultural supplies in flooded districts.[84] In 1937, Rs 3.4 million in direct relief and a further 1.2 million in *takavi* loans was sanctioned as hailstorm relief. In 1950, as we have seen, relief included food supplies air-dropped to affected tracts, with a total of Rs 8,342,969 allocated for financial relief.[85]

While it is difficult to gauge the adequacy or effectiveness of such relief on the basis of these brief accounts, the general attitude to acute distress post-1910 contrasts starkly with that in the late 19th century. In 1933, severe flooding prompted relief operations 'on an unparalleled scale': twenty-one relief centres were opened in Rohtak district alone, boats were requisitioned from neighbouring districts 'to rescue the marooned people,' Rs 21 lakhs of land revenue (tax) obligations were remitted, and Rs 9 lakhs seed loans distributed, along with Rs 114,500 gratuitous relief.[86] The contrast in outcome can be seen, for example, comparing autumn fever death rates in Jullundur district in 1875–1876 (chapter 5) with those in 1933–1934: a three-fold increase in autumn mortality in 1876 followed severe 1875 floods, compared with a negligible rise in 1934 (Table 11.4). From the 1910s, the central government also assumed increasing financial responsibility for famine

Table 11.4 Oct.–Dec. fever death rate, crude death rate (per 1,000), July–Sept. rain (inches), Jullundur district, Punjab, selected years

	July–Sept. rain (in)	*Oct.–Dec. FDR*	*CDR (per 1,000)*
1875	49.0	10.7	32.6
1876	18.4	29.0	58.4
1877	16.3	5.2	24.2
1878*	35.0	43.8	72.0
1900*	35.9	10.6	37.6
1908*	20.5	13.5	38.8
1933	31.6	5.4	25.4
1934	10.2	5.5	27.2

* 'scarcity'/famine years
Source: See Table 4.1.

relief in the form of a famine insurance scheme, again in contrast to a similar 1878 fund that was diverted to general debt reduction under the Lytton/Strachey administration to cover military campaigns in Afghanistan.[87]

Two famines compared: Hissar district, 1938–1940 and 1899–1900

To what extent were the new policies effective in dealing with severe and extensive harvest failure? The 1920s and early 1930s were years of relatively favourable rainfall and harvests in Punjab. Severe drought, however, returned to the subcontinent in the late 1930s. Few references to famine conditions in 1938–1940 appear in colonial famine historiography texts; yet all-India harvest shortfalls in both 1938 and 1940 were exceeded only in the 'great' famines years of (1896–1897 and 1899–1900) and 1907–1908 (Table 10.1). Drought was especially severe in southeastern Punjab, in Hissar district extending over four years, 1936–1939, the longest period of drought on record (Table 11.5), with monsoon rainfall falling to 1.6 inches in 1938 and to 1.1 inch the following year. Crop output in 1938 and 1939 reached only 9 and 16 per cent, respectively, of normal harvests. '[W]ithin living memory,' the Public Health Commissioner observed in 1939, 'famine has never been so intense or so prolonged as it has been during this latest visitation.'[88]

Gratuitous relief and general suspension of land revenue demand preceded formal declaration of famine, followed by establishment of village-level works, and ultimately large relief works. Tasks were

Table 11.5 Oct.–Dec. fever death rate (per 1,000), crude death rate (per 1,000), July–Sept. rain (inches), Hissar district, 1938–1940, 1898–1900

	July–Sept. rain (in)	Oct.–Dec. FDR (per 1,000)	CDR (per 1,000)
1939–1940 Famine			
1938	1.6	5.1	31.7
1939	1.1	5.6	42.0
1940	13.0	8.3	37.8
1899–1900 Famine			
1898	4.8	6.6	27.7
1899	0.7	6.4	29.3
1900	15.7	32.4	96.4

Source: See Table 4.1.

repeatedly lowered in response to changing conditions of the population.[89] Hissar district death rates did rise by 67 per cent in 1939 to 42 per 1,000 population, but this was a small fraction of the 1900 toll when one-tenth of the population perished (Table 11.5).

Relief measures in 1899–1900, by contrast, were manifestly deterrent.[90] Fines for short work were frequent; non-working children received 15 per cent of the adult wage, less than 400 calories, despite extremely high mortality among them. Further efforts to 'driv[e] off such as were not in absolute want' were taken in April 1900 in the face of mortality already four times the pre-famine level.[91] Few received a discharge dole, with only a few village works established in a single district (Rohtak).[92] Many thus faced a period of little or no food between dismissal and the autumn ripening of *kharif* crops, and death rates soared further with the return of malaria.

What is so striking in the official accounts of the 1899–1900 famine is the seeming equanimity of the administration in the face of the mounting deaths tolls. In its subsequent official report on the famine, the Punjab government remarked upon the minimal increase in crime, suggesting this was 'partly due to the very large extent to which whipping was resorted to by the Courts in preference to imprisonment during the famine.'[93] The resort to whipping as a means of social control during times of famine – to control 'offences committed for the purpose of getting the advantage of prison food for a time' – was not a new phenomenon in India in 1899–1900,[94] nor for that matter in other societies historically, if for self-evident reasons rarely documented. What is remarkable here is how starkly the practice reflected unmet need – and as well, the degree to which higher level officials were enured to the wretched implications of human starvation.

This grim comparison is not meant to suggest that measures in 1939–1940 were adequate.[95] Nor does the experience in 1899–1900 Punjab represent all pre-1900 relief. What it does highlight, however, is the shift away from deterrence as the central informing principle of relief policy after 1901, and thus in levels of unmet need (starvation) between the two periods.

Agriculture taxation and credit policies after 1900

Changes in famine relief practices after 1901 were not limited to conditions on the large relief works. Administration of tax relief and agricultural loans underwent similarly important shifts. In the immediate wake of the 1900 'Great Famine,' more than 8 million rupees of uncollected taxes were remitted in Punjab, on order from the Government of

India. Substantial changes in flexibility of tax demand also occurred.[96] Suspensions amounting to several million rupees annually were granted on an increasingly frequent basis during years of locally poor harvests (Table 11.6),[97] amounting by the 1930s to 10 per cent of demand. Much greater emphasis was placed on timely granting of suspensions: where delays occurred after 1910, officials were singled out for criticism.[98] Important changes in the timing of land revenue collection also took place after 1901: in Punjab, suspended taxes were no longer recouped in the first subsequent good harvest,[99] nor first instalments demanded before the marketing of crops when prices were at their lowest.[100] Suspensions were converted to remissions sooner.[101] In new canal colonies, revenue collection was partially converted to a fluctuating system, one where taxes were set somewhat higher as a proportion of the net harvest but varied year to year according to actual output. '[U]niversally popular,' the system was sanctioned increasingly for non-canal natural inundation regions. In 1898–1899, 1.7 million rupees were collected as fluctuating land revenue; by the mid-1920s this figure reached almost half of all land revenue demand.[102] These years also saw marked decline in coercive methods employed to collect land revenue, annual collection warrants declining from over 45,000 in the 1880s to less than 6,000 by 1920.[103] In 1928 land revenue assessment in the province was formally reduced to a maximum of one-quarter net produce, although with rising prices since the turn of the century this lower rate to a large extent had already been in effect.[104]

Changes in agricultural loans *(takavi)* policy followed a similar trajectory. Advances across the non-famine 1885–1895 decade averaged barely 300,000 rupees a year, whereas by the late 1920s agricultural loans routinely reached between 1 and 4 million rupees a year, now granted for flood losses as well (Table 11.6). It would be difficult to exaggerate the importance of affordable credit to subsistence peasant households. 'The decisive factor in Indian agriculture during the twentieth century, and probably in the last quarter of the nineteenth as well,' observed Daniel Thorner shortly after Independence, 'has been the chronic extreme shortage of capital of the great bulk of the cultivating peasantry.'[105] If this 'extreme shortage' was problematic to agricultural development during good harvest years, it held catastrophic consequences in years of harvest loss. Maharatna notes that the area harvested in 1900 in Punjab with return of good rains was considerably lower even than that in the drought year of 1899, suggesting a marked effect of capital depletion on subsequent productivity.[106]

Table 11.6 *Takavi* loans (in 100,000 Rs), Punjab, 1885–1930 (Land Improvement Loans Act, XIX of 1883 and Agriculturists' Loans Act, XII of 1884)

1885–1890	2.9*	1909–1910	26.0
1890–1895	2.6*	1910–1911	18.9
		1911–1912	20.2
1890–1891	3.2	1912–1913	7.6
1891–1892	n.a.	1913–1914	9.6
1892–1893	3.9	1914–1915	4.5
1893–1894	2.7	1915–1916	9.4
1894–1895	1.9	1916–1917	2.9
1895–1896	4.1	1917–1918	3.9
1896–1897	9.9	1918–1919	15.4
1897–1898	n.a.	1919–1920	20.3
1898–1899	17.3	1920–1921	39.2
1899–1900	32.7	1921–1922	24.4
1900–1901	44.5	1922–1923	7.8
1901–1902	10.4	1923–1924	7.0
1902–1903	18.0	1924–1925	19.5
1903–1904	2.6	1925–1926	16.4
1904–1905	19.9	1926–1927	13.2
1905–1906	11.9	1927–1928	24.3
1906–1907	4.0	1928–1929	19.2
1907–1908	31.6	1929–1930	45.7
1908–1909	35.3	1930–1931	12.8

* Six-year mean
Source: *Annual Reports, Punjab Land Revenue Administration*; J. Lindauer, S. Singh, *Land Taxation and Indian Economic Development* (Delhi: Kalyani Publ., 1979), 362–366.

In themselves, these changes hardly amounted to concerted agricultural development policy. They nonetheless reduced gaps in acute crisis relief which, because now available for less severe harvest failure, helped moderate the vicious cycle of famine- indebtedness and capital depletion.

Interpreting post-1920 famine control

Despite the significance of the post-1920 escape from major famines, the role of early 20th century changes in South Asian famine relief policy remains relatively invisible. '[G]eneral expansion of the economy,' Michelle McAlpin has concluded, 'was definitely the most important [factor] in mitigating the effects of crop failure' in the Bombay

Presidency. Economic growth meant 'fewer and fewer people needed to turn to the government for total relief.'[107] Bhatia, too, has suggested greater mobility and alternative employment opportunities largely explain the decline in famine mortality in the early years of the 20th century. By the 1920s and 1930s, he has concluded, 'the nature of the problem had undergone a change and the Codes had become practically obsolete.'[108]

Climatic factors also are cited in the timing of famine control, the droughts at the turn of the century considered anomalously severe. More favourable rains between 1920 and 1940 were associated with 'greater stability of agricultural production.' Agriculture was stagnant during this period, Guha observes, but it was stable.[109] Yet as seen in the case of Punjab, severe and prolonged drought returned in the later 1930s – but without the earlier death tolls. In part, this may reflect declining volatility of foodgrain prices compared with the later 19th century.[110] Maharatna, for example, notes a much smaller spread in grain prices in relation to drought and harvest failure in various regions of the subcontinent after 1901: Bombay jowar prices in 1876–1877 rose more than 300 per cent, from 26 to eight seers per rupee, whereas a major drought in 1911 saw an increase one-third this size.[111] And in Punjab, the increase in foodgrain price levels over the course of the 1938–1939 famine was marginal.[112] Further expansion of irrigation post-1903 no doubt also contributed to stabilising crop output, and prices in turn. However, the increase in irrigated area was modest in India as a whole, rising from 15.2 per cent of cultivated area in 1901 to 25.6 per cent by 1939,[113] much occurring in Punjab province itself. Yet famine declined across the subcontinent.

Nascent public intervention in foodgrain markets

Local 'scarcity' relief post-1920 likely moderated the immediate hunger impact of price swings occurring in smaller rural markets. But so also, arguably, did beginning intervention in the foodgrain market. The decision by the GOI to intervene directly in the grain market was first taken in 1918, one forced upon the administration with the catastrophic effects of war-time hyper-inflation, continuing British military demands for Indian grain exports despite severe harvest failure,[114] and provincial governments' desperate and unauthorised state bans on grain exports.[115] By late September 1918, the central government had been compelled to import rice from Burma and appoint a Foodstuffs Controller, prohibiting all foreign grain exports on private account.[116] Only at the close of the war in December 1918, however – and in the face of a famine-fuelled influenza hecatomb – did the GOI revoke earlier commitments for exports of Indian wheat to the UK.[117] In response to the dire food crisis, modest Australian wheat imports to India were contracted by the Royal Commission on Wheat Supply (UK) in Britain, and the GOI introduced a rigid system of internal controls.[118] Under declarations of 'general and severe privation,' limited famine relief measures were organised, including approval of 'cheap grain shops' initiated by private individuals,[119] a measure sternly proscribed by the GOI during all previous famines.[120] In 1922, the Indian Fiscal Commission formally recommended temporary export duties 'sufficiently high to check or prevent exports' whenever foodgrain prices rose to 'dangerous heights,'[121] and in 1924–1925, India became a net importer of foodgrains for the remainder of British rule.

Though not comparable to measures later undertaken in World War II, acknowledgement of the State's obligation to intervene brought a new factor to play in market behaviour. To what extent public expectation of government intervention contributed to dampening down speculative reflexes in local markets and price hypervolatility between the wars is difficult to gauge, though some impact seems probable.[122]

Also important in reducing vulnerability to starvation, Bhattacharya points to 1909 as marking beginning recovery in real wage levels in Punjab after three decades of decline.[123] In the past, periods of severe harvest failure saw wage rates fall not only in real terms, relative to soaring foodgrain prices, but in nominal terms as well, compounding 'entitlement' collapse.[124] After 1907–1908, harvest failure no longer invariably triggered plummeting wage rates, a pattern first remarked upon by officials during the 1907–1908 U.P. famine, as seen above. Maharatna has also suggested a possible role for pre-emptive and regularised drought relief measures in supporting wage levels during periods of poor harvests.[125] Beginning wage stability across drought periods undoubtedly was related also to increased mobility and access to alternate employment. During the 1952–1953 famine in Mysore and Maharashtra states, for example, 15 per cent of households in surveyed villages were found to have migrated in search of work compared with 3.8 per cent before the famine. Yet by comparison, almost one-quarter of the famine-affected population was employed on village-level relief works, and two-thirds of the 25,877 surveyed households had access to village ration ('fair price') shops.[126]

Few writers, to be sure, suggest a single determinant in South Asia's escape from famine. Most acknowledge a combination of factors, including famine relief, together converging to eliminate great famines after 1920. But key questions regarding the *timing* of specific factors remain. With respect to Punjab, both 'favourable weather gods' and economic modernisation are unconvincing explanations for the escape from famine. Drought and crop failure as severe as that marking the 1890s continued across the first two decades of the 20th century. Good rains and harvests did return in the early 1920s. But the later 1930s experienced severe drought, unprecedented in duration. 'Great' famine mortality, however, did not.[127] Moreover, the abruptness of the decline in malaria lethality after 1908 in Punjab is difficult to explain in the gradualist terms suggested by 'economic modernisation.' Indeed, much of the major infrastructure development was already in place by the final years of 19th century, in advance of the great famines at the turn of the century. There can be little doubt, as McAlpin suggests, that fewer people needed 'total' relief after 1908.[128] Yet this is exactly what would be expected if agricultural support was helping to pre-empt collapse of the agricultural economy during periods of harvest failure.

Conclusions

The vast famine relief works organised under the principles of the 1880 Famine Commission Report undoubtedly saved many lives among those who sought relief upon them during the major famines of the late 19th century. Total expenditure on relief was large with over 3 million persons on relief in 1896–1897. And efforts of local officials in individual instances were heroic. Yet, framed by classical economic principles of non-interference in the economy, the 1883 Code was destined to compound capital drain out of the agricultural economy, in turn arguably increasing vulnerability to famine.[129] Bound by ideological constraints, the vicious cycle of escalating need, costs, and punitive deterrence so visible by the late 1890s, arguably were inevitable consequences.

The turning point in the escape from famine in South Asia, in practical terms, came later, in the first two decades of the 20th century: first, with the 1901 Commission's commitment to pre-emptive relief; then, with the decisions, in the wake of the 1907–1908 U.P. famine, to make relief routinely available for harvest failure beyond just years of catastrophic crop losses, and ultimately the price of foodgrains ('scarcity') in itself a 'test' of need. This later history reveals how technically easy it was to prevent mass starvation given the infrastructural base that existed by the second half of the 19th century.[130]

Underlying these changes was a fundamental shift in the concept of 'famine.' The 1880 Famine Commission Report avoided offering a definition of famine except in purely procedural terms framed around the 'test work' test of need: '[i]f such test works attract labourers in large numbers, then it may be considered proved that distress exists.'[131] In framing its 1888 provincial Famine Code, the Punjab administration offered its own definition, incorporating 1880 Famine Commission principles:

> When a *natural* calamity has affected a material portion of the population of any locality so that the poorer *classes* will perish *from starvation* unless the general resources of the State are applied to their relief, a famine is said to exist.[132]

Unremarkable at first glance perhaps, this definition restricted government responsibility in three crucial ways. By limiting famine to 'natural' calamities, it excluded price-induced epidemic starvation. By referring broadly to 'the poorer classes,' it restricted relief, in practice, to catastrophic episodes of agricultural collapse where starvation ('perishing') was widespread, extending beyond the most poor, labouring classes. And finally, in its emphasis on starvation as primary cause of famine mortality, it retained the 1880 report's artificial distinction between starvation deaths and mortality due to associated epidemics.

Over the course of the first two decades of the 20th century, all three definitional restrictions were jettisoned. The 1901 report categorically rejected the distinction between starvation deaths and epidemic mortality, setting the task to be aspired to as prevention of *any* increase in mortality. After the 1907–1908 famine, relief was no longer restricted to widespread harvest failure, and as well began to be granted on the basis of 'scarcity' *per se* – grain prices 40 per cent or more above normal levels. By implication, famine was now considered, if unofficially, a failure of the state rather than an act of god. It would be only in the aftermath of the 1943–1944 Bengal famine, however, that serious effort was given to making price control a central aspect of official famine prevention policy, feasible administratively only with establishment of large buffer stocks, a coordinated policy that awaited the post-Independence era.[133]

Limitations to 'Relief'

The regularisation of drought and flood relief did not, of course, constitute agricultural development. In spite of the substantial increase in *takavi* advances, such sums were available only in response to acute crisis and thus did little to remedy the general absence in Indian agricultural production of affordable credit. Likewise, though tax suspensions became far more frequent after 1910, over half the taxation demand in the province remained fixed from year to year.[134] It is hardly the case, therefore, that relief measures had been transformed into enlightened agricultural policy. Pervasive chronic hunger (undernourishment) unquestionably continued across India, and for subgroups may well have worsened as foodgrain production stagnated and per capita foodgrain availability declined from between 447 and 497 grams per day in 1911 to an estimated 373 grams by 1941.[135]

Extremely low consumption levels among the poor remained, the 1952 Agricultural Labour Enquiry finding that among 'households living on Rs 100 a year or less, grain consumption amounted to 11 ounces per capita (312.5 grams), equivalent to a daily diet of 1,150 calories.'[136] Presumably, this figure reflects a household average of child and adult consumption levels;[137] nonetheless, such levels suggest that the bottom decile of the population faced endemic semi-starvation, with little capacity for regular work.[138] Recent South Asian anthropometric research also indicates little if any increase in adult stature from the late 19th century to the 1940s: a 0.7 centimetre increase between 1914 and 1940, improvement concentrated largely in higher caste groups.[139] This suggests that the prevalence of marked undernourishment (chronic hunger) remained widespread through to mid-20th century.

In this context, more effective management of acute food crises was the minimum possible response of the British Raj to a worsening agricultural situation across the country. Colonial land tenure and lack of affordable credit for the vast majority of smallholders and tenant cultivators continued to block the required intensification of foodgrain production that otherwise ought to have accompanied modest growth in population after 1920.[140] Under the continuing shadow of the Malthusian premise that equated growth in food production to increased land area, official 'development' was channelled largely to Punjab's 'empty' *doab* lands, canal expansion masking agricultural stagnation for the greater subcontinent, with urban migration deemed a safety valve[141] and 'a malaise of underprivilege linger[ing] on.'[142] 'Once the land-revenue policies were fixed,' Thorner observed in 1955,

> the policy of the state in respect to Indian agriculture was largely hands-off. There was no serious effort by the government of India to make the landowning groups take interest in the productive side of agricultural operations. . . [T]he net effect of British rule was to change drastically the social fabric of Indian agriculture

but to leave virtually unaffected the basic process of production and the level of technique. The upper strata of the new agrarian society benefitted handsomely. . . . Capital needed for the development of agriculture was siphoned off, and the level of total output tended toward stagnation.[143]

By 1946, only 25 per cent of private capital formation lay in the agricultural sector, despite comprising two-thirds of the labour force.[144] In such a context, better management of epidemic starvation (famine), paradoxically, appears to have allowed the administration to engage in a policy of brinkmanship, as the food situation was allowed to slip still further into the state of inadequacy so apparent in the final years leading up to Independence in 1947.[145]

Yet the significance of relief policy changes post-1901 ought not to be overshadowed by this deeply problematic trajectory of food production. Rather, their impact needs to be gauged in relation to what preceded them. In terms of the purposes of this study, what seems evident is that post-1901 government intervention did offer increasingly effective short-term relief during acute agricultural crises, substantially reducing the frequency, duration, and extent of epidemic starvation in the subcontinent.[146] Modernisation of economic infrastructure clearly made it easier to organise effective pre-emptive relief measures and ensure adequacy of local foodgrain supplies – and made such measures less costly than they had been in 1873–1874 Bengal. This enabling effect would remain unactualised, however, in the absence of measures to ensure *access* to those supplies through employment generation that protected individual purchasing power. '[I]t is plausible,' Drèze observes,

> that the improvement of communications towards the end of the nineteenth century did make a major contribution to the alleviation of distress during famines. However . . . this factor alone could hardly account for the very sharp reduction in the incidence of famines in the twentieth century. . . . Even today, it is clear that the high level of market integration in India would be of little consolation for agricultural labourers if government intervention did not also protect their market command over food during lean years . . . by generating purchasing power in affected areas.[147]

No less important, post-1901 relief policy changes helped stem the cumulative drain of capital and labour out of the agricultural economy that recurrent frank famine had, up to that time, ordained.[148]

A fuller understanding of the role of public intervention in India's escape from famine awaits more detailed accounts of post-1901 relief in regions beyond Punjab. This overview, however, suggests that the economic modernisation thesis on its own is an incomplete explanation of famine control in South Asia.

Vilyatpur

The significance of changes in drought and flood relief policies is suggested as well in a 1974 study of a village in Punjab's Jullundur district between 1848 and 1969.[149] Tom Kessinger's study of Vilyatpur, a village largely insulated from classic famine, sheds important light on endemic (non-famine) hunger and early 20th-century shifts in subsistence precarity, expressed demographically in household formation.

The two major groups making up the village were hereditary servants *(sepidars)*, mainly dalit, known as Chamars, and the Sahota (Jat) landowning households to whom they were attached. Employing jamabandi land records, Kessinger determined that of the nine Chamar households resident in the village in 1848, five had died out by 1900, whereas 17 of the 52 Sahota households were no longer traceable. Some of the latter had migrated permanently to the canal colonies, but others had apparently died out as well, with one-fifth owning less than two acres of land and dependent on wage labour.[150]

The effects of 'insecure life,' Kessinger observed, 'had pronounced consequences for village social structure.' In 1848, 57 per cent of household heads were 25 years of age or younger when they assumed succession, compared with 17 per cent in 1958. Many 19th-century households, he adds, 'ha[d] been constantly in peril – there being only a single adult male descendant in each generation.'[151] The effect of this shift in survival is apparent also in caste profile changes. Constituting only 9 per cent of village adult males in 1848, Chamar men made up 15 per cent in 1922 and 28 per cent by 1958. These figures do not take into account canal colony and overseas emigration of Sahota households, and thus do not necessarily reflect changes in caste survival rates relative to one another. Nevertheless, the proportionate increase suggests substantially improved survival rates for Chamar males relative to pre-1900 conditions.[152]

In considering how these changes came about, Kessinger noted the general 'disappearance of contagious disease . . . after 1918,' but suggested this was 'difficult to explain' because 'there was no wholesale introduction of Western public health methods in rural Punjab.' An answer, he offered, lay perhaps 'in better nutrition related to developments in village agriculture,' a question to which the remainder of the study was directed.[153]

Agricultural development from the turn of the 20th century, he showed, involved intensification of production achieved largely by employing existing agricultural methods. Double-cropping rose steadily after 1910: from 31 per cent of cultivated acreage in 1848, to 61 per cent by the early 1940s. With 'accelerated' population growth after 1911, *per capita* cultivated area declined by half to 0.46 acres by 1951, yet increased output was 'sufficient not only to sustain village agriculture in the face of this pressure, but to yield a rising standard of living for most residents.' Greater double-cropping helped reduce slack portions of the agricultural year. Non-agricultural work also increased after 1910 – in brick kilns, housing construction, and whitewashing activities – growth accompanied by the emergence of rural towns.[154] Historically, wage levels of full-time labourers were a 7 per cent share of the harvested crops. Off-season labour was also regulated through *begar*, forced labour without payment. By the early 20th century, a nascent loosening of unipolar power relationships was taking place, evident in the struggle by *sepidar* households for ownership of housing plots.[155] Beginning access to outside employment for the traditional servant castes from the 1920s brought a degree of bargaining power such that increasingly wages were negotiated on an annual, then daily, basis.[156]

Initial South Asian mortality decline after 1920 generally has been interpreted in terms of economic 'modernisation' combined with famine control. As an explanation for the beginning rise in life expectancy in Jullundur district, however, some qualification is needed. '[F]ew deaths were ever attributed to famine in Jullundur,' Kessinger noted. But the district's well-irrigation assets, he added, did not protect against famine prices.

> Jullundur's merchants and cultivators are so accustomed to adequate crops even in the worst years, that they sold everything not needed for immediate consumption during famines to take advantage of the inflated prices in afflicted areas. This caused difficulty in the district when a scarcity extended over several years because there were no reserves for the local nonagricultural population to draw on.[157]

Nor, it could be added, did well-irrigation protect against flood-triggered crop losses and associated agricultural paralysis. Indeed, pre-1920 malaria epidemics were as intense as those experienced elsewhere in the province; and average mortality levels in the district were no lower than for those districts subject to famine (Table 11.7).[158]

It would appear on the surface, Kessinger noted, that by the final years of the colonial period little had changed in Vilyatpur. Permanent wells numbered only 33 in the 1930s compared with 30 in 1848; the first diesel-powered pump was introduced only in 1944. Much of the colonial road and rail transportation network was already in place well before the turn of the century.[159] Increased productivity after 1920 came in part through improved seeds, but access to agricultural credit remained limited.[160] Remittances by Sahota emigrants did increase, as did recruitment in the army, but both were limited primarily to Sahota households, and earnings were generally

Table 11.7 Annual crude death rate (per 1,000), minus plague mortality, Jullundur district, and mean for 24 plains districts, Punjab, 1875–1908

| Year | Mean, 24 | | Year | Mean, 24 | |
	Jullundur district	Plain district		Jullundur district	Plain district
1875	32.6	26.9	1892	43.8	50.2
1876	58.4	30.2	1893	31.1	29.0
1877	24.2	20.6	1894	56.1	38.3
1878	72.0	37.8	1895	30.6	29.4
1879	34.3	38.8	1896	30.5	30.8
1880	25.2	27.1	1897	25.7	31.3
1881	29.9	30.7	1898	30.6	31.6
1882	21.3	27.2	1899	28.5	29.8
1883	22.5	25.4	1900	37.6	50.9
1884	38.2	37.5	1901	38.3	36.0
1885	26.6	28.3	1902	35.6	36.6
1886	28.2	27.8	1903	37.5	40.0
1887	29.5	36.0	1904	27.5	30.9
1888	31.1	31.0	1905	29.1	31.6
1889	34.0	32.1	1906	29.2	32.3
1890	39.5	49.8	1907	29.7	32.6
1891	24.6	29.4	1908	38.7	50.1
Mean 1875–1908 CDR (minus plague)				33.6	31.6

Source: Ann. Rpt. Sanitary Commissioner, Punjab, 1875–1908

directed to land purchases rather than capital investment. Kessinger observes,

> [t]he absence of sanitation, the use of animal and human power for most tasks, the simplicity of tools and techniques, and the *monotony of the diet*, clothing, and housing – especially for landless laborers – all suggest that there has been little improvement in the quality of life. And yet, though relatively poor and backward, present conditions do not preclude the possibility that the general state of things was worse in the past.[161]

Of any changes observed, he suggests, 'transformation in the conditions of work for the Chamar agricultural laborers [was] the most dramatic,' with 'more chamar-agricultural labourers . . . fully employed at better rates of pay than ever before,' the only caste and occupational group to find 'without exception or qualification . . . the present better than the past.'[162]

But beyond real wage recovery (Figures 3.4a-b), and double-cropping expansion,[163] additional improvements in employment and food security, not considered by Kessinger, were also taking shape post-1920: pre-emptive relief of flood and drought hardship, and of scarcity prices. Increasingly flexible tax collection and direct food relief during floods likely reduced seasonal and year-to-year gaps in access to food and indebtedness, and, in turn, cumulative capital depletion.[164] It is also probable that such changes contributed substantially to the very different mortality outcome observed in the severe floods of 1933–1934 compared, for example, with 1875–1876 (Table 11.8).[165]

Kessinger's reference to 'monotony of diet' inadvertently points to a link he does not quite succeed in making between increased household survival and improved food security. 'Monotony' of diet, by which he appears to infer *qualitative* nutrient deficiency, was not the paramount historical problem. Gaps in minimum daily *quantity* of staple foodgrains was. Kessinger's data on improved household survival suggest a historic shift in human subsistence from often one meal per day, and episodically none, to increasing access to two, and away from a pre-modern existence 'constantly in peril.'[166]

Situated in 'irrigation-secure' Jullundur district, socio-economic conditions in this single village were hardly representative of the province, much less the wider subcontinent. Nonetheless, they offer insights into endemic forms of hunger, beyond outright famine, notably those bound up with conditions of work in the larger meaning of

Table 11.8 July–Sept. rain (inches), crude death rate, Oct.–Dec. fever death rate (per 1,000), Jullundur district, Punjab, 1875–1876, 1892, 1933–1934

Year	July–Sept. rain (in)	CDR	Oct.–Dec. FDR (per 1,000)
1875	49.0	32.6	10.7
1876	18.4	58.4	29.0
1892	25.0	43.8	15.4
1933	31.6	35.4	5.4
1934	10.2	27.2	5.5

Source: See Table 4.1.

the term. Despite their specificities, they illuminate demographically the import of changes in subsistence (in)security taking place in this period – and the probable contribution of post-1908 drought and flood relief policies to household survival, and to decline in malaria lethality as well.

Twentieth-century malaria history offers a further opportunity to examine the role of acute hunger in Punjab malaria mortality with the subsequent interruption in malaria transmission through the 1950s residual insecticide spray program in East Punjab, a subject to which we now turn.

Notes

1 Curzon to Hamilton, Apr. 22, 1901, cited in John. L. Hill, 'A.P. MacDonnell and the Changing Nature of British Rule in India 1885–1901,' in R.I. Crane, N.G. Barrier, eds., *British Imperial Policy in India and Sri Lanka, 1858–1912: A Reassessment* (New Delhi: Heritage Publishers, 1981), 58.
2 *Report of the Indian Famine Commission 1901* (Calcutta: Government Printing Office, 1901), 2 [hereafter *FCR* 1901].
3 *Report of the Indian Famine Commission* (London: HMSO, 1880), pt. 1, 40 [hereafter *FCR* 1880].
4 *FCR* 1901, 61–62 [emphasis added]. Official famine mortality statistics ended with return of the monsoon rains, thus excluded autumn malaria deaths; *The Punjab Famine of 1899–1900*, (Lahore: Punjab Revenue Department, 1901), Vol. 2, Appendix IX, 180–181 [hereafter, *FCR* (Punjab), 1901].
5 *FCR* 1901, 72.
6 Hill, 'MacDonnell and the Changing Nature of British Rule,' 59–60.
7 *FCR* 1901, 105, 17–19, 10.

8 Ibid., 19, 15, 23.
9 Ibid., 22.
10 Ibid., 11–13, [emphasis added].
11 Ibid., 16, 12.
12 Secretary of State to Governor in Council of Bombay, 4 (Legislative), dated Dec. 26, 1878. *Despatches to Bombay*, India Office Records, Vol. L/ PJ/3/1498, 266, as cited in S. Ambirajan, 'Malthusian Population Theory and Indian Famine Policy in the Nineteenth Century,' *Population Studies*, 30, 1, Mar. 1976, 5–14, at 10.
13 *FCR* 1901, 106, 16, 47.
14 Ibid., 22.
15 Ibid., 18, 24.
16 'The tasks should be low at the outset, as low as half the ordinary famine task – it may often be necessary to go even lower – and should be gradually raised as the new-comers improve in dexterity and physical condition'; ibid., 31–33.
17 Ibid., 28, 33, 31, 34.
18 Ibid., 49, 52, [emphasis added].
19 Ibid., 52–53.
20 Ibid., 54.
21 Ibid., 39–42.
22 Ibid., 48–49.
23 Ibid., 71–72, 82. Depopulation figures ranged from 5.6 per cent in Bombay to 12 per cent in Ajmer.
24 D. Kumar, 'The Fiscal System,' in D. Kumar, ed., *Cambridge Economic History of India* (Cambridge: Cambridge University Press, 1983), Vol. 2, 905–944, at 916 [hereafter *CEHI*].
25 *PLRA* 1896–1897, 33.
26 J. Lindauer, Sarjit Singh, *Land Taxation and Indian Economic Development* (New Delhi: Kalyani Publishers, 1979), 362–366.
27 *FCR* 1901, 85.
28 *PLRA* 1877–1878, Extracts from Commissioners' and Deputy Commissioners' Reports, 2 [hereafter, Exts].
29 Lindauer and Singh, *Land Taxation*, 362–366.
30 M.B. McAlpin, *Subject to Famine: Food Crises and Economic Change in Western India, 1860–1920* (Princeton: Princeton University Press, 1983), 190, 211–212. For an alternate view, see A.K. Bagchi, 'Land Tax, Property Rights and Peasant Insecurity in Colonial India,' *Journal of Peasant Studies*, 20, 1, Oct. 1992, 1–49, at 6–10.
31 *FCR* 1901, 71–72, 82; H.K. Trevaskis, *The Punjab of Today* (Lahore: 'Civil and Military Gazette' Press, 1931), 161.
32 *Report on the Marketing of Wheat in India* (Simla: GOI Press, 1937), cited in E.T. Stokes, 'Agrarian Relations: North and Central India,' *CEHI*, 36–86, at 85.
33 *1902 Land Revenue Policy of the Indian Government* (Calcutta: Office of the Superintendent, 1902), 12–20. Bhattacharya cites the Punjab revenue rate as 33 per cent of the cash rental; 'The Logic of Tenancy Cultivation: Central and South-east Punjab, 1870–1935,' *IESHR*, 20, 2, Apr.– June 1993, 121–170, at 169. Other local 'cesses', including the salt tax,

amounted in 1870 to one-third the land revenue rate; W.W. Hunter, *The India of the Queen and Other Essays* (London: Longmans, Green, 1903), 173–174.

34 *PLRA* 1877–1878, Exts., 5; *PLRA* 1878–1879, Exts., 2.

35 *PLRA* 1896–1897, Exts., 26; *FCR* 1901, 107–111.

36 S.S. Thorburn, 'Agricola Redivivus,' *The Asiatic Quarterly Review*, XXXII, July 1901; cited in W. Digby, *Prosperous British India* (London: Unwin, 1901), 299–300; S.S. Thorburn, *The Punjab in Peace and War* (Edinburgh: Blackwood, 1904), 242–243. See also, *PLRA* 1886–1887, Exts., 8; *PLRA*, 1883–1884, Exts., 1.

37 *FCR* 1901, 81. B.M. Bhatia noted that in the Bombay Presidency over 99 per cent of the assessment was collected in the famine year of 1896–1897; *Famines in India* (Bombay: Asia Publishers House, 1963), 190–192.

38 *FCR* 1901, 81, 107–111; Lindauer and Singh, *Land Taxation*, 362–364.

39 *FCR* 1901, 85, 81. On land revenue demand and indebtedness, see also, E. Whitcombe, *Agrarian Conditions in Northern India* (Berkeley: University of California Press, 1972), at 14–15, 147–160.

40 Bhatia suggests utilisation of loan legislation depended on the exceptional energies of individual district collectors in surmounting bureaucratic impediments; *Famines in India,* 192–196.

41 *PLRA* 1894–1895, 44; Digby, *Prosperous British India*, 300.

42 *FCR* 1880, 75–76.

43 *FCR* 1901., 84–85.

44 Ibid., 107.

45 See for example, J.M. Neeson, *Commoners: Common Right, Enclosure and Social Change in England, 1700–1820* (Cambridge: Cambridge University Press, 1993).

46 See ch. 10, note 17.

47 Concern for agricultural reform marked MacDonnell's career in India, helping formulate the Tenancy Act of 1885, and personally overseeing 1896–1897 U.P. famine relief. After retiring in 1901 from the Indian Civil Service, MacDonnell worked, ultimately unsuccessfully, for political devolution in Ireland as permanent under-secretary in Dublin; L. Perry Curtis, 'MacDonnell, Antony Patrick,' *DNB*, 1844–1925, doi: 34714.

48 *FCR* 1901, 92. Romesh Dutt addressed similar questions; in *Open Letter to Lord Curzon on Famines and Land Assessment in India* (London: Paul Kegan, 1900). See also, P. Gray, 'Famine and land in Ireland and India, 1845–1880: James Caird and the Political Economy of Hunger,' *The Historical Journal*, 49, 1, 2006, 193–215.

49 Despite honours and adulation for MacDonnell's contributions to famine relief policy, Hill concludes the 1901 FCR 'made no significant impact' on the larger agrarian issues. 'Only minor legislative palliatives were offered by the Government of India to reverse the decay of rural society and its agrarian base'; 'MacDonnell and the Changing Nature of British Rule,' 77, 66–67.

50 *Report of the Indian Irrigation Commission* (London: HMSO, 1903), 121.

51 *FCR* 1901, 21.

52 Bhatia, *Famines in India*, 292–294.

53 *Season and Crops Report* (Punjab), 1901–1902, 1940–1941.

54 A.R Vasavi, 'The Millet Drought': Oral Narratives and the Cultural Grounding of Famine-Relief in Bijapur,' *South Indian Studies*, 2, July–Dec. 1996, 205–233 at 218.

55 The 1907 U.P. *kharif* crop was 31 per cent of normal compared with 39 per cent in 1896, with comparable *rabi* harvests, at 60 per cent normal; Government of the United Provinces of Agra and Oudh, *Narrative and Results of the Measures adopted for the Relief of Famine during the Years 1907 and 1908*, Resolution No. 2107/I, Oct. 14, 1908, 19, 18, 32; [hereafter *FCR* (U.P.) 1908].

56 *FCR* (U.P.) 1908, 100–102, 21, 29.

57 Ibid., 85, 74.

58 Ibid., 37.

59 Ibid., 37, 42.

60 A. Maharatna, 'Regional Variation in Demographic Consequences of Famines in Late 19th and Early 20th Century India,' *EPW*, June 4, 1994, 1399–1410.

61 A. Maharatna, *Demography of Famines* (New Delhi: Oxford University Press, 1996), 88, Figure 2.16.

62 Maharatna, 'Regional Variation,' 1407–1408, Table 11.

63 J. Chaytor White, 'Report on the Outbreak of Malarial Fever in the United Provinces During the Period September to December 1908,' *RMSI*, 1, 2, Mar. 1930, 114–130.

64 Bhatia, *Famines in India*, 236.

65 *FCR* (U.P.) 1908, 150.

66 Ibid. 1908, xvi, 72, 86; H.S. Srivastava, *The History of Indian Famines, 1858–1918* (Agra: Sri Ram Mehra, 1968), 321.

67 *FCR* (U.P.) 1908, 42, 105–109.

68 Maharatna, *Demography of Famines*, 116–117.

69 *FCR* (U.P.) 1908, 26.

70 Ibid., 41–44; Maharatna, 'Regional Variation,' Table 9, 1406.

71 *Season and Crops Report* (Punjab), 1907–1908, 6.

72 The reluctance to resort to test work relief in Punjab in late 1907 and 1908 is curious. In part, it may be explained by a shortage of labour 'owing to the ravages of plague' over the previous several years. But also, continuing fear of plague may have deterred some from attending the test works, given the association of relief works with epidemic disease.

73 S.R. Christophers, 'Malaria in the Punjab,' *Sci. Mem. Off. Med. San. Dep.*, 46 (Calcutta: Superintendent Government Printing Office, 1911), 127, 109.

74 Srivastava, *History of Indian Famines*, 316–319; G. Blyn, *Agricultural Trends in India, 1891–1947* (Philadelphia: University of Pennsylvania Press, 1966), 334.

75 A 'scarcity district' was one 'where distress was not so severe as to necessitate the change of test works into relief works although some relief was required in the form of aid, and in some cases civil works and gratuitous relief'; *Circular*, 16–40–1, GOI, Department of Rev. and Ag. (Famine) from Secy. to Government of India to Local Governments, Simla, the Aug. 23, 1915, as cited in Srivastava, *History of Indian Famines*, 290.

76 Srivastava, *History of Indian Famines*, 345, 311–314. Earlier relief efforts included provision of fodder but only with 'established' famine.

77 K.S. Singh, 'The Famine Code: The Context and Continuity,' in J. Floud, A. Rangasami, eds., *Famine and Society* (New Delhi: Indian Law Institute, 1993), 139–162, at 143; Srivastava, *History of Indian Famines*, 326.
78 *India in the year1919*, 68. As late as the 1896–1897 famine, the Bombay government intervened to block Bombay municipal committees from opening fair price shops; Bhatia, *Famines in India*, 241, 288–289.
79 Srivastava, *History of Indian Famines*, 316.
80 *PLRA* 1921–1922, 3.
81 *The Punjab Famine Code* (revised) (Lahore: Department of Revenue & Agriculture, 1930), para. 65. By 1913, the Bengal Famine Code allowed for gratuitous relief before declaration of a state of famine, the latter now triggered where gratuitous relief reached half of 1 per cent of the local population for a period of two months or more. Post-Independence, Singh notes, some States eliminated altogether the test work method of assessing need; 'The Famine Code,' 143.
82 Data appear by individual village and household, including numbers of houses damaged or destroyed, cattle lost, fodder and crops destroyed; *PLRA* 1923–1924, 3.
83 *PLRA* 1924–1925 Proc., 1.
84 *PLRA* 1928–1929, 6.
85 *PLRA* 1936–1937, 2; Dir. Gen. H. Services, GOI, *Report for the Quadrennium, 1949–1952*, 34–35.
86 *PPHA* 1933, 16; 'Review of the reports on the operations for the relief of distress caused by floods in the Amballa division during Sept. 1933,' *Supplement to the Government Gazette, Punjab*, Jan. 25, 1935, 11–12.
87 P. Bandyopadhyay, *Indian Famine and Agrarian Problems: A Study of the Administration of Lord George Hamilton, Secretary of State for India, 1895–1903* (Calcutta: Star Publishers, 1987), 95–127; also, Srivastava, *History of Indian Famines*, 374–376.
88 *PPHA* 1939, 1.
89 Reports of scurvy led to the provision of sprouted gram in addition to ordinary foodgrains; *PPHA*, 3; *PLRA*, 1939–1940, 4.
90 *FCR* (Punjab), 1900, Vol. 1, 24, 96–99; Bandyopadhyay, *Indian Famine and Agrarian Problems*, 63–67, 226.
91 Ibid., xxii. For a demographic account, see D. Guz 'Population Dynamics of Famine in Nineteenth Century Punjab, 1896–1897 and 1899–1900,' in T. Dyson, ed., *India's Historical Demography: Studies in Famine, Disease and Society* (London: Curzon Press, 1989), 197–221; also, A. Maharatna, *Demography of Famines* (New Delhi: Oxford University Press, 1996), 60–63.
92 *FCR* (Punjab) 1900, Vol. 1, 25, 10.
93 Ibid., 35.
94 See, for example, A. Mukherjee, 'Scarcity and Crime: A Study of Nineteenth Century Bengal,' *EPW*, 28, Feb. 6, 1993, 237–243, at 24; Srivastava, *History of Indian Famines*, 137; *Settlement Report, North West Provinces and Oudh, 1877–1879*, 3–4; K. Currie, 'British Colonial Policy and Famines: Some Effects and Implication s of "Free Trade" in the Bombay, Bengal and Madras Presidencies, 1869–1900,' *South Asia*, 14, 2, 1991, 23–56 at 43.
95 A former assistant Director of the Nutrition Laboratory at Coonoor, R. Passmore calculated that the purchase of salt and condiments would

reduce the maximum wage to 2,700 calories, and that walking 12–16 miles daily to relief works required a further 500 calories, concluding that the famine codes 'have neglected the basic physiology of work'; 'Famine in India,' *Lancet*, Aug. 1951, 303–307, at 306.

96 Resolution by the Governor General of India in Council, 1, Jan. 16, 1902, in *Land Revenue Policy of the Indian Government* (Calcutta: Office of the Superintendent Government Printing Office, 1902).

97 Lindauer and Singh, *Land Taxation*, 362–366.

98 *PLRA* 1916–1917, 2.

99 *PLRA* 1901–1902, Exts., 2–3.

100 N. Bhattacharya, 'Agrarian Change in Punjab, 1880–1940,' unpublished PhD dissertation, Jawaharlal Nehru University, 1985, 78.

101 Bhattacharya, 'Agrarian Change in Punjab, 1880–1940,' 77–78.

102 *PLRA* 1924–1925, 2; *PLRA* 1907–1908, 5.

103 *PLRA* 1884–1885, 12; *PLRA* 1920, Statement X; Trevaskis, *Punjab of Today*, 159. From 1901, open criticism of the harshness of tax collection appears in official reports; *PLRA* 1901–1902, 9.

104 *PLRA* 1916–1917, 2; J.M. Douie, *Punjab Settlement Manual*, 4th ed. (Lahore: Govt Printing Press, 1930), 44. Making up 53 per cent of total revenues in 1901, by 1937–1938 land revenue contributed only one fifth; Kumar, 'The Fiscal System,' *CEHI*, 928. Factors underlying post-World War I decline in land revenue demand is explored in E. Stokes, 'Agrarian Relations,' *CEHI*, 83.

105 D. Thorner, 'Long Term Trends in Output in India,' in S. Kuznets et al., eds., *Economic Growth: Brazil, India, Japan* (Durham: Duke University Press, 1955), 123–124. Interest rates of 35–38 per cent are frequently quoted; also, a traditional monthly rate of one anna on the rupee (75 per cent annually).

106 A. Maharatna, *Demography of Famines* (New Delhi: Oxford University Press, 1996), 84. D. Rajasekhar, 'Famines and Peasant Mobility: Changing Agrarian Structure in Kurnool District of Andhra 18710–11900,' *IESHR*, 28,2, 1991, 121–150 at 137.

107 McAlpin, *Subject to Famine*, 189–190. For critical reviews, see S. Guha, 'Review,' *IESHR*, 23, 1986, 237–239; C.N. Bates, 'Review,' *Modern Asian Studies*, 19, 1985, 866–871; and A. Appadurai, 'How moral is South Asia's Economy?' *Journal of Asian Studies*, 43, 2, May 1984, 481–497.

108 Bhatia, *Famines in India*, vii, 308; B.M. Bhatia, 'Famine and Agricultural Labour in India,' *Indian Journal of Industrial Relations*, 10, 1975, 575–594, at 591.

109 S. Guha, 'Mortality Decline in Early Twentieth Century India: A Preliminary Inquiry,' *IESHR*, 28, 4, 1991, 371–392, at 385; S.K. Ray, 'Weather and Reserve Stocks for Foodgrains,' *EPW*, Review of Agriculture, Sept. 1971, A131-A142, cited in Guha, 'Mortality Decline in Early Twentieth Century India.' See also S.R. Sen, *Growth and Instability in Indian Agriculture* (New Delhi: Ministry of Food and Agriculture, 1967). Klein also notes the post-1901 shift to pre-emptive famine relief, yet assumes the revised Codes remained largely 'untested' in light of 'relatively benign [weather] in the interwar years'; 'When the Rains Failed: Famine, Relief, and Mortality in British India,' *IESHR*, 21, 2, 1984, 185–214, at 205, 207.

110 'J.M. Hurd, 'Railways,' in D. Kumar, ed., *CEHI*, Vol. 2, 737–761, Graph 8.2.

111 Maharatna, *Demography of Famines*, 113, 45, 59.

112 *Seasonal and Crops Report* (Punjab), 1938–1940. The 1938–1939 harvest shortfall was accompanied by 2.9 million tons grain imports that year and 1939–1940, compared with exports of 0.4 million tons during the 1899–1900 famine year; Blyn, *Agricultural Trends*, 334.

113 V. Anstey, *The Economic Development of India* (London: Longmans, Green, 1952), 616, Table X; K.E. Whitcombe, 'Irrigation,' *CEHI*, 677–736.

114 Crop loss was similar to 1896–1897; Blyn, *Agricultural Trends*, 334.

115 This account draws heavily on David Arnold's, 'Looting, Grain Riots and Government Policy in South India 1918, *Past and Present*, 84, 1979, 111–145 at 129, 137–140. See also, Bhattacharhya, 'Agrarian Change in Punjab, 1880–1940,' 373–374.

116 Arnold, 'Looting, Grain Riots,' 139–141; L.F. Rushbrook Williams, *India in the Year 1919* (Calcutta: Superintendent Government Printing Office, 1920), 66.

117 Arnold, 'Looting, Grain Riots,' 139; *India in the Year 1919*, 65–66. For analysis of influenza lethality in relation to 1918 harvest failure patterns, see I. Mills, 'Influenza in India During 1918–1919,' in Dyson, ed., *India's Historical Demography*, 222–260 at 229.

118 *India in the Year 1919*, 67.

119 Ibid., 68; Srivastava, *History of Indian Famines*, 322.

120 Bhatia, *Famines in India*, 241.

121 *Report of the Indian Fiscal Commission, 1921–1922* (Simla: n.p., 1922), 119.

122 Arnold notes a marked decline in foodgrain riots in Madras Presidency from the early 1920s; 'Dacoity and Rural Crime in Madras, 1860–1940,' *Journal of Peasant Studies*, 7, 2, 1979, 140–167.

123 N. Bhattacharya, 'Agricultural Labour and Production: Central and South-East Punjab, 1870–1940,' in K.N. Raj et al., eds., *Essays on the Commercialization of Indian Agriculture* (New Delhi: Oxford University Press, 1985), 105–152, at 143–145. See also, S. Guha, 'Some Aspects of Rural Economy in the Deccan 1880–1940,' in Raj et al., eds., *Essays on the Commercialization of Indian Agriculture*, 210–246, at 226.

124 *PPHA* 1900, 3.

125 *FCR* (U.P.) 1908, 27. See above at note 56, p. 339.

126 V.M. Dandekar, V.P. Pethe, *A Survey of Famine Conditions in the Affected Regions of Maharashtra and Mysore, 1952–1953* (Bangalore: Gokhale Institute, 1972), 7, 34.

127 Between 1868 and 1908, Punjab experienced eight years of monsoon rainfall under 10 inches; between 1909 and 1940, seven years (Table 4.1). See also, K.C.S. Acharya, *Food Security System of India: Evolution of the Buffer Stocking Policy and its Evaluation* (New Delhi: Concept Publishers, 1983), 25–27.

128 McAlpin, *Subject to Famine*, 190.

129 Sanjay Sharma highlights long-term detrimental impacts of the 1837–1838 famine in the North-Western Provinces, in *Famine, Philanthropy*

and the *Colonial State* (New Delhi: Oxford University Press, 2001), 191–206, 68.

130 Assuming political stability, famine control was feasible even in the relative absence of modern industrial technology; P.E. Will, B. Wong, *Nourish the People: The State Civilian Granary System in China, 1650–1850* (Ann Arbor: University of Michigan, 1991).

131 Department of Revenue & Agriculture (Punjab), 152, Oct. 5, 1888, *The Punjab Famine Code*, 13.

132 Ibid., 1 [emphasis added].

133 For details, see ch. 15. See also, R.N. Chopra, *Evolution of Food Policy in India* (New Delhi: Palgrave Macmillan, 1981); Acharya, *Food Security System of India*; H. Knight, *Food Administration in India 1939–1947* (Stanford: Stanford University Press, 1954). A buffer stock grain storage system had been urged, unsuccessfully, by dissenting 1880 Famine Commission members, James Caird and H.E. Sullivan; FCR 1880, 88–92.

134 Lindauer and Singh, *Land Taxation*, 109–112.

135 A. Heston, 'National Income,' in D. Kumar, ed., *CEHI*, Vol. 2, 376–462, at 410, Table 4.6. Estimates by Blyn are slightly higher; *Agricultural Trends in India*.

136 *Agricultural Labour: How They Work and Live* (New Delhi: All-India Agricultural Labour Enquiry, 1952), cited in D. Narain, *Distribution of the Marketed Surplus of Agricultural Produce by Size-Level of Holding in India* (Bombay: Asia Publishers House, 1961), 36–37. Specific consumption levels reported in the 1952 enquiry may be subject to some level of error; D. Thorner, 'The Agricultural Labour Enquiry: Reflections on Concepts and Methods,' *Economic Weekly*, June 23, 1956, 759–766. Nonetheless, the general pattern supports the view of marked deficiency.

137 An early 1940s rural Bengal survey found 10.7 per cent of the population with per capita annual incomes below 100 rupees, R.B. Lal, S.C. Seal, *General Rural Health Survey, Singur Health Centre, 1944* (Calcutta: All-India Institute of Hygiene and Public Health, GOI Press, 1949), 95.

138 A similar finding has been estimated for the bottom 10 per cent of the pre-Revolutionary population in France; R. Fogel, 'Second Thoughts on the European Escape from Hunger: Famines, Chronic Malnutrition, and Mortality Rates,' in S.R. Osmani, ed., *Nutrition and Poverty* (Oxford: Clarendon Press, 1992), 243–280.

139 A.M. Guntupalli, J. Baten, 'Inequality of Heights in North, West, and East India 1915–1944,' *Explorations in Economic History*, 43, 2006, 578–608, Figs. 12–14. For similar findings, see L. Brennan, J. McDonald, R. Shlomowitz, 'Long-Term Change in India Health,' *Journal of South Asian Studies*, 24, 1, 2003, 51–69.

140 P. Mohapatra, 'Coolies and Colliers: A Study of the Agrarian Context of Labour Migration from Chotanagpur, 1880–1920,' *Studies in History*, 1, 2, n.s., 1985, 297–299; E. Boserup, *The Conditions of Agricultural Growth* (Chicago: Aldine, 1965), 98–100; G. Omvedt, *The Political Economy of Starvation: Imperialism and the World Food Crisis* (Bombay: Leela Bhosale, 1975), 27–35.

141 *Report of the Royal Commission on Agriculture in India* (London: HMSO, 1928), Vol. 10, 88, cited in J.H. Perkins, *Geopolitics and the*

Green Revolution: Wheat, Genes, and the Cold War (New York: Oxford University Press, 1997), 100.

142 P. Robb, 'New Directions in South Asian History,' *South Asia Research*, 7, 2, Nov. 1987, 133.

143 Thorner, 'Long Term Trends in Output,' 127.

144 Stokes, 'Agrarian Relations in North and Central India,' 85.

145 In the absence of fundamental land tenure reforms, devolution of famine relief to local sub-district levels also served to strengthen the hold of the rural elite over the lives of the landless, and the scope for patronage, a legacy that extends to the modern period; K. Mathur, N, Gopal Jayal, *Drought Policy and Politics in India* (New Delhi: Sage, 1993); P. Sainath, *Everybody Loves a Good Drought* (New Delhi: Penguin, 1996), 17–24.

146 Increased attention to agricultural stress is reflected in Census figures: between 1860 and 1902, 11 famines and 14 'scarcity' years are recorded as occurring in British territory; comparable figures for 1903–1946 are 22 famines and 29 scarcities; *Census of India, 1951*. Vol. I, Part 1-A, Appendix IV, 'Famine and Pestilence: Part A – List of Famines and Scarcities,' 265–270.

147 J. Drèze, 'Famine Prevention in India,' in J. Drèze, A. Sen, eds., *The Political Economy of Hunger* (Oxford: Clarendon Press, 1990), Vol. 2, 13–122, at 24.

148 Ibid., 33.

149 T. Kessinger, *Vilyatpur 1848–1969, Social and Economic Change in a North Indian Village* (Berkeley: University of California Press, 1974).

150 Ibid., 64, 98, 95, 42, 116, 29, 63. Many weaver and Brahmin households also died out; in the latter case, perhaps related to Sikh conversion of most Sahotas in the late 19th century; ibid., 98, 42.

151 Ibid., 84, 88, Table 10.

152 Ibid., 95, 164, 123.

153 Ibid., 87.

154 Ibid., 119, 115, 104, 218. Bhattacharya notes that nearly half of the 51,000 industrial workers in Punjab in 1928 were seasonal workers in cotton ginning factories, employed during slack agricultural periods; 'Agricultural Labour and Production,' 105–152, 129.

155 Kessinger, *Vilyatpur*, 127.

156 Ibid., 56–57, 123–129, 217; Bhattacharya, 'Agricultural Labour and Production,' 118.

157 Kessinger, *Vilyatpur*, 87.

158 For details, see chs. 5 and 11.

159 Kessinger, *Vilyatpur*, 34, 155, 137, 15–16, 202; Hurd, 'Railways,' in *CEHI*, Vol. 2, at 745.

160 Kessinger, *Vilyatpur*, 121–122, 107–109, 138. See also, S. Singh, 'Agricultural Science and Technology in the Punjab in the Nineteenth Century,' *Indian Journal of History of Science*, 17, 2, 1982, 191–204.

161 Kessinger, *Vilyatpur*, 209 [emphasis added].

162 Ibid., 217, 209, 124, 219.

163 Bhattacharya, 'Agricultural Labour and Production,' 143–134.

164 Well before the late 19th-century 'great' famines, revenue officials had identified famine-level foodgrain prices as a prominent cause of indebtedness in Jullundur district; *Final Report of the Revised Settlement of the*

Jullundur District in the Punjab (Lahore: Punjab, Revenue Department, 1892), 45.

165 See ch. 5.

166 Kessinger, *Vilyatpur,* 84. Lardinois estimates between 7.5 per cent and 38.8 per cent of villages were deserted in 10 districts during the late 18th-century East India Company military occupation of Tamil South India; R. Lardinois, 'Deserted Villages and Depopulation in Rural Tamil Nadu c. 1780–1830,' in Dyson, ed., *India's Historical Demography,* 16–48, Appendix to ch. 2.

12 Acute hunger and malaria lethality

'Test cases' post-1940

Among the factors contributing to annual malaria death rates in colonial Punjab – those affecting transmission rates, and those influencing malaria lethality (acute hunger and quinine access) – only one can be seen to have changed demonstrably for the rural population of the province after 1908, that of mass destitution. Both the suddenness with which major famines were controlled in the early years of the 20th century, and the effectiveness of famine prevention evident in Hissar district in 1939–1940, suggest that decline in epidemic starvation through routine public intervention measures was a central factor. Additionally, increasingly routine flood relief measures after 1920 appear to have moderated the acute hunger consequences of excess rainfall and hastened agricultural recovery in all regions of the province.

More definitive evidence of the role of famine control in epidemic malaria decline comes from several instances of what might be considered almost 'control-study' contexts: first, the tragic World War II circumstances of epidemic starvation triggered by war-time hyperinflation and administrative preoccupation; and second, the virtual elimination of malaria transmission a decade later through DDT spray programs from the early 1950s.

Malaria without the famine code

After an interval of almost three decades, overt famine would return to the Indian subcontinent in the early 1940s, ushered in, as in 1917–1918, with the circumstances of a war-time economy. It would be in the northeastern region of the subcontinent, under malarial conditions quite different from Punjab, that the power of acute hunger underlying malarial lethality would be demonstrated most starkly in the closing years of colonial rule. Much has been written about the 1943–1944 Bengal famine in which over 2 million Bengalis perished. In 1981, Amartya Sen reclaimed key insights into its causes: starvation was triggered primarily by the soaring cost of foodgrains rather than food availability decline. As well, his study importantly highlighted that the 'gigantic' rise in mortality mirrored almost exactly the 'normal' seasonal mortality of non-famine years, 'just linearly displaced severely upwards.'[1]

In earlier work, I have explored the central role of starvation underlying the dramatic rise in malaria lethality, the leading cause of death in Bengal in 1943.[2] Certainly also, the Bengal famine is an abject example of the consequences of 'scarcity' in the absence of the Famine Code and relief measures, as war-time imperial priorities led the government to ignore appeals from district officials for the declaration of famine in the province and application of routine relief operations. Bengal, however, was not the only site of heightened malaria mortality over the course of World War II. One year earlier, famine and epidemic malaria had returned to Punjab as well.

Unlike in Bengal, the 1942 Punjab epidemic was preceded classically by drought, with fever mortality following return of the rains. Once again, harvest failure was most severe in the southeast of Punjab province (Table 12.1). Barely recovered from record-level drought two years earlier, harvest failure was superimposed upon war-time hyper-inflation, wheat prices rising 300 per cent by 1942. Death rates rose throughout the province, but were highest in districts also struggling

Table 12.1 Oct.–Dec. fever death rate (per 1,000), % normal July–Sept. rain, 11 plains districts, (East) Punjab, 1941, 1942

District	Oct.–Dec. FDR (per 1,000)			% normal July–Sept. rain	
	1941	1942	1908	1941	1942
Hissar	5.8	27.5	19.4	19	187
Rohtak	6.3	22.4	23.7	49	186
Gurgaon	4.9	18.9	17.2	54	144
Karnal	6.2	24.1	18.3	60	150
Amballa	5.4	17.1	12.8	46	225
Hoshiarpur	5.4	7.4	14.7	82	130
Jullundur	3.5	8.4	13.5	70	120
Ludhiana	4.9	11.5	14.6	70	165
Ferozepur	6.6	13.9	16.1	56	138
Amritsar	4.5	3.6	18.9	99	113
Gurdaspur	7.5	11.3	13.0	115	204

Source: *PPHA*, 1941–1946; *Season and Crops Report*, Punjab, 1941–1942; ch. 4, Table 4.1.

Table 12.2   Famine relief (10,000 Rs) sanctioned by the Punjab Government,*
              1921–1951

	Rs		Rs
1921–1922	44.3	1936–1937	3.6
1922–1923	0.7	1937–1938	12.9
1923–1924	0.0	1938–1939	332.3
1924–1925	13.2	1939–1940	701.4
1925–1926	8.7	1940–1941	258.7
1926–1927	5.0	1941–1942	41.8
1927–1928	1.2	1942–1943	20.7
1928–1929	19.7	1943–1944	5.2
1929–1930	44.4	1944–1945	129.8
1930–1931	83.5	1945–1946	150.7
1931–1932	25.8	1946–1947	33.7
1932–1933	5.0	1947–1948	0.8
1933–1934	9.1	1948–1949	1.3
1934–1935	0.3	1949–1950	231.9
1935–1936	1.0	1950–1951	834.3

* 1948–1951, East Punjab (India).
Source: *Stat. Abst.*, 1920–1921 to 1948–1949; Dir. Gen. Health Services, *Rpt. for the Quadrennium, 1949–1952*, 34.

with drought. Five per cent of the Hissar district population succumbed over the course of the year, with autumn 1942 fever death
rates reaching levels recorded in pre-1909 epidemics.

The nature and extent of famine relief measures in the province
in 1942 are difficult to gauge from the scanty administrative reports
published across the war period. As was the case druing World War
I, European military needs drained district administrations of experienced staff. Direct famine relief expenditure in 1941–1942 was later
reported as Rs 625,569,[3] one-half rupee *per capita* over the two-year
period, and total expenditure amounted to less than one-twelfth that
for the 1939–1940 famine period (Table 12.2), suggesting that much
of the destitution in 1942 went unrelieved.[4] The sudden reappearance
of marked malaria lethality in Punjab province after an interval of
25 years is further evidence of a central role for acute hunger in the
region's malaria mortality history. It also casts doubt on changes in
malaria parasite virulence as an explanation of post-1920 epidemic
decline.[5]

Malaria control: (East) Punjab, 1951–1960

Additional insights into the role of famine control in epidemic malaria
decline, albeit the inverse of those above, are offered in the context of

malaria transmission control one decade later and its impact on general mortality levels. Following initial trials in several industrial and plantation populations,[6] two DDT-based anti-malarial 'demonstration units' were established by Indian malaria researchers in (East) Punjab in 1950, under the existing State Malaria Organization. Several thousand villages in Karnal and Gurgaon districts were included, involving a population of 0.4 million.[7] The pilot project brought 'a striking reduction' in child spleen and parasite rates, and on that basis, a control program was initiated in 1953–1954 across the State as part of the wider National Malaria Control Programme (NMCP) under the Indo-American Point-IV Agreement. In the following analysis of the impact of the residual insecticide spray program, only 11 of the 23 plains districts in the earlier 1868–1940 analysis are included, those composing the plains districts of the post-Partition Indian State of (East) Punjab. This area, nevertheless, encompasses a large number of the districts subject to serious epidemics in the colonial period.

Four malaria control units were created in 1953 for operation in nine of the State's 13 districts. The program commenced in July of that year, with DDT-sprayed once or twice during the malaria season. In the first year of operations (1953–1954), 2,526 villages with a population of 1.6 million were covered. Over the following year (1954–1955), the number of units was increased to seven, with the program extended to one-quarter (3.3 million) of the State's population. Further surveys followed in April–May 1955, and the program was expanded to the remaining population beginning in June 1955.[8]

In some districts, such as Karnal, the majority of villages were covered by late 1955. In others, such as Hoshiarpur, wide coverage does not appear to have been achieved until 1959–1960. Data on DDT coverage, by district, across the 1950s decade were subsequently reported in the 1961 Punjab Census district reports, which includes annual numbers of houses sprayed, 'persons living in houses sprayed with DDT,' and expenditures incurred (Table 12.3).[9] These accounts are of varying levels of completeness and consistency, particularly figures for population covered, and the latter are not included in Table 12.3. Despite such deficiencies, the Census data nevertheless convey a general profile as to the timing of the program's extension across the State.

Published data on spleen and malaria parasite rates across program implementation unfortunately are limited. Within the first year of the program, D.R. Mehta reported the spleen rate in DDT spray areas as below 10 per cent in November 1954 compared with 40 per cent or more preceding the spray program.[10] Infant parasite rates of 0.2 per cent in the initial year of the program (1953–1954) were reported as 0.07 per cent one year later.[11] By 1958–1959, the average spleen rate

Table 12.3 Annual DDT spray program expenditure (10,000s Rs) *, no. of houses sprayed (10,000s),* crude death rate, crude birth rate (per 1,000), infant mortality rate (per 1,000 live births), 11 plains districts, Punjab State (India), 1951–1960

HISSAR district

Year	CDR	IMR	CBR	Houses (10,000s)	Rs (10,000s)
1951	15.0	96.4	45.7		
1952	16.1	113.6	41.8		
1953	17.1	124.0	40.6		
1954	14.3	96.1	43.2	n.a.	1.0
1955	13.2	86.3	47.1	n.a.	3.4
1956	16.2	93.5	45.8	n.a.	3.6
1957	13.6	79.2	49.1	14.3	8.0
1958	17.1	82.5	49.9	16.9	14.1
1959	12.1	69.7	49.8	21.1	21.6
1960	14.7	88.7	50.4	23.0	21.8

AMBALLA district

Year	CDR	IMR	CBR	Houses (10,000s)	Rs (10,000s)
1951	15.0	116.9	40.1		
1952	16.1	128.0	40.2		
1953	17.1	133.0	37.9	n.a.	1.0
1954	14.3	115.7	41.2	5.9	4.3
1955	13.2	99.4	44.9	9.4	5.1
1956	16.2	123.1	43.2	12.5	5.3
1957	13.6	94.1	41.5	12.5	5.3
1958	17.1	114.9	45.4	15.5	16.8
1959	12.1	96.1	38.1	16.7	19.5
1960	14.7	102.8	43.6	18.6	25.8

ROHTAK district

Year	CDR	IMR	CBR	Houses (10,000s)	Rs (10,000s)
1951	14.3	98.4	45.4		
1952	19.2	117.3	45.7		
1953	19.2	111.5	45.7	n.a.	3.1
1954	13.8	93.3	45.3	n.a.	7.1
1955	14.5	87.0	49.5	n.a.	8.1
1956	16.2	109.1	47.3	n.a.	5.6
1957	14.9	99.1	48.3	n.a.	7.9
1958	16.2	101.1	47.7	6.5	4.9
1959	11.8	76.2	46.0	17.1	23.0
1960	15.0	75.2	46.0	15.7	22.8

HOSHIARPUR district

Year	CDR	IMR	CBR	Houses (10,000s)	Rs (10,000s)
1951	20.9	172.5	42.2		
1952	20.0	153.5	40.6		
1953	20.5	165.1	36.7		
1954	15.7	136.6	39.7	n.a.	4.9
1955	15.2	130.9	42.6	n.a.	4.4
1956	13.6	163.5	39.1	n.a.	6.6
1957	15.4	143.7	34.3	n.a.	5.8
1958	17.3	155.2	36.6	5.3	4.9
1959	13.7	135.9	34.2	21.7	22.4
1960	15.9	140.3	35.5	20.5	24.7

GURGAON district

Year	CDR	IMR	CBR	Houses (10,000s)	Rs (10,000s)
1951	18.0	119.1	45.0		
1952	23.2	131.3	46.6		
1953	22.9	130.5	48.2	n.a.	5.4
1954	16.6	110.4	46.9	11.6	7.6
1955	17.7	114.8	50.3	13.3	9.6
1956	18.3	118.2	50.0	15.3	9.8
1957	17.9	98.9	49.8	18.4	12.1
1958	20.3	112.0	50.7	17.2	15.4
1959	15.1	97.4	49.0	21.8	20.0
1960	17.0	118.7	46.1	20.8	23.7

JULLUNDUR district

Year	CDR	IMR	CBR	Houses (10,000s)	Rs (10,000s)
1951	15.7	130.2	41.0		
1952	13.1	128.4	39.3		
1953	16.0	127.9	37.8		
1954	13.0	117.7	38.3	6.1	3.0
1955	13.2	109.5	41.1	12.7	3.2
1956	15.0	109.3	38.7	14.8	4.6
1957	13.0	103.8	35.1	15.5	4.4
1958	14.1	108.8	35.0	15.3	16.0
1959	12.1	102.1	33.8	15.8	21.7
1960	13.3	96.7	33.6	15.9	23.3

KARNAL district

Year	CDR	IMR	CBR	Houses (10,000s)	Rs (10,000s)
1951	14.1	103.9	40.9		
1952	16.4	118.0	44.5		
1953	19.8	135.8	42.4	n.a.	5.7
1954	14.4	107.8	46.4	8.3	9.1
1955	13.7	97.1	47.6	13.2	10.5
1956	16.5	103.0	45.7	11.1	8.4
1957	15.1	95.7	49.9	15.1	10.5
1958	17.3	115.4	48.9	13.8	16.4
1959	12.9	92.0	47.8	15.5	22.2
1960	15.4	91.2	49.3	17.0	24.0

LUDHIANA district

Year	CDR	IMR	CBR	Houses (10,000s)	Rs (10,000s)
1951	13.1	121.0	29.9		
1952	13.1	125.6	33.5		
1953	14.2	124.2	32.6	n.a.	1.0
1954	11.7	109.3	41.8	n.a.	3.4
1955	12.1	104.6	46.5	n.a.	7.6
1956	13.6	116.3	45.7	n.a.	3.1
1957	12.8	106.7	45.2	n.a.	3.9
1958	13.6	115.9	45.2	n.a.	0.0
1959	12.1	109.1	43.5	16.4	16.9
1960	12.6	114.9	44.2	16.6	18.5

FEROZEPUR district

Year					
1951	17.8	139.2	34.1		
1952	16.1	128.1	42.2		
1953	16.9	131.1	41.1	n.a.	
1954	13.0	113.4	41.4	5.8	2.5
1955	12.9	115.2	42.4	13.2	4.8
1956	13.8	113.8	42.0	13.3	7.9
1957	11.8	108.2	39.4	13.1	8.6
1958	12.5	111.9	39.6	14.7	9.5
1959	10.5	95.9	39.9	16.4	0.0
1960	11.4	72.6	35.7	15.0	27.1

AMRITSAR district

Year					
1951	15.9	121.4	35.9		
1952	15.1	115.7	40.0		
1953	16.8	129.1	39.6	n.a.	2.0
1954	13.0	120.8	40.1	n.a.	6.3
1955	12.7	115.5	41.0	n.a.	9.0
1956	13.0	124.8	38.7	n.a.	9.2
1957	12.0	110.4	34.2	14.8	8.5
1958	11.5	104.5	34.2	14.5	16.4
1959	10.1	92.2	33.3	19.0	27.9
1960	11.2	101.6	34.4	16.6	24.9

GURDASPUR district

Year					
1951	16.6	134.8	36.4		
1952	15.7	130.3	41.8		
1953	17.5	141.8	39.2	n.a.	3.7
1954	12.9	116.9	39.4	9.6	6.1
1955	12.6	106.9	42.5	14.0	7.1
1956	16.0	128.0	42.6	16.5	10.2
1957	11.7	107.7	35.9	0.0	10.4
1958	13.4	115.7	36.9	0.0	0.0
1959	11.2	109.9	34.7	15.1	17.7
1960	12.5	110.1	34.4	13.9	18.8

Source: *Census of India, 1961*, Punjab, District Handbooks.

* DDT spray operations are reported from July of one year to June of the next; here, recorded as the year of the first six-month period (July–Dec.).

for the State as a whole had fallen to 1.5 per cent and infant and child parasite rates in 1958–1959 were observed to be nil.[12] By comparison, falciparum parasite rates in young children reported in mid-1930s Karnal district were 27.0 per cent in the malaria season and 7.5 per cent in the pre-malaria season.[13] The apparent rapid decline in malaria indices was accompanied by a substantial drop in clinical cases of malaria diagnosed at government hospitals and dispensaries: 511,775 malaria cases in 1951 compared with 380,496 in 1954,[14] at a point where only one-quarter of the population had been included in the program.

The immediacy of the program's impact on malaria transmission is suggested as well in observed changes in the seasonal pattern of fever deaths. As seen in chapter 4, autumn fever deaths dominated the pre-1909 pattern of fever mortality in the province, a profile that changed after 1920 to approximately equal October and May–June fever mortality peaks (Figures 4.3a-b). The latter seasonal profile was still evident in 1952 (Figure 12.1). After 1953, however, the seasonality of fever deaths shifted again: the state-wide autumnal rise was further reduced, with May–June 1954 and 1955 fever deaths now proportionately more prominent.[15] Given that transmission conditions in 1954 likely were favourable with slightly above average rains, the near disappearance of the autumn fever curve also suggests substantial decline in malaria transmission in the region.[16]

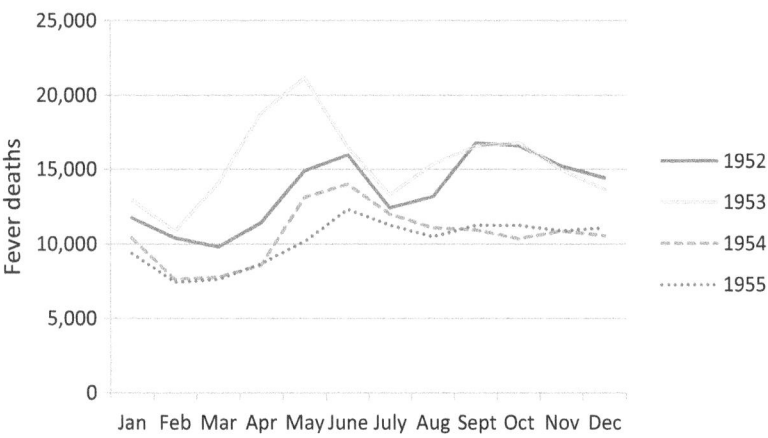

Figure 12.1 Monthly distribution of fever deaths, Punjab State (India), 1952, 1953, 1954, 1955

Source: *Health Statistics of India, 1951–1953*, 134–135, Table 20; *Health Statistics of India, 1954–1955*, 165–166, Table 18.

Mortality trends under the National Malaria Control Programme

What impact did the near elimination of malaria transmission in the 1950s have on mortality levels in Punjab State? A notable stepwise decline in CDR (crude death rate) occurred in 1954 (Table 12.4), from 18.5 deaths per 1,000 in 1953 to 13.9 per 1,000 in 1954, with a further marginal decrease to 13.8 per 1,000 in 1955.[17] Yet the contribution of the spray program to this improvement is unclear for several reasons.

First, the 1954 dip in mortality was not limited to the autumn months of the year. The 1.1 per 1,000 decline in Oct.–Dec. fever death rate between 1953 and 1954 constituted only one-quarter of the total (annual) mortality decline of 4.6 per mille between these two years. It might be suggested that interruption in malaria transmission may have had a broader impact on general mortality levels with the elimination of a major endemic disease. But such an impact would be expected to affect mortality levels *after* the autumn 1954 malaria season, an effect not evident in 1955.

Second, by late autumn 1954, only one-quarter of the population was covered by the DDT spray program.[18] It is possible that the greater portion of the malaria mortality burden in the State was mitigated at this time if, as Mehta suggests,[19] villages chosen initially for the program were those of greater endemicity. Yet CDR decline in 1954 is seen in all districts (Figures 12.2 a-k), including those

Table 12.4 Mean crude death rate, annual and Oct.–Dec. fever death rate (per 1,000), infant mortality rate (per 1,000 live births), Punjab State (India), 1951–1960*

	CDR	Oct.–Dec. FDR	IMR*
1951	16.5	3.3	122.7
1952	17.1	3.6	125.9
1953	18.5	3.5	131.6
1954	13.9	2.4	112.4
1955	13.8	2.5	106.3
1956	15.8	2.5	118.0
1957	14.0	3.0	103.7
1958	15.3	3.1	111.7
1959	12.2	2.2	96.2
1960	13.9	2.9	99.2

* IMR data represent the 11 plains districts only.
Source: *Health Statistics of India, 1951–1953*, 111, Table 15; *Health Statistics of India, 1954–1955*, 166, Table 18; *Census of India, 1961*, Punjab, District Handbooks.

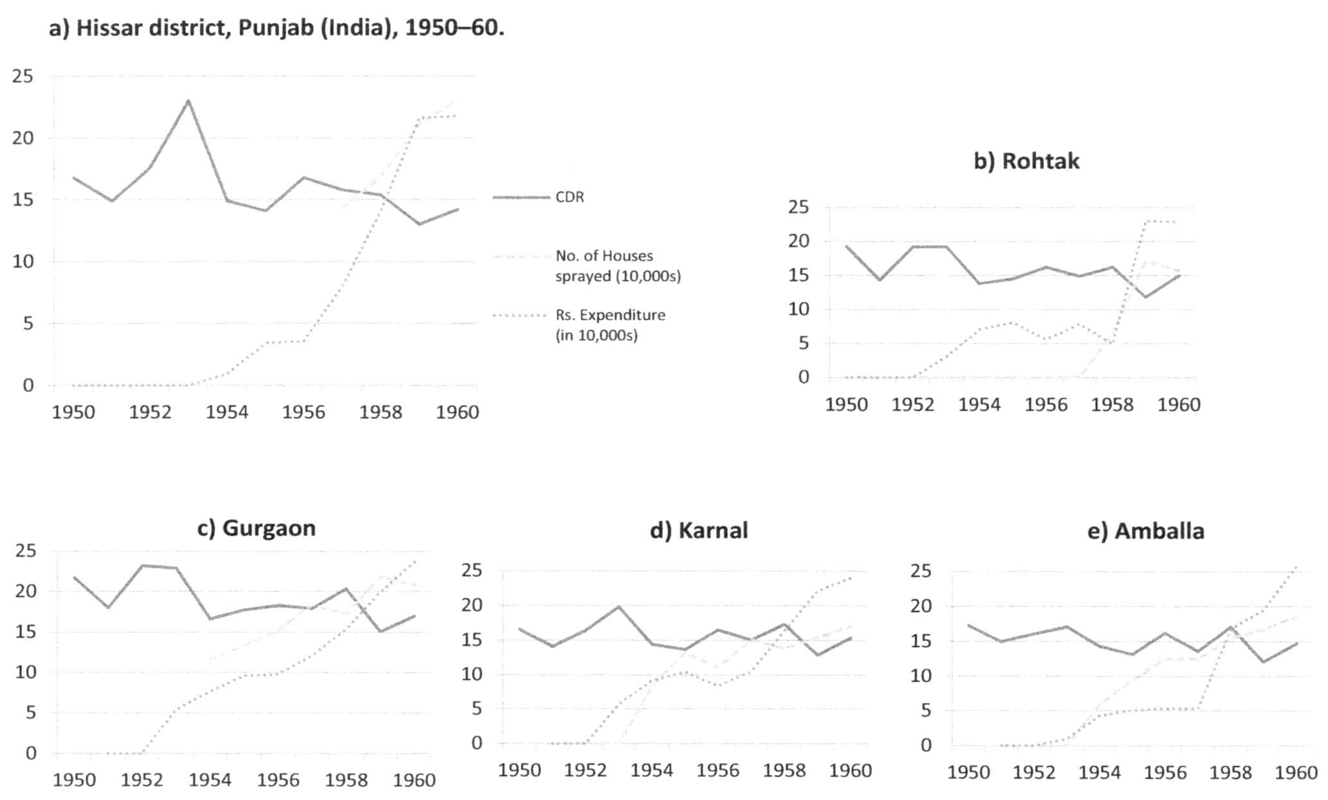

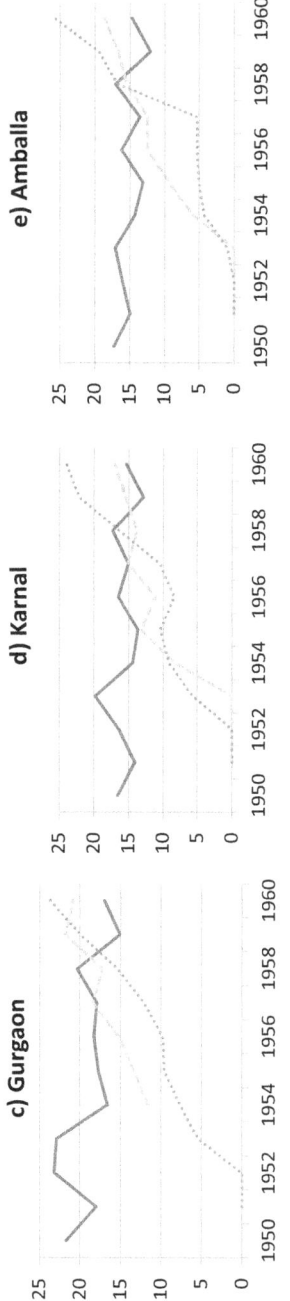

a) Hissar district, Punjab (India), 1950–60.

b) Rohtak

c) Gurgaon

d) Karnal

e) Amballa

CDR

No. of Houses sprayed (10,000s)

Rs. Expenditure (in 10,000s)

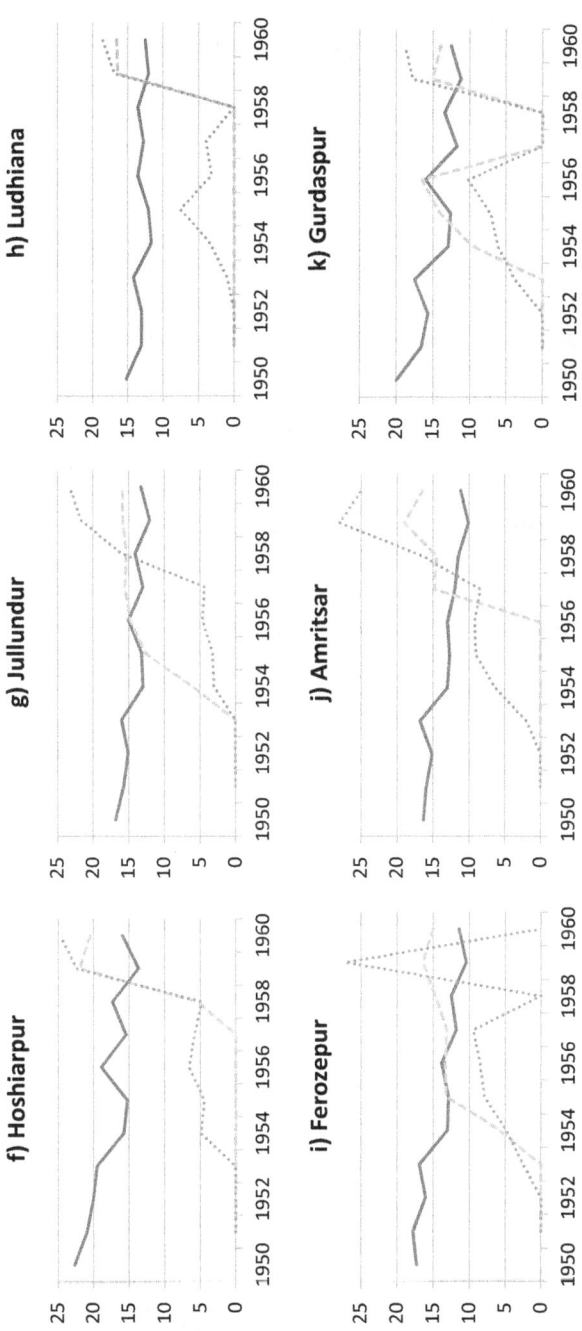

Figure 12.2a–k Annual crude death rate (per 1,000), no. of houses DDT-sprayed (10,000s), Rs expenditure (in 10,000s), by district, 1950–1960, 11 plains districts, Punjab State (India)

Source: *Census of India, 1961*, Punjab. District Handbooks.

where expenditure on the program in 1954–1955 was limited. In Hissar district, for example, appreciable DDT spraying appears to have begun only in 1955–1956 (Figure 12.2a),[20] yet a marked decline in CDR is also seen in the district in 1954. Indeed, a flattening of the district's autumn fever death rate curve is evident only after 1956 (Figure 12.3).

Finally, no decline in crude death rate or infant mortality (IMR) is apparent in the first year of the program in those districts where spray operations were initiated in July 1953, in the six districts (Gurgaon, Gurdaspur, Rohtak, Karnal, Ferozepur, and Amritsar) that appear to have received most of the initial program funding (Table 12.3, Figures 12.2).[21] Instead, mortality levels rose in 1953, as in the rest of the State, though DDT coverage for some, perhaps all, of these districts likely proceeded through much of the 1953 transmission season. Together, this suggests that other factors were contributing to the 1954 CDR decline across the State.

Malaria mortality across the colonial period was typically highest amongst young children. Infant mortality rate trends thus offer an important further gauge of spray program impact. Infant death rates can be seen to have followed closely those of the general population (Figure 12.4), with 1954 again standing out as the point of most substantial decline across the decade. But as with overall mortality (CDR), the decline is seen in all districts (Table 12.3), including those where DDT coverage, judging by houses sprayed and program expenditure,

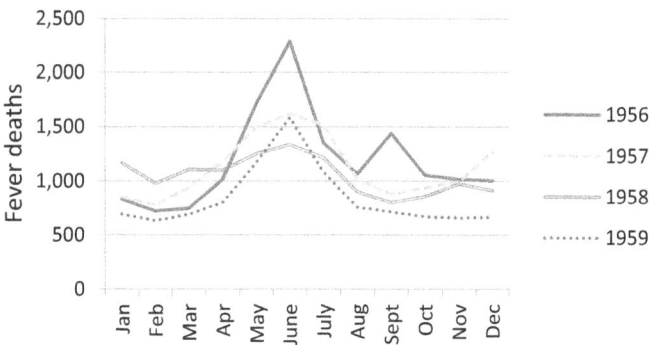

Figure 12.3 Fever deaths, by month, Hissar district, Punjab State (India), 1956–1959

Source: *Report on the Public Health in the Punjab State during the year 1956. . . 1960*, Chandigarh: Controller of Printing & Stationary, Punjab, 1962.

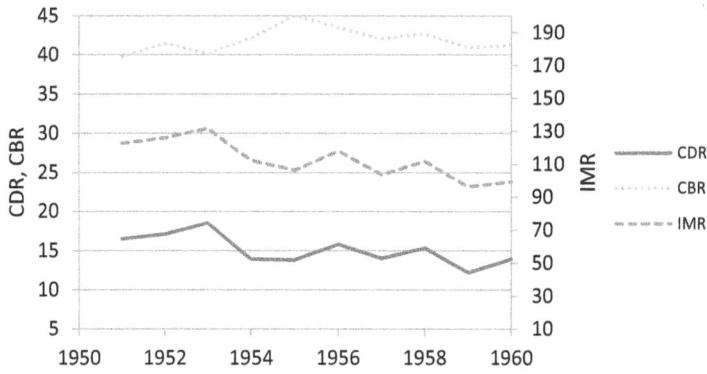

Figure 12.4 Mean annual crude death rate, crude birth rate (per 1,000), infant mortality rate (per 1,000 live births), 11 plains districts, Punjab State (India), 1951–1960

Source: *Census of India, 1961*, Punjab. District Handbooks.

appears to have been still very limited. The decline in infant mortality in 1954 is associated temporally with initiation of the DDT program, yet in districts such as Ferozepur, considerable expansion of houses covered the following year shows no further impact (Table 12.3). Many questions remain, then, regarding the contribution of DDT to the stepwise decline in mortality rates across the State in 1954.[22]

Economic conditions in early 1950s Punjab

Initiation of residual insecticide spraying in Punjab State, in fact, coincided with major economic shifts. The early 1950s were years of famine in Bombay State and Mysore in 1953.[23] Though on the periphery of the major famine tracts, drought affected Punjab's southeastern region in 1951 and continued a second year in Hissar and Ferozepur districts (Table 12.5).

Further compromising livelihood and food security at this time were major changes in food distribution policies. The 1952–1953 period saw the lifting of foodgrain rationing and price controls in Punjab, programs that had been put in place in the final years of World War II. Monthly wheat prices were still under government price control, but prices of the generally cheaper foodgrain crops such as gram, bajra, and jowar rose steeply in 1952 and early 1953. When the price ceiling for gram was removed in June of 1952, for example, market prices

Table 12.5 July–Sept. rain (inches),* by district,** Punjab State (India), 1951–1954

	1951	1952	1953	1954	1868–1944 average
Hissar	**6.5**	**8.6**	12.7	12.6	10.5
Rohtak	**8.2**	19.7	18.0	11.8	13.6
Gurgaon	**10.4**	19.4	18.5	12.6	17.7
Karnal	**11.6**	26.7	20.5	14.3	20.2
Amballa	16.5	20.7	23.7	24.2	20.8
Hoshiarpur	22.3	24.3	25.3	32.9	22.6
Jullundur	12.7	23.7	20.8	20.6	17.4
Ludhiana	14.7	16.4	14.9	20.3	17.3
Ferozepur	**8.2**	**6.9**	10.9	12.0	10.4
Gurdaspur	**15.9**	21.1	29.6	27.1	21.9

*deficit districts, in bold; **Amritsar data unavailable
Source: *Census of India, 1961*, Punjab, District Handbooks; Table 4.1; *Season and Crop Report*, 1941–1944.

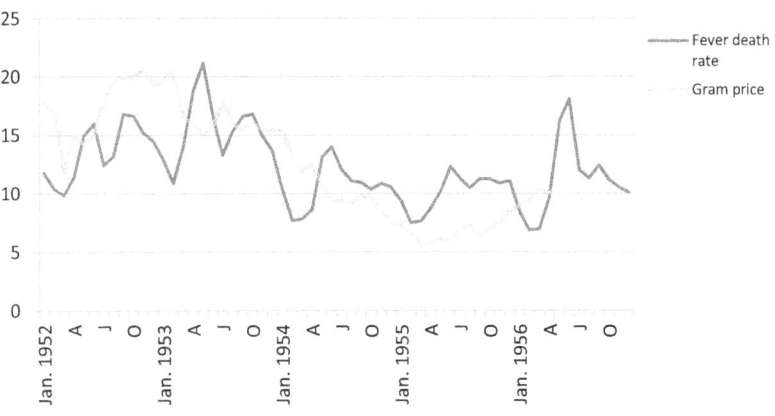

Figure 12.5 Mean monthly fever death rate, 11 plains districts; monthly gram price (Rs/maund, Ludhiana), Punjab State (India), 1952–1956

Source: *Health Statistics of India, 1951–1953*, 134–135, Table 20; *Health Statistics of India, 1954–1955*, 165–166, Table 18; *Census of India, 1961*, Punjab. District Handbooks.

rose over 80 per cent by year's end (Figure 12.5).[24] Across this same period, the size of the 'rationed population' in (East) Punjab was reduced by two-thirds, from 5.8 million in December 1952 to 1.8 million one year later.[25]

Reported mortality levels in the state can be seen to have followed the rise in prices with a three- to five-month lag: fever death rates climbed in the early months of 1953 to peak in April–May of 1953 at 60 per cent above 1951 levels, then plummeted in the final days of 1953 following the bumper harvests and falling prices.[26] In the event, the good harvests of 1953 coincided with cessation of government grain procurement at guaranteed prices. Together, this caused foodgrain prices to plunge further, in the case of gram, falling to one-third their 1952–1953 level by the end of 1954.[27] Market prices generally recovered in 1955–1956, but with the return of indifferent harvests, price behaviour became increasingly volatile, prompting re-institution of a modified system of foodgrain price controls and government procurement policy in the State in 1957.[28]

Interpretation

Initiation of the DDT-based malaria spray program in (East) Punjab in 1953 and its expansion in 1954 thus coincided with a period of marked fluctuation in grain prices and public foodgrain distribution, economic conditions that confound assessment of the spray program's impact on mortality patterns. Several general observations, nevertheless, can be made. Drought-related agricultural unemployment and 'scarcity' prices undoubtedly underlay the initial rise in general mortality levels seen in 1952 in the State, crude death rates rising most in the drought-affected southeastern districts (Figures 12.2a-c). The further rise in the death rate in early 1953 likely was related to continuing high foodgrain prices exacerbated by the lifting of price controls and a decline in the population covered by the foodgrain subsidy program, developments that combined to further undermine food security in the autumn months of 1953. These economic conditions appear to have overridden any potential mortality impact of the initial 1953 DDT spray operations. The marked fall in staple foodgrain prices in 1954 likely played a very substantial role in the drop in the crude death rate that year, an interpretation consistent with the general fall in deaths rates recorded across the State, including Hissar district where DDT use appears to have been the lowest of any district.

As to the role of DDT in death rate trends through the remainder of the 1950s decade, there appears to be little consistent relationship at district level between further CDR decline and timing of spray program expansion. In a number of districts, mortality decline is largely limited to the year 1954, with limited subsequent improvement in mortality indices. The reported proportion of houses covered in Jullundur district, for example, increased from approximately 38 per cent in 1954 to 75 per cent in 1955, but the district registered no decline in crude death rate in that, or subsequent, years (Figure 12.2g).

Interestingly, in a number of the southeastern districts (Hissar, Rohtak, Amballa), both infant and general mortality levels in 1954 were similar to those recorded in 1951. Under-reporting of deaths in 1951 is unlikely since birth rate figures for that year are high, in the 40s per 1,000 population (Table 12.3). This suggests that the 1954 stepwise decline in these districts may largely reflect recovery from 1952–1953 economic (climatic, administrative, market) stresses.

Certainly, some malaria deaths among infants and young children, and stillbirths, were averted in 1950s Punjab with DDT's abrupt interruption of malaria transmission in the state. But the greatest drop in infant mortality between 1953 and 1954 (27.9 points) took place in Hissar district where 1954 DDT coverage appears to have been lowest; nor is decline evident in 1953 among the initial DDT districts. Thus, the contribution of the spray program to mortality decline appears to have been quite limited relative to that of improved foodgrain access in 1954 with plummeting price levels. Moreover, DDT-averted malaria deaths in 1954 were dwarfed by the earlier decline in malaria mortality between 1920 and 1950, considered further below. Future research with extant NMCP records may well shed more light on this interesting decade. But on the basis of available Census data, other interpretations of the impact of malaria transmission control in the state seem implausible.[29]

Limited impact of the DDT-based malaria control program on mortality levels in Punjab (India) may also be a function of the epidemiological phenomenon referred to as 'competing risk': some, possibly many, of the infant deaths averted in 1954 due to interrupted autumnal malaria transmission may simply have been postponed to different seasons of the following year. Those children most at risk of succumbing to malaria infection whose deaths were averted in 1954, by virtue of undernourishment-compromised immune capacity, would also have been particularly vulnerable to other seasonal infections at subsequent times of the year.

This is not to suggest that food security in (East) Punjab State was ideal, or even good, in the 1950s. Endemic and seasonal levels of acute hunger no doubt remained, particularly amongst the landless and young children. In the 1960s, 4.2 per cent of children 12–36 months of age in Narwangal district villages were observed to weigh less than 60 per cent of their expected weight-for-age; and an additional 20 per cent, weighed between 60 and 69 per cent of normal level.[30] But epidemic incidence of semi- and frank starvation so prominent in the pre-1910 era no longer plagued the region.

Post-World War II mortality decline in Punjab

The limited decline in crude death rate levels in East Punjab with the 1950s control of malaria transmission stands in contrast also to the marked decline in mortality experienced in the decade immediately preceding the residual insecticide spray program. By 1951, the mean crude death rate for the 11 plains districts had declined by 38 per cent from pre-World War II (1930–1939) levels (Figure 12.6), and infant mortality rate by 29 per cent (Table 12.6).

Assessing causal factors is particularly complicated in the case of Punjab however because of disruption in vital registration following on the political events of the partition of British India on the eve of its Independence in late 1947. Punjab, along with Bengal, was directly affected by the territorial division associated with Partition, with the Republic of India retaining the 11 eastern plains districts of the former colonial province, while the western and west-central districts came to form Punjab State in Pakistan.[31]

In the brief two-year period, 1945–1946, before Partition, the crude death rate in eastern Punjab fell below 20 deaths per mille for the first time since initiation of vital registration eight decades earlier, much of

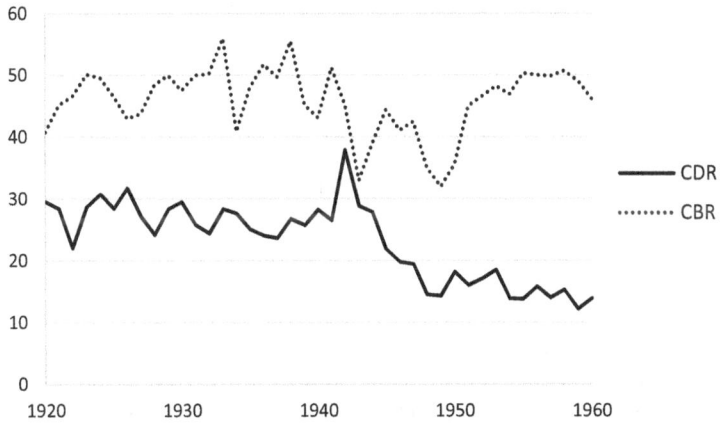

Figure 12.6 Mean annual crude death rate, crude birth rate (per 1,000), infant mortality rate (per 1,000 live births), 11 plains districts, (East) Punjab, 1920–1960 (plague deaths omitted)

Sources: 1920–1947: *PSCR, PPHA*; 1948–1950: Directorate General of Health Services, *Report for the Quadrennium, 1949–1952*, 28; *1951–1960: Census of India, 1961*, Punjab. District Handbooks.

Table 12.6 Mean crude death rate, crude birth rate (per 1,000), infant mortality rate (per 1,000 live births), 11 plains districts, (East) Punjab, 1940–1960

	CDR	IMR	CBR
1940	28.2	178.2	43.1
1941	26.5	215.4	51.2
1942	37.9	213.6	45.1
1943	28.8	190.0	33.0
1944	27.8	173.1	39.0
1945	21.9	145.1	44.4
1946	19.8	133.6	41.1
1947	19.4	154.1	42.5
1948	14.5	130.3	35.0
1949	14.3	131.5	32.0
1950	18.2	160.3	35.6
1951	16.0	122.7	45.0
1952	17.1	125.9	46.6
1953	18.5	131.6	48.2
1954	13.9	112.4	46.9
1955	13.8	106.3	50.3
1956	15.8	118.0	50.0
1957	14.0	103.7	49.8
1958	15.3	111.7	50.7
1959	12.2	96.2	49.0
1960	13.9	99.2	46.1

Source: 1940–1947: *PPHA*; 1948–1950: Directorate General of Health Services, *Report for the Quadrennium, 1949–1952*, 28; *1951–1960*: 1961 Census, Punjab, District Handbooks.

the drop apparent in 1945 itself. The decline does not appear to have been spurious, a function of a sudden fall in vital registration coverage, because a similar decrease is not evident in crude birth rates for these two years.[32]

A second period of marked decline in crude death rates in these same districts, now Punjab state (India), can be seen in 1948 and 1949. Here, however, the decline is accompanied by lower birth rates as well. An explanation thus appears to lie largely in the partial disruption of vital registration related to the chaotic conditions associated with the mass migration of Muslim and Hindu populations between the two regions of the now divided Punjab. Indeed, the sharp decline in 1948 vital rates is most marked for those districts (Ferozerpur, Amritsar, and Gurdaspur) bordering the Partition line with (West) Punjab state in Pakistan (Table 12.7).[33]

Resumption of birth rate levels to pre-Partition levels is evident for most (East) Punjab districts by 1951. This suggests that civilian security conditions are likely to have recovered one year earlier, taking into account an estimated one year lag between the return of social stability, marriage and pre-crisis conception rates, and subsequent births. Vital registration of deaths, therefore, is likely largely to have recovered as well at this time, returning to approximate pre-Partition levels of completeness in 1950.[34] Notably, however, the levels to which recorded mortality rates 'rebounded' in 1950–1951 are considerably lower than those for birth rates (Figure 12.6). The trend of mortality decline first apparent in 1945 appears, in fact, to have been maintained into the early 1950s.

The scale and speed of the 1945–1951 crude death rate decline in (East) Punjab offers important additional perspective for interpreting the region's malaria mortality history. Despite near eradication of malaria transmission in the state in the mid-1950s, the rate of decline after 1951 was much less steep. Indeed, in many of the 11 plains districts, little further decline is evident relative to crude death rate levels recorded in 1951 (Table 12.7). Even for those districts where crude death rates continued to decrease through the 1950s decade, the decline was considerably less prominent than in 1945–1951.

What explains the exceptional improvement in life expectancy in Punjab between 1945 and 1951? Given the marked shortages of antimalarial drugs and other medicines through the war, it is unlikely that improvement in curative care could explain much of the fall in mortality in 1945: reported quantities of quinine and synthetic antimalarials (mepacrine and quinacrine) distributed in the province totalled 3.94 million tablets,[35] much of this directed to urban facilities: in 1947, quinine distributed through public health agencies in East Punjab was reported as 946 pounds in urban areas, 387 in rural;[36] the figure for quinine in 1953–1954 was 1,779 pounds, amounting in *per capita* terms to less than half the level distributed during the 1908 epidemic.[37]

The new anti-malarial drug, chloroquine, a 4-amino-quinolone with fewer side effects than quinine and mepacrine, would become cheaply available in India in the later 1950s. But as late as 1954–1956, Ministry of Health reports make no mention of its distribution through government health facilities.[38] Some unspecified amount of chloroquine, on the other hand, does appear to have been made available through the DDT spray program itself, but the first reference to distribution of anti-malarial drugs within the program appears in 1953–1954.[39] As for rural access, the Punjab State government in 1953 was still reporting difficulty in attracting medical practitioners to work in rural dispensaries, and many remained unstaffed.[40]

Table 12.7 Annual crude death rate, crude birth rate (per 1,000), by district, 1941–1960, 11 plains districts, (East) Punjab*

	Hissar		Rohtak		Gurgaon		Karnal		Ambala		Hoshiarpur		Jullundur		Ferozepur		Ludhiana		Amritsar		Gurdaspur	
	CDR	CBR	CDR	CBR	CDR	CBR	CDR	CBR	CDR	CBR	CDR	CBR	CDR	CBR	CDR	CBR	CDR	CBR	CDR	CBR	CDR	CBR
Mean CDR 1930–40	29.6		28.2		32.8		32.8		32.8		28.5		25.6		27.6		27.7		28.9		28.9	
1941	26.4	44.3	28.6	49.2	26.7	51.2	29.4	46.4	26.0	42.1	26.8	40.7	22.7	39.5	26.4	44.4	23.7	42.8	26.0	44.4	28.5	44.3
1942	54.9	38.5	44.6	41.2	38.4	45.1	46.8	41.8	37.9	39.5	27.1	40.6	25.5	38.8	54.9	39.2	30.3	40.0	24.7	39.2	31.4	43.5
1943	30.0	29.3	32.3	31.3	32.4	33.0	36.0	31.0	30.4	31.0	25.2	40.2	23.4	34.9	30.0	31.8	25.5	34.3	26.4	31.8	25.7	38.5
1944	32.3	44.8	28.1	38.8	31.5	39.0	30.8	39.1	27.9	37.7	26.3	39.5	22.8	36.2	32.3	42.7	23.3	39.8	25.1	42.7	25.1	41.6
1945	22.9	42.9	21.9	43.1	24.7	44.4	23.6	44.5	23.4	41.9	23.0	42.6	18.7	38.3	21.1	42.4	19.5	41.4	20.2	42.4	19.9	44.2
1946	19.1	44.5	16.7	42.4	19.2	41.1	18.3	42.0	19.4	39.7	23.4	40.6	18.6	37.2	19.4	37.5	19.3	38.1	22.3	37.5	21.6	43.2
1947	20.2	36.7	20.1	42.5	17.6	33.8	19.9	39.0	26.3	36.6	22.2	35.0	18.6	29.6	19.2	30.9	19.0	32.6	19.9	30.9	**10.4**	**22.9**
1948	14.2	**30.5**	15.4	39.8	20.4	**35.0**	17.5	**33.9**	16.7	**31.4**	15.5	**29.6**	12.2	**28.9**	11.3	**25.6**	12.5	41.4	11.1	**25.6**	13.0	**26.9**
1949	13.2	37.1	14.9	39.7	19.8	32.0	14.2	39.8	14.5	35.3	17.3	**35.0**	12.5	**31.2**	11.2	**30.5**	12.3	38.1	**13.1**	**30.5**	**14.3**	30.0
1950	16.8	37.9	19.3	40.9	21.7	**35.6**	16.6	35.8	17.3	36.9	22.7	**32.2**	16.8	32.0	17.3	30.1	15.2	**32.6**	16.3	30.1	20.0	29.3
1951	14.9	45.7	14.3	45.4	18.0	45.0	14.1	40.9	15.0	40.1	42.2	42.2	15.7	41.0	17.8	**34.1**	13.1	**29.9**	15.9	**34.1**	16.6	36.4
1952	17.6	41.8	19.2	45.7	23.2	46.6	16.4	44.5	16.1	40.2	20.0	40.6	15.1	39.3	16.1	42.2	13.1	**33.5**	15.1	42.2	15.7	41.8
1953	23.0	40.6	19.2	45.7	22.9	48.2	19.8	42.4	17.1	37.9	20.5	36.7	16.0	37.8	16.9	41.1	14.2	**32.6**	16.8	41.1	17.5	39.2
1954	14.9	43.2	13.8	45.3	16.6	46.9	14.4	46.4	14.3	41.2	15.7	39.7	13.0	38.3	13.0	41.4	11.7	41.8	13.0	41.4	12.9	39.4
1955	14.1	47.1	14.5	49.5	17.7	50.3	13.7	47.6	13.2	44.9	15.2	42.6	13.2	41.1	12.9	42.4	12.1	46.5	12.7	42.4	12.6	42.5
1956	16.8	45.8	16.2	47.3	18.3	50.0	16.5	45.7	16.2	43.2	18.9	39.1	15.0	38.7	13.8	42.0	13.6	45.7	13.0	42.0	16.0	42.6
1957	15.8	49.1	14.9	48.3	17.9	49.8	15.1	49.9	13.6	41.5	15.4	34.3	13.0	35.1	11.8	39.4	12.8	45.2	12.0	39.4	11.7	35.9
1958	15.4	49.9	16.2	47.7	20.3	50.7	17.3	48.9	17.1	45.4	17.3	36.6	14.1	35.0	12.5	39.6	13.6	45.2	11.5	39.6	13.4	36.9
1959	13.0	49.8	11.8	46.0	15.1	49.0	12.9	47.8	12.1	38.1	13.7	34.2	12.1	33.8	10.5	39.9	12.1	43.5	10.1	39.9	11.2	34.7
1960	14.2	50.4	15.0	46.0	17.0	46.1	15.4	49.3	14.7	43.6	15.9	35.5	13.3	33.6	11.4	35.7	12.6	35.7	11.2	35.7	12.5	34.4

Source: *Census of India*, 1951. Punjab. Part 1-A; *Census of India*, 1961, Punjab District Handbooks; *Annual Report of the Public Health Administration, Punjab*, 1930–1940.

* Figures in bold likely reflect relative under-registration

Nor is post-1944 mortality decline likely to have been related to pre-DDT vector control operations. In the late 1930s, a special malaria control organisation had been set up under an Assistant Director of Public Health, Malariology, with six units undertaking rural anti-larval operations in the province, a program that expanded post-war to 12 units. The work carried out, however, appears to have been extremely limited: the 1947 public health report recorded that 1,397 villages had been visited and a total area of 1,728.5 square feet 'filled up or drained.'[41] There were, on the other hand, major economic and public policy shifts affecting food security from the mid-1940s through to the early 1950s.

The Punjab economy in 1945–1946

The immediate post-war period was one of unprecedented, if short-lived, economic growth, triggered by post-war reconstruction and positive terms of trade for many regions of the non-industrialised world. Even before the war ended there had been direct 'benefits' of the war economy for Punjab province. Over the course of the war, Indian army troop strength tripled to 1.5 million, at least half of all combat troops recruited from Punjab.[42] In addition to direct employment, the provisioning of the Indian army (and British and American troops stationed in India) required enormous quantities of foodstuffs. Between 1941 and 1944, Defence Forces purchases of foodgrains increased four-fold to 699,000 tons a year, in addition to vegetables, meat, eggs, and milk. As one of the few foodgrain surplus regions of British India, Punjab was well placed to reap the commercial benefits. Punjab cultivators with surplus grain were guaranteed assured prices and markets even before procurement policies were set in place in 1946.[43] In his late 1940s narrative account of rural Punjab, Darling also described a new 'affluence' related to greater work opportunities, rising wages, and improved bargaining power, reflected classically in an emerging servant-availability 'problem.'[44] Nor was the late-war economic boom limited to Punjab. In his 1954 account of 1940s food administration in India, H.F. Knight observed that 'the increase in the money value of crops during the war allowed the farmer to pay his land revenue and his debts with the sale of a smaller quantity of grain than before, with the result that he and his family could eat more food, and thus send a smaller quantity to market.'[45]

There was, of course, a much darker side to the war economy as well, to which Punjab was by no means immune. Extreme price inflation accompanied the war-time economic surge, as we have seen, in

Punjab in 1942. The war had acutely exacerbated an already dire food security situation in the country. Three decades of stagnation in overall foodgrain production and declining *per capita* levels, in turn, had left the subcontinent increasingly dependent on foreign imports of staple foodgrains. With the 1942 Japanese occupation of Burma and abrupt curtailment of rice exports to India, the British Raj found itself facing a food crisis of profound dimensions.

The consequences of a war economy were played out most starkly in Bengal, as seen above. Bengal, however, was not the only food deficit region at the outbreak of World War II. Throughout much of southern India, the food situation also was desperate, foodgrain prices by late 1942 having reached 'scarcity' levels in all regions. By late 1943, the horrors of famine in Bengal had forced the central government to take complete control over staple foodgrain distribution across India. Indeed, the Madras government had already proceeded on its own.[46] Over the final two years of the war, a comprehensive program of price control and food distribution took shape, and by 1945, a population of 50 million in 516 cities and towns in British India was covered by food rationing.

Precariousness of overall foodgrain supply deepened further, however, in the final days of the war with consecutive years of poor harvests in 1945 and 1946. South Asian crop conditions coincided, moreover, with poor agricultural harvests globally, reducing prospects for imports and further fuelling inflation.[47] By September 1946, open market wheat prices across the subcontinent were almost 400 per cent above August 1939 levels. In the face of even greater harvest shortfalls post-war, the ration system was further expanded to a population of over 150 million in 771 towns and rural areas by October 1946, and 159.5 million by early 1947, at this point covering just over half the population of British India.[48]

Punjab foodgrain controls and hunger endemiology

As a foodgrain-surplus region of British India, Punjab initially had resisted central government efforts for procurement and controlled prices. That indisposition would be overcome with the poor harvests of 1945 and 1946 and deepening food shortages. Facing increasing food anxiety within Punjab itself, the provincial government introduced a comprehensive system of monopoly procurement of wheat in April 1946. Within the year, all surplus foodgrains were under government control through the province's 500 grain markets: '[a]ll movement of wheat by rail or road was prohibited, except between village and market, or under government permit.' A system of direct food rationing, begun initially in three Punjab cities in 1944, was expanded to all towns and cities, covering a population of 3 million of the province's 28 million population, a system that would remain in place through to 1952–1953.

Rationing was not extended to the rural population of Punjab, unlike in the southern deficit provinces and States of Travancore and Cochin. However, a network of Fair Price Shops ('Relief Quota Shops') ensured access to foodgrains at controlled prices for 3.55 million of the rural Punjab population.[49] As well, market price controls and price guarantees at favourable levels to rural producers contributed to greater price stability, and more assured price-access at village level.[50] For the rural poorest, access to staple foodgrains is likely to have improved simply through reduction of seasonal fluctuations in foodgrain prices. At the same time, active government support associated with the post-war Grow More Food Campaign may well have increased agricultural employment.[51]

Hastily organised, the food procurement and rationing system that emerged across India in the final years of British rule was not without problems, particularly in Bengal where the relative absence of a rural administrative structure made implementation that much more difficult and open to abuse.[52] Yet in June 1946, assessment by the American Famine Mission under Theodore W. Schultz found

> a highly successful system of rationing and enforced procurement of foodgrains. . . . No country in the world, with perhaps the exception of Russia, has gone so far in controlling basic food distribution. . . . Popular provincial governments and skilled public administrators together have accomplished extraordinary results.[53]

Briefly terminated in 1952–1953, as seen above, the program would be re-introduced in modified form in 1957.

Thus, the economic boom of the later war years in Punjab province corresponded also to a period of unprecedented public intervention in foodgrain supply and distribution. Rationing and food price controls, prompted by the sheer depth of the late-war food crisis, ensured that at least some of the benefits of the post-war economic boom reached some of the least food secure. Hardly lavish, nor even minimally adequate, the official ration amounted to at most 16 ounces of foodgrain (wheat or rice) per adult a day, reduced to 12 ounces through the peak crisis period of 1945–1946 – and in southern India, even less. But for those most vulnerable, for whom access to basic food was most precarious, this amount, at controlled prices, assured real if limited access to staple grains, quite possibly shifting many households from zero meals a day to at least one, through the annual 'lean' or 'hunger' seasons when prices were high and employment and earnings low or negligible.[54] Accompanying this shift, Knight later observed, was public articulation of the notion of 'equal sacrifice,' containing also an embryonic notion of a 'right' to food.[55]

For agriculturalists, post-war economic conditions were favourable in a number of spheres. Between 1938 and 1948, the real burden of the agricultural revenue demand declined by an estimated 75 per cent, largely the effect of war-time inflation. But the country's financial situation had also been transformed. From one of major pre-war debt, by the end of World War II, the Reserve Bank of India had accumulated foreign assets, owed mainly by Britain, of over Rs 17,000 million.[56] Few food consumption studies were undertaken across this period, but on the basis of those available, Sinha in 1961 concluded that 'cultivators during the post-war period [were] eating more than they did in the pre-war years.' Dietary survey data from the post-war 1949–1950 period show a 10–12 per cent increase in cereal consumption for West Bengal and Hyderabad, and additional increases in vegetables, oils, and milk, compared with levels observed in 1934–1938.[57] For Punjab, there is evidence of a shift from millets and gram towards wheat consumption, generally a more expensive grain. There also appears to have been increased consumption of vegetables, oils/ghee, and sugar, altogether increasing total calorie consumption above levels recorded in the 1930s.[58] Though these data in the case of Punjab represent cultivator households rather than the landless, the shift away from nearly complete dependence on grains suggests a broader improvement in caloric consumption and food security in the province.[59]

'An abrupt period of discontinuity'

Post-war economic growth was not limited to Punjab, or even South Asia. European reconstruction had triggered a surge in demand for raw materials and primary products, and a corresponding shift in terms of trade between the industrialised and developing countries through the later 1940s.[60] The economic boom was associated with a marked drop in general mortality levels in many global regions. In Egypt, crude death rates fell from 27.7 in 1945 to 17.7 by 1952. Major declines were seen across Latin America and Africa as well in the immediate post-war years, corresponding to a period of 'unusually rapid economic growth.'[61]

For India as a whole, between the 1921–1930 and 1941–1950 decades, the crude death rate fell by 31 per cent, infant mortality by 28 per cent. Much of this improvement was concentrated in the immediate post-war period, amounting to one 'of the fastest CDR declines of the modern era,' Dyson and Murphy observe, improvement that 'took up to a century to achieve in nineteenth-century Europe.'[62] To a limited extent, the post-World War II accelerated mortality decline in South Asia represented catch-up with an earlier trend of modest decline evident from the 1920s, a pattern reversed with World War II price inflation. But it also reflected a real jump in survival rates in the later 1940s above the pre-existing trend. In Punjab, for example, life expectancy in Ludhiana district rose by 12 years across the 1940s decade, much of that increase occurring between 1945 and 1950.[63] 'A very sizeable fraction of all mortality decline since World War II [to 1990],' Dyson and Murphy observe, 'occurred in an abrupt period of discontinuity which ended around 1952.'[64]

The period of favourable terms of trade would draw to a close by the early 1950s, as also that of rapid mortality decline, in Punjab and in developing countries generally.[65] In some (East) Punjab districts, more modest levels of decline are evident through the 1950s. But, as seen earlier, it is difficult to relate temporally even this later decline to DDT-based interruption of malaria transmission.[66] Expressed another way, the contribution of malaria transmission control in rising survival rates was vastly overshadowed by that of food distribution policies and increased employment levels for the food-insecure across the post-World War II decade.

In the post-1920 era, no longer were acute food crises allowed to proceed to mass starvation ('epidemics of death') in British India – except where imperial priorities and preoccupations of war interceded. Along with pre-empting epidemic destitution, famine relief policies post-1920 began to stem the recurring capital drain from agriculture, thus possibly moderating to some extent levels of *endemic* destitution alongside its epidemic form. The sheer depth of the World War II food crisis further forced the establishment of some minimal food-access 'floor' for at least some among the most food-insecure portion of the population. In light of the close pre-World War I relationship between destitution and malaria lethality, these two major shifts in public policy – control of epidemic *acute* hunger and some portion of its endemic form – may well explain the absence of a demonstrable effect on crude death rate levels in Punjab with the interruption in malaria transmission in the 1950s.[67]

Malaria rebound

With the decline in external funding of the National Malaria Eradication Programme in India in the late 1960s, malaria transmission rebounded rapidly in much of South Asia, including in Punjab. The annual parasite incidence (API), a general measure of malaria prevalence, was as low as 0.02 per 1000 in Punjab (India) in 1965, but by 1978 it had climbed back to 55.9 per 1,000 in Haryana (the post-Independence State, formerly southeast Punjab).[68] In some districts falciparum malaria prevalence reached 327.6 per 1,000 population.[69] A 2004 estimate suggests annual malaria incidence in India as high as 70 million, taking into account a high rate of 'inapparent' (subclinical) infection.[70] Yet despite the return to high rates of both vivax and falciparum infection amongst a largely non-immune population, modest mortality decline continued through the late 1960s, 1970s and 1980s.[71]

Some have attributed the absence of an identifiable increase in general death rate levels with malaria's return to improved access to treatment.[72] Availability of anti-malarial drugs no doubt was better in India by the 1970s than two decades earlier. But timely access to basic medical care in rural India was by no means universal or even necessarily good in these later post-Independence decades.[73] Malaria in South Asia by the mid-20th century, it appears, had lost most of its historical 'terror,' as it also had in Italy by the late 1920s.[74]

Most, but not all. The profile of malaria morbidity and mortality evident in contemporary India appears to correspond closely to that of the colonial period, the human toll concentrated geographically and socio-economically among populations most marginalised, most subject to destitution, and with least access to basic treatment. And as in the earlier colonial period, it is a handful of health workers and activists who have undertaken the technically and professionally challenging task of documenting this socio-economic profile underlying much of malaria's continuing human cost.[75]

Notes

1 A. Sen, *Poverty and Famines: An Essay on Entitlement and Deprivation* (Oxford: Clarendon Press, 1981), 216; Famine Inquiry Commission, India, *Report on Bengal* (New Delhi: Government of India, 1945), 123. Maharatna suggests a possible role for immunological factors in explaining regional differentials in 1943 Bengal malaria mortality. He points to proportionately greater famine mortality increases in previously 'healthier' districts where endemic malaria levels were lower, positing that greater pre-famine acquired immunity levels in the less-healthy districts offered

relative protection from malaria; *The Demography of Famines* (New Delhi: Oxford University Press, 1996), 220. He also notes, correctly, that climatic conditions were unchanged in 1943, but not the corollary: that malaria transmission was probably also unchanged. Thus, it is unclear why higher acquired immunity would abruptly offer increased protection there in 1943 when it did not in years before. More likely, changes in relative protection stemmed from factors unrelated to malaria *transmission*, but rather from changes in host *response* to its endemic presence, either through differential treatment access (unlikely), or a shift in relative *susceptibility* to malaria between the two groups of districts. For discussion of differing vulnerability to famine-hyperinflation among Bengal districts in 1943; see S. Zurbrigg, 'Regional Differentials in 1943 Bengal Malaria Mortality: A Comment,' *Uncoupling Disease and Destitution: The Case of South Asian Malaria History*, in preparation.

2 S. Zurbrigg, 'Did Starvation Protect from Malaria? Distinguishing Between Severity and Lethality of Infectious Disease in Colonial India,' *Social Science History*, 21, 1, 1997, 27–58.

3 *Stat. Abst*, 1949.

4 Aggressive relief measures were undertaken in Bombay and Madras provinces in Dec. 1942; A.R. Vasavi, 'The 'Millet Drought'' Oral Narratives and the Cultural Grounding of Famine-relief in Bijapur,' *South Indian Studies*, 2, July–Dec. 1996, 205–233; A. Maharatna, *The Demography of Famines: An Indian Historical Perspective* (New Delhi: Oxford University Press, 1996), 222–234.

5 Guilmoto remarks on the often highly speculative character to the thesis of changing microbe virulence in epidemic analysis; 'Towards a New Demographic Equilibrium: The Inception of Demographic Transition South India,' *IESHR*, 28, 3, 1992, 247–289, at 276.

6 WHO-initiated demonstration projects were located in the Sagar area of Karnataka, the U.P. Terai, Orissa, and Wynaad Taluk, Kerala; R. Rao, *Anophelines of India*, 1st ed. (New Delhi: Malaria Research Centre, ICMR, 1984), 152. A U.S.-aided trial was undertaken in Bombay province; D.K. Viswanathan, T. Ramachandra Rao, 'Control of Rural Malaria with D.D.T. Indoor Residual Spraying in Kanara and Dharwar Districts, Bombay Province. First Year's Results,' *IJM*, 1, 4, Dec. 1947, 503–542.

7 D.R. Mehta, 'Malaria Control in the Punjab (India) with Special Reference to the National Malaria Control Programme,' *IJM*, 9, 4, Dec. 1955, 327–342, at 335.

8 Mehta, 'Malaria control in the Punjab,' 335–336, 338; *Report on the Public Health Administration of the Punjab State, 1955*, 26 [hereafter, PPHA].

9 *Census of India, 1961*. Punjab. District Handbooks, No. 1, Hissar; __, No. 2, Rohtak; __, No. 3, Gurgaon; __, No. 4, Karnal; __, No. 5, Amballa; __, No. 9, Hoshiarpur; __, No. 10, Jullundur; __, No. 11, Ludhiana; __, No. 12, Ferozepur; __, No. 13, Amritsar; __, No. 14, Gurdaspur.

10 Mehta, 'Malaria Control in the Punjab,' Appendix I, 342; M. Yacob, S. Swaroop, 'Malaria and Spleen Rate in the Punjab,' *IJM*, 1, 4, Dec. 1947, 469–487.

11 Directorate of National Malaria Eradication Programme, *Malaria and its Control in India* (New Delhi: Directorate General of Health Services, GOI, 1986), 43.

12 *Health Statistics of India, 1958–1959* (New Delhi: India. Ministry of Health, Directorate General of Health Services, n.d.), 249, Table 48.

13 E.P. Hicks, S. Abdul Majid, "A Study of the Epidemiology of Malaria in a Punjab District," *RMSI*, 7, 1, 1937, 1–43, 40.

14 Mehta, 'Malaria control in the Punjab,' 338.

15 *Health Statistics of India, 1951–1953* (New Delhi: Director General of Health Services, Ministry of Health, GOI Press, 1958), 134–135, Table 20; *Health Statistics of India,1954–1955*, 165–166, Table 18; *Ann. Rpt on the Public Health in the Punjab State during the Year 1956 (1957, 1958, 1959, 1960)* (Chandigarh: Director, Health Services, Punjab), Annual Form X. Unfortunately, monthly data do not appear to be available for individual districts in the public health reports for the years 1951–1955, a period of district boundary and reporting changes.

16 Monthly fever mortality data at district-level were unavailable to the author for the years 1948–1955; thus, it has not been possible to track Oct.–Dec. fever death rates for individual districts across the key 1953–1954 period.

17 *Health Statistics of India, 1951–1953*, 111, Table 15; *Health Statistics of India, 1954–1955*, 166, Table 18; *Census 1961*, Punjab. District Handbooks, note 43.

18 Mehta, 'Malaria control in the Punjab,' 335, 338.

19 Ibid., 335.

20 For initial districts, 1953–1954 expenditures ranged between Rs 30–56,000; the initial 1954–1955 expenditure for Hissar district is reported as Rs 9,551. In reporting district spleen rates, Mehta omits Hissar altogether; 'Malaria control in the Punjab,' 342.

21 Almost half the Gurgaon and Karnal district population was recorded as 'living in DDT-sprayed houses' in 1953–1954; District Handbooks, Table 27.

22 A second, smaller dip in both vital rates is seen in many districts in 1959. In this case, unlike 1954, the decline does not generally correspond to program expansion, with the exception of Hoshiarpur district.

23 *Census 1951*, 61.

24 *Census of India, 1961*. Punjab District Handbooks: Ludhiana, Jullundur, Amballa, Ferozepur, Table 10; Gurgaon, Table 9.

25 [Republic of India]. *Food Situation in India, 1939–1953* (New Delhi: Directorate of Economics and Statistics. Food Economics Branch, 1954), 76–79.

26 *Health Statistics of India (1951–1952–1953)*, 134–135.

27 *Census of India, 1961*. Punjab, District Handbooks.

28 R.N. Chopra, *Evolution of Food Policy in India* (New Delhi: Palgrave Macmillan, 1981), 85–87, 76–77; J. Mooij, *Food Policy and the Indian State: The Public Distribution System in South India* (New Delhi: Oxford University Press, 1999), 68.

29 The impact of economic conditions on malaria mortality trends is an issue raised in relation to post-World War II Sri Lanka, analysis that also has questioned the assumed primacy of the DDT spray program in post-war mortality decline. On this, see H. Frederiksen, 'Malaria Control and Population Pressure in Ceylon,' *Public Health Reports*, 75, 10, Oct. 1960, 865–868; __, 'Determinants and Consequences of Mortality Trends in Ceylon,' *Public*

Health Reports, 76, 8, Aug. 1961, 659–663. See also, C. Langford, 'Reasons for the Decline in Mortality in Sri Lanka Immediately After the Second World War: A Re-Examination of the Evidence,' *Health Transition Review*, 6, 1996, 3–23, 15; Zurbrigg, *Uncoupling Disease and Destitution*.

30 A.A. Kielmann, C. McCord, 'Weight-For-Age as an Index of Risk of Death in Children,' *Lancet*, 311 (8076), June 10, 1978, 1247–1250.

31 In the analysis that follows, 1920–1960 data relate to the 11 eastern plains districts.

32 A characteristic birth rate decline, however, is seen in 1943 in the famine-affected districts following famine conditions in eastern Punjab in 1942. See also Dyson and Das Gupta, 'Demographic Trends in Ludhiana District,' 89.

33 These three districts show 1948 crude birth rates in the mid-20s per 1000 population, levels that may also reflect some actual decline accompanying the insecurities of mass migration; Dyson and Das Gupta, 'Demographic Trends in Ludhiana District,' 95.

34 Two districts are exceptions, with birth rates remaining low in 1951 (Ferozepur) and 1951–1953 (Ludhiana), suggesting possible under-registration also of deaths in these years.

35 *GOI-PHC*, 1945, 15–16.

36 *Stat. Abst., India, 1950* (Calcutta: GOI Press), 63; *PPHA* 1947, Appendix I, 39, *Statistical Appendices to the Annual Report of the Director-General of Health Services for the Year 1947*. Part I, 1950, 48, 50.

37 Directorate General Health Services, 'Ministry of Health,' *Annual Report, 1953*, 130.

38 Directorate General Health Services, 'Ministry of Health,' *Report for 1954–1956*, 204.

39 Mehta, 'Malaria control in the Punjab,' 338.

40 'Directorate General of Health Service,' *Annual Report, 1953*, 30.

41 *Report of the Public Health Administration of East Punjab for the year 1947*, 3, 28–29. Mehta characterised pre-1950 antimalaria measures in Punjab as 'very restricted'; 'Malaria control in the Punjab,' 334.

42 H.F. Knight, *Food Administration in India, 1939–1947* (Stanford: Stanford University Press, 1954), 158.

43 Ibid., 229, 136.

44 M.L. Darling, *At Freedom's Door* (London: Oxford University Press, 1949), 90, 67.

45 Ibid., 14.

46 Maharatna, *The Demography of Famines*, 224–225.

47 'By . . . 1945, there was a widespread belief that the cessation of hostilities would be followed by economic depression . . . It was thus thought necessary that the war expenditure should be replaced by other expenditure . . . based on a five-year plan. . . . The enhanced purchasing power arising from war and post-war inflation . . . led . . . to still higher prices'; *Census of India, 1951*, ch. I, Section III, 'Growth of Population,' 42–43. Savings bank deposits in Orissa increased twenty-fold to Rs 1,20,61,110 between 1945 and 1949; ibid.

48 Knight, *Food Administration in India*, 215, 307–308, 189.

49 *Census of India, 1951*, Vol. I. India, Part I-A, 316–317.

50 In April 1944, the GOI offered guaranteed prices, committed to buying all wheat in Punjab and Sind at Rs 7 and 8. This, and a similar plan

in Bombay 'proved a very steadying influence when acute shortage reappeared in 1946'; *Indian Year Book, and Who's Who* (Bombay: Bennett, Coleman and Co., 1947), 349; cited in Knight, *Food Administration in India*, 213.

51 Knight, *Food Administration in India*, 122–148.
52 In Calcutta alone, Darling estimated there were 'not less than a million bogus rations cards.' Black market activity, he observes, was also widespread in Punjab; *At Freedom's Door*, 40–41, 320–321.
53 Knight, *Food Administration in India*, 253.
54 A similar increase in life expectancy occurred in Britain during both world war periods with food rationing and unemployment decline; J. Drèze, A. Sen, *Hunger and Public Action* (Oxford: Clarendon Press, 1989), 182.
55 Sinha, *Food Administration in India*, 265.
56 E. Stokes, 'Northern and Central India,' in D. Kumar, ed., *Cambridge Economic History of India* (Cambridge: Cambridge University Press, 1983), vol. 2, 36–85 [hereafter *CEHI*]; D. Kumar, 'The Fiscal System,' in D. Kumar, ed., *CEHI*, 905–945.
57 R.P. Sinha, *Food in India: An Analysis of the Prospects for Self-Sufficiency by 1975–1976* (Bombay: Oxford University Press, 1961), 16; S.M. Roy, 'Food Consumption in India,' *Agricultural Situation in India*, Vol. 7, 1952, as cited in Sinha, *Food in India*, 17.
58 Ibid., 17.
59 Set against this was slight decline in industrial wages between 1931–1932 and 1950–1951; V.K.R.V. Rao, 'Changes in India's National Income,' *Supplement to Capital*, Dec. 16, 1954, as cited in Sinha, *Food in India*, 11.
60 T. Dyson and M. Murphy, 'Macro-Level Study of Socioeconomic Development and Mortality: Adequacy of Indicators and Methods of Statistical Analysis,' in J. Cleland, A. Hill, eds., *The Health Transition: Methods and Measures* (Canberra: Australian National University, 1991), Health Transition Series No. 3, 147–164, at 151. See also, E. Boserup, 'The Role of the Primary Sector in African Development,' in L. Mats, ed., *The Primary Sector in African Development* (London: Croom Helm, 1985); G.K. Helleiner, *Peasant Agriculture, Government and Economic Growth in Nigeria* (Homewood IL: Irwin, 1966), 30.
61 Dyson and Murphy, 'Macro-Level Study,' 148; T. Dyson, M. Das Gupta, 'Demographic Trends in Ludhiana District, Punjab, 1881–1981: 'An Exploration of Vital Registration Data in Colonial India,' in Ts'ui-jung Liu et al., eds., *Asian Population History* (Oxford: Oxford University Press, 2001), 79–104, at 95.
62 Dyson and Murphy, 'Macro-level study,' 153, 148.
63 Dyson and Das Gupta, 'Demographic Trends in Ludhiana,' 95.
64 Dyson and Murphy, 'Macro-level study,' 147.
65 Ibid.
66 Other post-Independence development programs affecting food security and mortality levels were pursued: in Hissar, for example, irrigated area rose from one-eighth of cropped area to one-third by 1961; *Census of India, 1961*. Punjab. District Census Handbook, Hissar, 66–67.
67 Whether this was so in less economically fortunate states in India remains a question for future analysis.

68 Directorate of National Malaria Eradication Programme, *Malaria and its Control in India*, 172, Table 55.

69 V.P. Sharma et al., 'Studies on the True Incidence of Malaria in Kharkhoda (District Sonepat, Haryana) and Kichha (District Nainital, U.P.) Primary Health Centres,' *IJM*, 20, June 1983, 21–34, at 31; V.P. Sharma, K.N. Mehrotra, 'Malaria Resurgence in India: A Critical Study,' *Social Science Medicine*, 22, 1986, 835–845.

70 V.P. Sharma, 'Battling the Malaria Iceberg with Chloroquine in India,' *Malaria Journal*, 6, 2007, 105. See also, R.S. Yadav et al., 'The Burden of Malaria in Ahmedabad City, India: a Retrospective Analysis of Reported Cases and Deaths,' *Annals of Tropical Medicine and Parasitology*, 97, 8, 2003, 793–802; WHO, *World Malaria Report*, 2009.

71 Similar late 1960s malaria rebound occurred in Sri Lanka; Department of Census and Statistics, *The Population of Sri Lanka* (Colombo: Govt of Sri Lanka, 1974), Table 2.19.

72 D. Bradley, 'Malaria: Old Infections, Changing Epidemiology,' *Health Transition Review*, 2, 1992, Suppl. 137–152, at 151.

73 I.P. Singh, 'Malaria Raj in Rajasthan,' *Health for the Millions*, Nov.–Dec. 1994, 41–51, 46–47, 58–59. K. Mankodi, 'Political and Economic Roots of Disease: Malaria in Rajasthan,' *EPW*, Jan. 27, 1996, PE-42–48, at 47.

74 N.H. Swellengrebel, 'Some Aspects of the Malaria Problem in Italy,' in LNHO. Malaria Commission, *Report on its Tour of Investigation in Certain European Countries in 1924*, C.H. 273, Geneva, Mar. 26, 1925, Annex 11, 168–171.

75 See, for example, V.P. Sharma, 'Malaria and Poverty,' *Current Science*, 84, 2003, 513–515; M. Shiva, 'Mewat Calling: A Brief Report of the Malaria Outbreak in Mewat,' *Health for the Millions*, Mar.–Apr. 1997, 11–12; K.K. Mathur et al., 'Epidemic of Malaria in Barmer District (Thar Desert) of Rajasthan During 1990,' *IJM*, 29, Mar. 1992, 1–10; K. Mankodi, 'Political and Economic Roots of Disease: Malaria in Rajasthan,' *EPW*, Jan. 27, 1996, PE-42–48; M. Pai et al., 'Malaria and Migrant Labourers,' *EPW*, Apr. 19, 1997, 838–842; A. Kumar et al., 'Malaria Related to Construction in Panaji, Goa,' *IJM*, 28, Dec. 1991, 219–225; V. Kamat, 'Resurgence of Malaria in Bombay *(Mumbai)* in the 1990s: A Historical Perspective,' *Parassitologia*, 42, 2000, 135–148, 2000, at 145; R. Tripathy et al., 'Clinical Manifestations and Predictors of Severe Malaria in Indian Children,' *Pediatrics*, 120, e454–460, 2007; L. Lobo, *Malaria in the Social Context: A Study in Western India* (New Delhi: Routledge) 165, 170.

13 Conclusion

The poorer classes have been much distressed for food, and have suffered unusual hardships in consequence. The [high fever mortality rate] . . . is the result of widespread poverty and distress for food which have reduced the bodily strength of the people to such a degree as to render them incapable of resisting the assaults of any disease going.
– *Punjab Sanitary Commission Report*, 1878, pp. 28–29.

Compiled as a key technique of imperial control over the Indian subcontinent, the annual vital registration records of colonial South Asia offer historians exceptional insights into conditions of living and the determinants of premature mortality in the region. No one in the Indian Medical Service analysed this wealth of data more effectively than S.R. Christophers, whose work empirically confirmed the commonplace relationship between malaria lethality and 'scarcity.'[1] Ironically perhaps, it would be this most loyal servant to the British Raj who helped steer the India Office ultimately away from its disastrously ideological doctrine of foodgrain *laissez-faire*.

S.R. Christophers's 1911 *Malaria in the Punjab* is an epidemiological account of the role of acute hunger (semi- and frank starvation) in the 'fulminant' malaria epidemics that afflicted the northwest plains of British India. Through detailed spatial mapping of autumn epidemic fever mortality, he demonstrated the primacy of broad economic factors at play, beyond either rainfall or physiography, in the region's 'fulminant' malaria epidemics. These factors he interpreted as prevailing agricultural hardship – epidemic human destitution – in many cases compounded by post-drought flooding. Fever mortality in years such as 1908 was similar in its seasonal timing to that in non-epidemic years, revealing 'only a great exaggeration of normal stress.'[2] The physiologic mechanisms underlying the 'exalted' lethality of malaria under famine conditions, he inferred, involved starvation-induced suppression of immune capacity, but possibly also secondary dose effects. Delayed recovery – inability to clear parasites from the bloodstream – among the famished, he hypothesised, possibly led to heavier infection levels in subsequent feeding mosquitoes, and, in turn, higher sporozoite doses inoculated in succeeding cycles of human transmission.[3] And yet here, too, the mortal impact fell largely on the famished.

Employing modern methods of statistical analysis, this study has re-examined, and corroborated, Christophers's 1911 findings regarding the central role of 'scarcity' in Punjab's epidemic malaria history between 1868 and 1908. His conclusions are further borne out with extension of the quantitative analysis to the 1909–1940 period of epidemic decline and to subsequent years, including the 1950s decade that saw the virtual elimination of malaria transmission in the region. This study thus belongs to the field of historical *endemiology*: analysis of trends in the mortality burden of diseases routinely present in populations. It contrasts with more classic *epidemic* history where the focus is generally on diseases exceptional in their epidemiology and inherent virulence such as bubonic plague or pandemic influenza, introduced irregularly into populations from external sources.

The significance of the distinction is considerable. As an endemic disease, the seasonal mortality toll of malaria in the Indian subcontinent was shaped by broader socio-economic factors beyond ecological conditions of vector transmission. Malaria *mortality* historiography is, therefore, also, at its core, an exploration of a region's larger ecological, subsistence, and political histories – if more complex for this reason.

The particular ecology of the northwest plains of the Indian subcontinent offers an important opportunity to track with some confidence malaria death rates across the colonial period. This, in turn, allows analysis of trends in malaria mortality in relation to yearly malaria transmission levels, human host destitution (acute hunger), and access to curative treatment, and thus to elucidate the relative contribution of each in the region's malaria history. Preceding by more than three decades the DDT-based malaria eradication program of the 1950s, the decline in epidemic malaria in Punjab sheds renewed light on the role of staple-food precarity in malaria's historical mortality burden.

A link between hunger and malaria lethality was well recognised in 19th-century British India, understood certainly by those directly affected, but also by provincial sanitary administrators whose annual reports from the 1880s were framed by harvest conditions and grain-price data. *Malaria in the Punjab*, then, was simply empirical confirmation of such a relationship. As seen in chapter 6, Punjab sanitary officials articulated the hunger-malaria nexus in classic predispositionist terms: '[t]he comparative scarcity of food' preceding the 1892 epidemic, 'reducing as it did the physical powers of the poorer classes, was doubtless a predisposing cause of the excessively severe outbreak of fever.'[4] Though rare to appear in official records, the primacy of hunger was expressed by the food-insecure themselves, in villagers' ardent late 19th-century appeal for irrigation over authorities' concerns with 'fever': 'GIVE US BREAD, if Providence wills we may die of fever.'[5]

A 'more complex' epidemiology

In modern epidemic theory, the concept closest to pre-20th-century understanding of predisposition is that of synergism – two factors in combination producing an effect greater than the sum of their individual effects. In its general use, however, the term arguably fails to convey the centrality of acute hunger in transforming endemic malaria infection into its historically 'fulminant' form. For a 20th-century audience with little direct experience of mass destitution, 'synergy' is more likely to be understood as enhancing lethality rather than largely determining it, the latter expressed in Christophers's depiction of malaria as 'merely reap[ing] a harvest prepared for it by the famine.'

Christophers recognised the linguistic limitations to modern epidemiological terminology. 'The word epidemic, applied as it is to outbreaks of disease on a small scale,' he advised, 'does not sufficiently characterise such vast exhibitions of the power of zymotic disease. . . . Large epidemics usually have a more complex epidemiology.'[6] The malaria 'death storms' mapped by him required instead an earlier, presanitationist interpretation: epidemic mortality appearing simultaneously over large areas unexplained by person to person 'contagion' and considered, in 19th-century zymotic terms, to originate instead under atmospheric conditions conducive to fermentation. It was this vast spatial character that Christophers invoked to convey the 'fulminant' malaria witnessed in Punjab – phenomena that would soon come to be referred to as 'regional' epidemics – but with his *zymonic* neologism highlighting a different spatial determinant involved, one economic rather than miasmic in nature, though also atmospheric in origin: harvest failure and paralysis of livelihood.

If *Malaria in the Punjab* offered a 'more complex' epidemiology, it was one only remotely recognisable to early 20th-century malaria researchers trained in sanitationist theory and newly aware of the vector role of anopheline mosquitoes in malaria transmission. Thus, Christophers was reclaiming an earlier understanding of epidemic disease that recognised the immense variation in clinical morbidity and mortality observed with common endemic infections. Four decades earlier, Sir Joseph Fayrer, Surgeon-General and President of the Medical Board at the India Office, had come to describe malaria in similar terms, as 'varying in intensity from the deadliest fever to the most transient disturbance of the general health,' the former shown in 'the great prevalence . . . of the fevers and bowel complaints which destroy or deteriorate millions . . . in some years almost challeng[ing] comparison with the Black Death.'[7] It was an understanding arrived at through practical experience. Fayrer in his 1882 tract on the *Fevers of India* quotes, in agreement, remarks by the Secretary to the head of the Bengal Medical Department, ' "I came out [to India] imbued with a belief in the truth of the views of European pathologists, but Indian experience has compelled me to recognize that those views . . . are too exclusive, and quite inadequate.' "[8] Recounting the malaria death tolls recently reported during the famine years of 1877–1879, Fayrer concluded that '[t]he fundamental cause of the great loss of life from fever [in India] was increased predisposition from scarcity of food.'[9]

Christophers no doubt was familiar with Fayrer's 1882 text. But his later zymonic attribution, penned in 1924, quite possibly was informed also by the malaria epidemic that had recently swept across post-World War I famine-afflicted Russia.[10] Though the latter was generally interpreted at the time in modern entomological terms, with an emphasis on vector transmission, the close relationship with prevailing epidemic typhus also suggested a central role for destitution (starvation). The Punjab inquiry, in other words, had led him to interpret 'fulminant' malaria in relation to the great mortalities of the past as 'death storms' from common, endemic infections rendered much more lethal under conditions of mass human debility. In this, he was straddling two epistemic eras, using modern scientific methods to demonstrate and incorporate pre-modern understanding of destitution in disease epidemic mortality patterns.[11]

Political significance

Malaria in the Punjab and its preceding sister report, *Malaria in the Duars*, are essentially expositions of epidemic and endemic acute hunger in colonial South Asia, in each case with starvation expressed epidemiologically through malaria lethality. Vital registration, initiated in the years immediately following the 1857 Indian Rebellion, had very quickly become a double-edged sword for the British Raj. It was a tool critical for tracking cholera, in particular, and for controlling outbreaks that threatened military control and imperial trade. But it also produced data that ultimately forced accountability for the Raj's own governance. For the relationship between epidemic mortality and acute hunger clearly was not limited to Punjab and the Duars labour camps. In his painstaking epidemiological account of the 1876–1877 famine, Madras Sanitary Commissioner William Cornish earlier had implored that 'abundance of food must be regarded by the Sanitarian much as the barometer is regarded by the Meteorologist. Cheap and plentiful food means health, and dear and scanty food, sickness and death.'[12] The detailed district graphs of monthly deaths and grain prices appearing in his 1878 annual report, he urged, 'place[d] before the statist and political economist factors of the very highest importance. They prove beyond the shadow of a doubt, the intimate connection between famine prices of food and mortality.'[13]

Yet empirical documentation of the 'intimate' scarcity-mortality connection was taking place at a point when the political impact of the incriminating mortality tables simultaneously was being offset by recent medical developments. Infectious diseases increasingly were being interpreted within specific nosological categories as localised pathological entities – and soon, microbial – distinct from conditions of the human host. The political convenience of the reductive shift would soon be evident in the pages of the 1880 Famine Commission Report itself, the enormous malaria mortality recorded in the final stages of 19th-century famines deemed to be climatic in origin and thus beyond the powers of the administration to control.[14] This position was reinforced in official reporting of famine mortality, where estimates of famine deaths included only those up to closure of famine relief works with return of the monsoon rains, and thus excluded ensuing autumn malaria deaths, often the greatest contributor to the overall famine toll. It was a trend Cornish had presciently decried three years earlier, warning in his 1877 sanitary report that

> [o]f late a fashion has sprung up of referring to mortality that unquestionably ought to be shown under the head of 'privation' or 'starvation' as due to disease, and in this way attention is diverted from the real fount and origin of excessive death-rates.[15]

This made it seem, Cornish suggested, 'that the epidemic diseases so prevalent during the [1876–1877] famine period were something apart from, and unconnected with the famine.'[16]

Macdonnell's 1901 Famine Commission Report categorically rejected this narrowed reading of famine mortality. But the two subsequent Punjab and Duars malaria inquiry reports went further, signalling the role of human destitution at a more general, endemic level, beyond officially declared 'famine.' Together, publication of the three reports marked a profound moral shift: from a view of malaria mortality as a natural process whereby the 'weaklings' were eliminated, to instead its perception as remediable neglect. In practical terms, the 1901 Famine Commission Report was acknowledgement that whipping no longer offered a sufficient means of social control in the face of needless starvation, while the later malaria reports directly implicated colonial economic governance in continuing endemic immiseration and 'underdevelopment' in British India.

Within less than a decade after Ronald Ross's 1897 confirmation of the role of mosquitoes in malaria transmission, the imperial government had been pushed to formally acknowledge the role of this neglect, with responsibility for malaria's toll now shifted from the miasmas and vectors of a tropical climate to the shoulders of the State. The admission that destitution lay at the core of the malaria burden was intended to counter increasingly insistent public calls for vector control on the part of senior members of the sanitary and medical administration. But it was aimed as well at continuing resistance on the part of plantation and industry owners to beginning government attempts to moderate their near-absolute powers under 19th-century indentured labour laws.

Demographic significance

Malaria's prominence in South Asian mortality history derives from several factors: first, the timing of annual malaria transmission coincided with peak famine starvation with return of the monsoon rains, and second, an epidemic efficiency where few amongst the famished escaped infection. While mortality from other endemic infections such as cholera, 'bowel disorders,' and smallpox, was also generally elevated over the course of a famine,[17] malaria often claimed the greatest number of lives and thus appears to have been a leading vehicle by which recurring subsistence crises limited population growth. Nor, it appears, was this prominence limited to Punjab, as seen in 1943–1944 Bengal. Yet colonial malaria researchers clearly also considered the Punjab region's malarial 'death storms' as exceptional (Figures 4.11a-d, 4.13). This, Christophers came to consider, was related to the compounding of drought-induced destitution by flood waters following return of the monsoon rains: the 'fine line' between too little and too much rain in the flood-prone northwest plains meant that economic variability year-to-year was particularly exaggerated.

Did this malaria 'fulminancy' mean generally higher mortality levels in Punjab compared with other regions of the subcontinent? Definitive assessment is beyond the scope of the present study. What this study does suggest, however, is that much of Punjab's pre-1920 malaria mortality, possibly most, was determined by destitution, endemic as well as epidemic. Flooding continued after 1920, and also its entomologically conducive effects. But fulminant malaria (with the exception of 1942) did not. Judging also from the failure of the 1950s DDT spray program to substantially influence general mortality trends, as seen in chapter 12, the lives saved by the virtual elimination of malaria transmission appear to have been extremely limited *relative to* the historical toll. This, of course, does not diminish the importance of individual lives saved with the abrupt 1950s interruption in malaria transmission, but rather serves to highlight the enormity of premature deaths at pre-modern (pre-1910) levels of life expectancy.

What is also clear is that post-1920 decline in malaria lethality (case fatality rate) was part of a broader demographic trend in the subcontinent, evident for other major infectious diseases as well. Guilmoto has shown a striking attenuation in lethality of cholera epidemics from the 1910s in south India, suggesting that this was not due to decline in 'frequency of epidemic outbreaks as the disease kept more or less its periodicity till the 1950s.' He notes a similar picture for smallpox, 'its cyclical character persisted though the crises' intensity diminished,' as has Ortega for cholera and total mortality in Bengal after 1920.

Epistemic significance

The history of malaria mortality in colonial Punjab raises substantial questions, epistemic in nature, as to what distinguishes 'famine' history from epidemic history. With the exception of the most severe depopulating famines where entire villages disappeared – conditions from which post-Rebellion Punjab was largely exempt – the distinction for the colonial period is unclear based on mortality figures. Malaria mortality and overall death rates in the province were as high in the epidemic years of 1890 and 1892 as in the 'great' famine year of 1899–1900 (Table 4.1). Relief measures may have moderated Punjab famine deaths to some extent in 1900. But a distinction between the two types of mortality crisis during this period can be seen as rather arbitrary where malaria was a leading trigger of mortality in both.

A further example of the difficulty in conceptually distinguishing epidemic and famine crises is seen in Jullundur, a district considered to be relatively protected from famine, yet with annual mortality rates similar to levels elsewhere in the province. The district's mean annual crude death rate (minus plague deaths) for the 1875–1908 period was slightly higher (33.6 per 1,000) than for the plains districts as a whole (31.6 per 1,000).[18]

The interpretive difficulties encountered in distinguishing epidemic and famine mortality can be seen as well in Kingsley Davis's 1951 *Demography of India and Pakistan*. Davis recognised that 19 million people were 'missing' in the 1901 Census of India, based upon very modest expectations of population growth rates prevailing at the time of the previous Census in 1891. However, in the apparent absence of epidemics, he could account for only 6 million of these deaths, those in the two famine years, 1896–1897 and 1899–1900, there being no exceptional, or major influenza, epidemic in the decade, and as yet only very limited plague deaths in the final years of the decade. Thus, 13 million 'excess' deaths were left unaccounted for, unremarked upon, and effectively invisible historiographically.[19]

One further example of the definitional difficulties can be seen in a comparison of pre-1910 Punjab mortality with that in 1943–1944 Bengal. By all indicators, the Bengal famine was a 'great' famine, with over 2 million 'excess' deaths in a single province, a leading portion malarial: the death rate rising 50 per cent to 30.0 per mille in 1943 from a preceding quinquennial average of 21.2.[20] And yet the 1943 famine crude death rate of 30.0 was a level that four decades earlier would have been considered a 'normal' *endemic* figure in Punjab (Table 13.1).[21]

Table 13.1 Annual Oct.–Dec. fever death, crude death rate (per 1,000), 24 plains districts, Punjab, 1890–1900

	Oct.-Dec. FDR	CDR (per 1,000)
1890	17.0	49.8
1891	6.5	29.4
1892	17.0	50.2
1893	6.6	29.0
1894	9.8	38.3
1895	5.9	29.4
1896	4.3	30.8
1897	9.8	31.3
1898	6.3	31.6
1899	5.0	29.8
1900	18.6	50.9

Source: *PSCR* 1890–1900.

Reclaiming endemiology

Most of the 'saw-tooth' mortality of 19th-century Punjab was not due to inherently virulent diseases. Nor, with the exception of 1878, 1897, and 1900, due to famine. Yet even before the outbreak of plague in 1897, mortality levels were sufficiently high from endemic diseases to substantially limit population growth. Moreover, as severe as the plague epidemic was for Punjab – claiming over 3 million lives, Punjab bearing the greatest per capita burden of any province – its toll was no greater than the cumulative 'normal' autumn malaria fever mortality over the same 33-year period.[22] Thus in crude numbers, the plague epidemic, running unimpeded through its 1897–1930 course, did not dominate the region's demographic regime more than malaria deaths over this same period – though the former occurred in more terrifying outbursts and claimed a greater proportion of adult lives.

This perhaps explains Christophers's emphasis on 'endemiology' – a term he used to highlight variation in clinical morbidity of most endemic infections. For in describing epidemic malaria as 'a great exaggeration of normal stress,' it appears he was also pointing out the significance of 'ordinary' (seasonal, for example) acute hunger in non-famine autumnal malaria mortality. The impact of 'normal' stress on mortality levels becomes evident – if inversely – in the mid-1940s drop in crude death rates in Punjab with alleviation of a portion of endemic acute hunger through post-World War II foodgrain control policies, as traced in chapter 12 (Figure 12.6). The larger historiographic point here is that much malaria mortality – 'ordinary' (endemic) autumnal epidemic rises related to acute hunger – fails to appear in most accounts of 'epidemic' history.

Here, a comparative European context may be useful. In analysis of historical 'great mortalities' in Europe, Otto Andersen provides a rare quantitative account of an 1831 malaria epidemic in Denmark, one likely 'zymonic' in spatial form but smaller in scale than that in post-World War I Russia. He describes epidemic mortality conditions in the endemically malarial lowland regions of Denmark that followed several years of flood-related agricultural stress triggered by hurricane destruction of dikes and exacerbated by 'wet and cold' summers.[23] Most of the 1831 epidemic deaths were considered malarial ('the cold fever'), mortality rising to 49.8 and 41.8 per 1,000 in affected dioceses from pre-1825 levels of less than 20 per 1,000.

In a sense, the Denmark epidemic was akin to that following the precipitous decline in agricultural productivity in the 19th-century Burdwan division of Bengal – except that in the Denmark case the triggering cause of interrupted livelihood was not a permanent one, as hurricane destruction of the drainage system was in time remediable. This account is of added interest because the malaria endemic to the Danish low-land dioceses was most certainly vivax malaria, not falciparum infection. Moreover, as marked as the epidemic mortality was in 1831, it was considerably lower than that recorded in the recurring 'saw-tooth' peaks prevailing a century earlier in the region before enactment of agricultural reforms in the late 18th century.[24] It raises again, in other words, questions of how 'great mortalities' are defined and conceptualised, and the relative invisibility of endemic acute hunger.

Eclipse of the 'Human Factor'

There is little to suggest Christophers later reconsidered his 'scarcity' conclusions to the 1911 Punjab study. In a contributing chapter entitled 'Endemic and Epidemic [Malaria] Prevalence' in Boyd's major 1949 compendium *Malariology* Christophers included a detailed overview of his 1911 conclusions along with original maps and graphs.[25] Yet a brief three years later, his study would be remembered in very different terms, his statistical 'correlations' cited as showing instead that the 'the periodic epidemics were associated with certain rainfall characteristics and with an inadequate immunity in the local population'[26] – remembered, in other words, as a function of malaria transmission and by implication, of an inherent virulence of the malaria *plasmodium* itself.

To the very limited extent that *Malaria in the Punjab*, and the broader epidemiological malaria research undertaken in this early period, figure in modern medical deliberations, the immunological reinterpretation of Punjab malaria epidemicity continues to prevail in the medical literature: the region is seen as an area of 'unstable' malaria, with highly variable transmission and fluctuating acquired immunity levels accounting for epidemic vulnerability historically.[27] It is a reading, moreover, that has also come to inform historical research more broadly as noted in chapter 1. In a highly influential 1983 symposium on nutrition in history, malaria came to be classified alongside inherently virulent microbes such as plague and smallpox as an infection where the 'nutritional influence on outcome' was minimal.[28]

The demise of the 'human factor' in Punjab malaria historiography and its reinterpretation in immunological terms is a subject beyond the scope of the present study.[29] But in very general terms, a central element has been loss of the distinction between 'exciting' (or 'precipitating') causes of epidemics related to infection transmission; and those factors 'predisposing' to a fatal outcome.[30] At the same time, basic concepts of hunger have also been lost. Bundled under the rubric of 'nutrition,' the varied physical and epidemiological aspects of hunger are often invisible.

'Seeing' states of hunger beyond famine

Recent research in nutritional anthropometric history has begun to reclaim some visibility of historical hunger, with secular trends in human stature an important marker of cumulative, endemic undernourishment:[31] figuratively speaking, reflecting substantial prevalence of one meal a day rather than two.[32] Present-day undernourishment in childhood manifests in continuing prevalence of stunting in the modern world, often termed 'chronic malnutrition.' To some extent, stature can be a marker of acute hunger as well. Recent South Asian analysis, for example, identifies greater stunting in those adult cohorts born during the famine years of 1918 and 1943, an observation that suggests famine's greatest stature impact occurs in infancy and *in utero* -- that period of greatest physiologic growth and nourishment need.[33] It is unclear, however, to what extent adult stature may reflect general incidence of acute hunger in a population, given the much greater associated mortality. There is little indication, for example, of substantial increase in height in post-1920 British India over the 40 years of control of famine.[34] This suggests stature captures acute hunger shifts – *gaps* in access (figuratively, zero meals per day) – considerably less well than average *levels* of calorie intake. And as discussed in chapter 1, this may help to explain the seemingly 'paradoxical' rise in life expectancy post-1920 in the face of continuing high stunting prevalence in the population.[35]

Endemic acute hunger takes many forms. It encompasses 'hunger seasons,' regular intervals of weight loss in the agricultural year where little employment is available and increasingly unremunerative work is resorted to in an effort to stave of frank starvation.[36] Studies in contemporary agricultural populations document pronounced rainy-season weight loss and infant/toddler failure to grow.[37]

Hunger is 'visible' indirectly in conditions of work. Most obvious historically are wage levels insufficient to meet minimal calorie requirement even if wholly directed to expenditure on the cheapest staple foods available – or well below, in relation to reproductive and productive labour demands. Beyond wage insufficiency are issues of intensity and hours of work demanded for a given wage, aspects of greatest import for women where profound time constraints often bore disastrous consequences for nourishing young children historically, and still do for some groups. Such constraints, and the absence of provision for child care, are reflected indirectly in women's resort to soothing their infants with opium for the 12 or more hours of their early 20th-century Bombay factory shifts, a practice routine also among women working in the factories of industrialising Britain before them.[38] In this case, infant undernourishment often verged on semi-starvation. Unsurprisingly, infant mortality in 1920 Bombay among households of one room or less was estimated to be 631 per 1,000 live born, a level comparable to that registered also in the poor wards of Philadelphia and New York 40 years earlier[39] – 'endemic' mortality levels greater than that of a single epidemic year of 'fulminant' malaria such as 1908 Punjab. Soothing unfed infants with opium was not an uncommon practice in rural Indian households as well, a 1920 report suggests.[40] Certainly, as recently as the 1970s, many young children of landless households in rural Tamil Nadu were commonly left without care or feeding throughout the long days of daily wage labour during planting and harvest seasons.[41]

The intense physiologic growth requirements in infancy mean frequent 'on-demand' feeding is essential. The extent to which such needs can, or cannot, be met amidst the physical and time demands of daily subsistence survival constitutes a very large, if generally unwritten, chapter of health history. In explaining the latest child death in her village, Meena, Veeranendal midwife, described labouring women's dilemma with simple certitude: 'No time! and no money!'[42] As a *dalit* agricultural labourer herself, she understood perfectly the poverty constraints women such as herself faced, but in typically astute fashion she articulated 'no time' as the even greater, if inherently related, barrier. Viewed from the standpoint of vital registration ledgers, the implications of conditions of work and livelihood are perhaps difficult to discern. Yet for women at subsistence levels, such conditions immediately determine whether the most elemental needs of their young children can be afforded, or not, within the larger constraints of household survival.

The most extreme forms of endemic subsistence precarity were faced by migrant workers, conditions that Christophers and Bentley summed up in the term 'Tropical Aggregation of Labour.' The early 20th-century Duars tea plantations were an extreme example of endemic semi-starvation, but such conditions were recognised as affecting 'shifting' populations in general. Here, to the extreme physical hardships of migration itself, employment precarity, and utter dependence on labour recruiters, was added the complete absence of social cohesion. Such conditions are graphically portrayed in the 1909 Duars report, if often invisible historiographically otherwise. Such forms of endemic acute hunger are also poorly incorporated within analyses of late 19th and early 20th century mortality decline in industrialising Europe or North America – and post-Independence South Asia.

Tracking trends in human hunger is necessarily an enormous subject. Here, only a fragment of that history has been explored. However, the broad outlines evident in economic and public policy shifts across the colonial period suggest the years immediately following the 1908 Punjab malaria epidemic were a turning point in vulnerability to starvation in its epidemic form, and to a beginning extent in endemic starvation as well. Difficult perhaps to identify in the colonial revenue ledgers, a shift in subsistence precarity can be glimpsed in other ways, as seen in chapter 11 in Vilyatpur village's changing household lineage patterns. It can also be seen in the decline in malaria fulminancy in the wider province.

Contemporary echoes of malaria's past

How can the history of malaria mortality decline in colonial Punjab be reconciled with contemporary experience of malaria mortality in sub-Saharan Africa where a substantial malaria mortality burden remains? One part of the explanation clearly lies in the distinctive (holoendemic) character of malaria transmission prevailing in many tropical regions of Africa. As a highly anthropophilic species, the prime mosquito vector in much of the region, *Anopheles gambiae*, feeds almost exclusively on humans, resulting in as many as 300 infective bites annually. Such extreme inoculation rates lead to high levels of protective *acquired* immunity among the adult population but intense infection rates in the as yet non-immune, primarily infants and young children, amongst whom the malaria mortality impact is considerable.[43]

Yet even under such intense transmission conditions, acute hunger may be seen to have further accentuated malarial lethality in recent African experience. Famines in Swaziland, Ethiopia, and more recently Madagascar were associated with prominent epidemic malaria mortality.[44] As in South Asia, peak seasonal hunger stress also coincides with peak malaria transmission and mortality rates during the rainy season.[45] Conversely, better control of famine since 1960 has been cited as contributing to substantial decline in malaria death rates, along with increasing access to chloroquine and more recently artemisinin-combined therapy.[46] Moreover, recent marked decline in malaria mortality and transmission indices in many African countries since 2001[47] coincides with the return of economic growth after two decades of stagnation; in several instances, this decline clearly predated ramped-up programs to control malaria transmission.[48] The region's exceptional entomological conditions, in other words, may not entirely explain the well-documented mortality burden from the disease in sub-Saharan Africa. Nor negate a role for acute hunger in intensifying its historical lethality in other regions of the world.

Contemporary experience of malaria in South Asia reveals continuities with the historical experience. Though malaria deaths in modern India are a tiny fraction of those recorded pre-1910, their social profile appears to be similar: malaria morbidity and mortality is concentrated among populations most marginalised, most subject to destitution, with least access to basic treatment. As ever, malaria's burden is a signifier of poverty, subsistence precarity, and political neglect, requiring measures that address broader socio-economic determinants. Greater attention to such wider factors may explain success in malaria transmission control in particular regions of the country. The southwestern state of Kerala is one example. A large portion of the state lies within the Western Ghat hills, a region that as recently as the 1940s was one of intense (hyperendemic) malaria transmission. Following the 1950s DDT spray program, annual malaria cases rebounded by the 1980s to between 3,000 and 10,000 in a population of 32 million, a substantial level though modest compared with some other regions of the country. Through systematic case detection, treatment, and local spraying where indicated, new cases by the mid-2000s had declined to several hundred annually, most imported from other states or returning migrant workers.[49]

The experience of Kerala, Sunil Amrith observes, suggests the current malaria problem in India is not primarily entomological, but rather related to a lack of publicly accountable primary health services.[50] But the larger South Asian historical experience also suggests a further aspect to Kerala's malaria control success. Fundamental food security programs and labour reforms, through the 1960s and 70s in the state may well have limited transmission rebound by virtue of the time and food resources so afforded, helping to ensure rapid recovery, the feasibility of treatment access, and compliance with subsequent basic control measures.

The larger history of malaria mortality decline in Punjab suggests no contradiction exists between 'saving lives' through access to treatment, and transmission control where appropriate, on the one hand, and rising life expectancy in whole populations through subsistence security, on the other. Indeed, access to treatment is eminently more important for the food-insecure, those most at risk of dying from the disease. If differing in their respective contributions to health history, the two are both fundamental rights, though the former is no substitute for the latter: an assured 'two meals a day' to satisfy hunger.

Notes

 1 S.R. Christophers, 'Malaria in the Punjab,' *Scientific Memoirs by Officers of the Medical and Sanitary Departments of the Government of India* (New Series), 46 (Calcutta: Superintendent Government Printing Office, 1911), 107 [hereafter, MP].
 2 MP, 13.
 3 S.R Christophers, 'Malaria: Endemiology and Epidemiology,' in W. Byam, R.G. Archibald, eds., *The Practice of Medicine in the Tropics* (London: Henry Frowde, Hodder, and Stoughton, 1922), Vol. 2, 1546–1554.
 4 *PSCR* 1892, 3, 16.
 5 *PSCR* 1895, 20. A modern parallel to the oft-quoted Tuscan proverb ('the best remedy for malaria is a full cooking pot') appears in the response of a rural Egyptian farmer to officials' malaria control efforts in the late 1930s to destroy his rice fields, who protested, 'By God, malaria is more merciful to us than you as malaria troubles us for a few days and we recover without medicines, but you want to kill us all of starvation.'; M.A. Farid, 'The Malaria Programme – from Euphoria to Anarchy,' *World Health Forum*, 1, 1–2, 1980, 8–33, at 9.
 6 S.R. Christophers, 'Commentary,' in C.A. Gill, ed., 'Some Points in the Epidemiology of Malaria Arising out of the Study of the Malaria Epidemic in Ceylon in 1934–1935,' *Trans. Roy. Soc. Trop. Med & Hyg.*, 29, 5, Feb. 1936, 427–480, at 466.
 7 Sir Joseph Fayrer, *On the Climate and Fevers of India*, Croonian Lecture, Mar. 1882, (London: J&A Churchill, 1882), 13.
 8 Ibid., 217–218.
 9 Ibid., 20.
10 L. Tarassevitch, *Epidemics in Russia Since 1914* (Geneva: LNHO, 1923).
11 C. Hamlin, *Public Health and Social Justice in the Age of Chadwick* (Cambridge: Cambridge University Press, 1998).
12 *Report of the Sanitary Commissioner for Madras* 1876, 12 [hereafter, MSCR]; *MSCR* 1878, opp. p. 8.
13 *MSCR* 1878, 9.
14 *Report of the Indian Famine Commission* (London: HMSO, 1880), pt. 1, 40. See ch. 11, 328–329.
15 *MSCR* 1877, 147. During these years, Hamlin observes, 'an older *physiological* conception of disease was giving way to an *ontological* one'; C. Hamlin, 'Could You Starve to Death in England in 1839? The Chadwick-Farr Controversy and the Loss of the "Social" in Public Health,' *AJPH*, 85, 6, 1995, 856–866. This made 'diseases "things" or entities that were separate from the patient'; M. Worboys, *Spreading Germs: Disease Theories and Medical Practice in Britain* (Cambridge: Cambridge University Press, 2000), 5.
16 MSCR 1877, Appendix I, xxx.
17 L. Sami, 'Starvation, Disease and Death: Explaining Famine Mortality in Madras, 1876–1878,' *Social History of Medicine*, 24, 3, 2011, 700–719.

A zymonic character to epidemic cholera mortality was also suggested by Christophers. 'Epidemics of this magnitude are, however, by no means confined to malaria. Immense cholera epidemics have been of frequent occurrence. They are ascribed to infections carried by pilgrims returning from the pilgrim *melas* at Hardwar . . . but there must be something more at the back of them than the mere fact of such dissemination, some condition peculiarly favourable to the spread of cholera in such years. . . . [If mapped] I believe they also would shew the same focal character as did the two epidemics of malaria whose distribution I have illustrated'; 'What Disease Costs India,' *IMG*, Apr. 1924, 196–200.

18 See above, chapter 12.

19 K. Davis, *The Population of India and Pakistan* (Princeton: Princeton University Press, 1951, 42; I. Klein, 'Population Growth and Mortality in British India Part II: The Demographic Revolution,' *IESHR*, 27, 1, 1990, 33–63, at 60.

20 Famine Inquiry Commission, *Report on Bengal* (New Delhi: Government of India, 1945), 108.

21 The recent characterisation of history divided into two distinct epidemiological eras perhaps reflects similar conceptual constraints: pre-modern history, namely, most of human history, viewed as dominated by highly virulent diseases; and more recent, early modern history, where common endemic infections instead were prominent, with effective quarantine measures and stable states in place at this point; A. Carmichael, 'Infection, Hidden Hunger, and History,' *JIH*, 14, 3, 1983, 249–264; S.J. Kunitz, 'Mortality Since Malthus,' 279–302, in R. Scofield, D. Coleman, *The State of Population Theory: Forward from Malthus* (Oxford: Basil Blackwell, 1986), 279–302.

22 Based upon a mean 'excess' Oct.–Dec. fever death rate of approximately 4 per mille; 'excess' estimated by subtracting mean autumn fever mortality in drought years; see ch. 6, n72. The 1918 influenza pandemic, on the other hand, was an exceptional 'pestilence, if its toll in Punjab was also markedly heightened by war-time famine conditions; I. Mills, 'The 1918–1919 Influenza Pandemic – The Indian Experience,' *IESHR*, 1986, 23, 1.

23 O. Andersen, 'A Malaria Epidemic in Denmark,' in H. Charbonneau, A. Larose, eds., *The Great Mortalities: Methodological Studies of Demographic Crises in the Past* (Liege: Ordina Editions, 1979), 33–49.

24 Ibid., 35. H.C. Johansen, 'The Standard of Living in Denmark in the Eighteenth and Early Nineteenth Centuries,' in R.C. Allen, T. Bengtsson, M. Dribe, eds., *Living Standards in the Past* (Oxford: Oxford University Press, 2005), 307–318.

25 S.R. Christophers, 'Endemic and Epidemic Prevalence,' in M.F. Boyd, ed., *Malariology* (Philadelphia: W.B. Saunders, 1949), 698–721.

26 G. Macdonald, 'The Analysis of Equilibrium in Malaria,' reprinted in L. Bruce-Chwatt, V.J. Glanville, eds., *Dynamics of Tropical Diseases: The Late George Macdonald* (London: Oxford University Press, 1973), 132.

27 M.J. Bouma, H. van der Kaay, 'The El Niño Southern Oscillation and the Historical Malaria Epidemics on the Indian Subcontinent and Sri Lanka: An Early Warning System for Future Epidemics?' *Tropical Medicine and International Health*, 1, 1, Feb. 1996, 86–96.

28 See ch. 1, p. 24

29 I explore the epistemic question as to how, conceptually and institution-ally, this paradigmatic transformation took place in S. Zurbrigg, *Uncoupling Disease and Destitution: The Case of Malaria*, in preparation.
30 It was his understanding this distinction that led Thomas McKeown to pursue broader determinants to mortality decline in Britain; *The Modern Rise of Population* (London: Edward Arnold, 1976), 73.
31 R. Fogel, *Explaining Long-Term Trends in Health and Longevity* (New York: Cambridge University Press, 2012).
32 See ch. 1, p. 28.
33 A.V. Guntupalli, J. Baten, 'The Development and Inequality of Heights in North, West, and East India 1915–1944,' *Explorations in Economic History*, 43, 2006, 578–608, at 592.
34 L. Brennan, J. McDonald, R. Shlomowitz, 'Long-Term Change in Indian health,' *South Asia: Journal of South Asian Studies*, n.s., 26, 1, 2003, 51–69.
35 For further discussion, see ch. 1, p. 32.
36 M.A. Chen, *Coping with Seasonality and Drought* (New Delhi: Sage, 1991). For a contemporary portrait of seasonal hunger by women land-less labourers in Midnapore district, West Bengal, see N. Mukherjee, A. Mukherjee, 'Rural Women and Food Insecurity: What a Food Calendar Reveals,' *EPW*, Mar. 12, 1994, 597–599.
37 M.G.M Rowlands et al., 'Seasonality and the Growth of Infants in a Gambian Village,' in R. Chambers, R. Longhurst, A. Pacey, eds., *Seasonal Dimensions to Rural Poverty* (London: Frances Pinter, Institute of Development Studies, 1981). 'For the special feeding needs of infants and small children, see ch. 1, p. 29.
38 Drs. Margaret Balfour, Shakuntala K. Talpade, 'Maternity Conditions of Women Mill-Workers in India,' *IMG*, May 30, 1930, 241–249. Christopher Hamlin cites an estimate by one witness to the 1840 Sanitary Commission hearings that half the children in Ashton-under-Lyne were being dosed with opiates; *Public Health and Social Justice in the Age of Chadwick* (Cambridge: Cambridge University Press, 1998), 231–232.
39 Ibid.; R. Floud, R. Fogel, B. Harris, Sok Chul Hong, eds., *The Changing Body: Health, Nutrition, and Human Development in the Western World since 1700* (Cambridge: Cambridge University Press, 2011).
40 D. Curjel, *Improvement of the Conditions of Childbirth* (Calcutta, 1918), Appendix G, cited in Samita Sen, *Women and Labour in Late Colonial India: The Bengal Jute Industry* (Cambridge: Cambridge University Press, 1999), 154, 173.
41 Personal observations during 1970s field work in villages of Ramanathapuram district, Tamil Nadu.
42 See note 41.
43 For further discussion, see J.A. Webb, *Humanity's Burden: A Global History of Malaria* (New York: Cambridge University Press, 2009), 27–41. See also ch.1, note 82.
44 R. Packard, 'Maize, Cattle and Mosquitoes: The Political Economy of Malaria Epidemics in Colonial Swaziland,' *Journal of African History*, 25, 1984, 189–212; R.E. Fontaine, A.E. Najjar, J.S. Prince, 'The 1958 Malaria Epidemic in Ethiopia,' *American Journal of Tropical Medicine and Hygiene*, 10, 795–803; M. Garenne, et al., 'The Demographic Impact of a

Mild Famine in an African City: The Case of Antananarivo, 1985–1987,' in T. Dyson, C.Ó Gráda, eds., *Famine Demography: Perspectives from the Past and Present* (Oxford: Oxford University Press, 2002), 204–217.

45 Rowland, 'Seasonality and the Growth of Infants.'

46 R.W. Snow, J.F. Trape, K. Marsh, 'The Past, Present and Future of Childhood Malaria Mortality in Africa,' *Trends in Parasitology*, 17, 12, Dec. 2001, 593–597.

47 W.P. O'Meara, et al., 'Changes in the Burden of Malaria in Sub-Saharan Africa,' *Lancet/Infectious Diseases*, 10, Aug. 2010, 545–555.

48 W.P. O'Meara, et al., 'Effect of a Fall in Malaria Transmission on Morbidity and Mortality in Kilifi, Kenya,' *Lancet*, 372, Nov. 1, 2008, 1555-1562.

49 K. Sandeep, 'Control, Eradication and Resurgence of Malaria in Kerala during the Post 50 Years,' *Kerala Medical Journal*, 1, 2, Dec. 2008; V.P. Sharma, K.N. Mehotra, 'Malaria Resurgence in India: A Critical Study,' *Social Science and Medicine*, 22, 1986, 835–845, 836.

50 S. Amrith, 'Political Culture of Health in India: A Historical Perspective,' *EPW*, Jan. 13, 2007, 114–121.

Appendix

List of sanitary commissioners/ directors of public health, Punjab province, 1868–1940

1868–1875	A.C.C. De Renzy
1876–1885	H.W. Bellew
1886–1887	A. Stephen
1888–1889	W.A.C. Roe
1889–1892	A. Stephen
1893–1897	W.A.C. Roe
1898–1906	C.J. Bamber
1907–1908	E. Wilkinson
1909	C.J. Bamber offg.
1910–1911	E. Wilkinson
1912–1913	S. Browning Smith
1914	C.J. Bamber
1915–1917	H. Hendley
1918–1923	W.H.C. Forster
1924	C.A. Gill
1925–1926	W.H.C. Forster
1927–1929	C.A. Gill
1930	K.A. Rahman
1931	C.A. Gill
1932	R.C. Malhotra
1933–1935	K.A. Rahman
1936	C.M. Nichol
1937	A.H. Butt
1938–1939	C.M. Nichol
1940	A.H. Butt

Bibliography

GOI. *Annual report of the Sanitary Commissioner with the Government of India*, (1867–1919), continued as *Annual report of the Public Health Commissioner with the Government of India* (1920–1946).

———, *Census of India, 1951*, Vol. VIII, Part 1-A; *Census of India, 1961*. Punjab: District Census Handbooks.

———, *Census of India, 1961*. Punjab: District Census Handbooks.

———, *Report of the Commissioners Appointed to Inquire into the Sanitary State of the Army in India*, PP, Vol. I, London: HMSO, 1863.

———, *Report of the Indian Famine Commission*, London: HMSO, 1880.

———, Famine Inquiry Commission (1880), 'Note on the Results of the Enquiries Made into the Mortality in the North-Western Provinces and Oudh,' Government N.W.P. and Oudh, 596, dated Mar. 17, 1879, in *Report of the Indian Famine Commission. Part 3, Famine Histories*, London: HMSO, 1885, 243–250.

———, *Report of the Indian Famine Commission*, Simla: Government Central Printing Office, 1898.

———, Famine Inquiry Commission, *Report on Bengal* (1945).

Confidential Circular No. 44 F. – 8.1, dated Aug. 17, 1887; Resolution of the Government of India, 96-F/6–59 dated Oct. 19, 1888. 'Conditions of the Lower Classes of People of India.' Resolution of the Government of India, 96-F/6–59 dated Oct. 19, 1888.

———, *Report of the Indian Famine Commission*, Calcutta: Government Printing Office, 1901.

———, *Land Revenue Policy of the Indian Government*, Calcutta: Office of the Superintendent, 1902.

———, *Report of the Indian Irrigation Commission*, 1901–1903, London: HMSO, 1903.

———, *Report of the Indian Fiscal Commission, 1921–1922*, Simla: n.p., 1922.

———, *Report of the Royal Commission on Agriculture in India*, London: HMSO, 1928.

———, *Report of the Health Survey and Development Committee*, Vol. I, New Delhi: GOI Press, 1946.

——, *Statistical Abstract Relating to British India*, London: HMSO, 1840–1920.

——, *Proceedings of the Imperial Malaria Conference held in Simla, October 1909.*

——, *Proceedings of the Imperial Malaria Committee held in Bombay on 16th and 17th November 1911*, reprinted in *Paludism*, 4, 1911, 1–129.

——, *Proceedings of the Third Meeting of the General Malaria Committee Held at Madras, November 18–20, 1912.*

——, *Proceedings of the Third All-India Sanitary Conference, Held at Lucknow, January. 1914.*

——, *Indian Sanitary Policy, 1914: Being a Resolution issued by the Governor General in Council on the 23rd of May 1914*, Calcutta: Superintendent Government Printing, India, 1914.

——, *Memorandum by the Sanitary Commissioner with the Government of India Regarding the Measures Taken for the Suppression of Plague and Malaria*, GOI Press, Department of Education, Sept. 22, 1911.

GOI. 'Director-General of Health Services,' *Report for the Quadrennium, 1949–1952.*

——, Directorate General Health Services, *Annual Report*, 1953–1956.

——, *Health Statistics of India, 1951–1953, 1954–1955, 1958–1959.*

——, Directorate of the National Malaria Eradication Programme, *Malaria and its Control in India*, 1, 1986.

Govt, Punjab. *Report on the Sanitary Administration of the Punjab* (1867–1921), continued as *Report on the Public Health Administration of the Punjab* (1922–1947).

——, *Report of the Land Revenue Administration of the Punjab.*

——, *Report on the Season and Crops of the Punjab* (1901–1943).

——, *Annual Report, Public Works Department, Irrigation Branch.*

——, *Public Works Department, Buildings and Roads Branch. Administrative Report.*

——, *Punjab Gazetteer.*

——, *Gazetteer of the Gurgaon District*, 1883–1884.

——, *Report on Malaria in the Punjab* (1913–1918).

——, Settlement Report, Amritsar District, 1910–1914; Jullundur District, 1892; Sirsa District, 1879–1883; Karnal District, 1872–1880.

——, *Report on the Famine in the Punjab in 1896–1897*, 1898.

——, *The Punjab Famine of 1899–1900*, Vols. 1–2, Lahore, 1901.

——, *The Punjab Famine Code*, Department of Revenue & Agriculture, 1888.

——, *The Punjab Famine Code* (revised), Department of Revenue & Agriculture, 1930.

Govt, Punjab State [India]. Director of Health Services, *Report on the Public Health Administration, Punjab, for the Year 1955* (1956–1960).

——, *Annual Report on the Public Health in the Punjab State during the Year 1956* (1957, 1958, 1959, 1960).

Govt, Madras. *Annual Report of the Sanitary Commissioner for Madras*, 1877, 1878.

Govt, United Provinces of Agra and Oudh. *Narrative and Results of the Measures adopted for the Relief of Famine during the Years 1907 and 1908*, Allahabad: Scarcity Dept., 1908.

*

Acharya, K.C.S., *Food Security System of India: Evolution of the Buffer Stocking Policy and its Evaluation*, New Delhi: Concept Publishers, 1983.

Acton, H.W., R. Knowles, 'Studies on the *Halteridium* Parasite of the Pigeon, *Haemoproteus Columbae, Celli & San Felice*,' *Indian Journal of Medical Research*, 1, 4, 1914, 663–690.

Agnihotri, I., 'Ecology, Land Use and Colonisation: The Canal Colonies of Punjab,' *Indian Economic and Social History Review*, 33, 1, 1996, 37–58.

Alamgir, M., *Famine in South Asia: Political Economy of Mass Starvation*, Cambridge, MA: Oelgeschlager, Gunn and Hain, 1980.

Ambirajan, S., 'Political Economy and Indian Famines,' *South Asia: Journal of South Asian Studies*, 1, 1, Aug. 1971, 20–27.

———, 'Malthusian Population Theory and Indian Famine Policy in the Nineteenth Century,' *Population Studies*, 30, 1, Mar. 1976, 5–14.

———, *Classical Political Economy and the British Rule in India*, Cambridge: Cambridge University Press, 1978.

Amrith, S., *Decolonizing International Health: India and Southeast Asia, 1930–1965*, Basingstoke: Palgrave Macmillan, 2006.

———, 'Political Culture of Health in India: A Historical Perspective,' *Economic and Political Weekly*, Jan. 13, 2007, 114–121.

Andersen, O., 'A Malaria Epidemic in Denmark,' in H. Charbonneau, A. Larose, eds., *The Great Mortalities: Methodological Studies of Demographic Crises in the Past*, Liege: Ordina Editions, 1979, 33–49.

Anderson, M., 'India, 1858–1930: The Illusion of Free Labour,' in D. Hay, P. Craven, eds., *Masters, Servants and Magistrates in Britain and the Empire, 1562–1955*, Chapel Hill/London: University of North Carolina Press, 2004.

Appadurai, A., 'How moral is South Asia's Economy?' *Journal of Asian Studies*, 43, 2, May 1984, 481–497.

Arnold, D., 'Dacoity and Rural Crime in Madras, 1860–1940,' *Journal of Peasant Studies*, 7, 2, 1979, 140–167.

———, 'Looting, Grain Riots and Government Policy in South India 1918,' *Past and Present*, 84, 1979, 111–145.

———, 'Famine in Peasant Consciousness and Peasant Action: Madras 1876–1878,' in R. Guha, ed., *Subaltern Studies III: Writings on South Asian History and Society*, New Delhi: Oxford University Press, 1984, 62–115.

———, *Colonizing the Body: State Medicine and Epidemic Disease in Nineteenth-Century India*, Berkeley: University of California Press, 1993.

———, 'Crisis and Contradiction in India's Public Health History,' in D. Porter, ed., *The History of Public Health and the Modern State*, Amsterdam: Rodopi, 1994, 335–355.

Aykroyd, W.R., B.G. Krishnan, 'Diets Surveys in South Indian Villages,' *Indian Journal of Medical Research*, 24, 3, Jan. 1937, 667–688.

Bagchi, A.K., 'Land Tax, Property Rights and Peasant Insecurity in Colonial India,' *Journal of Peasant Studies*, 20, 1, Oct. 1992, 1–49.

Baker, W.E., T.E. Dempster, H. Yule. *Report of a committee assembled to report on the causes of the unhealthiness which has existed at Kurnaul*, 1847); in Collected Memoranda on the Subject of Malaria, *Records of the Malaria Survey of India*, 1, 2, Mar. 1930, 1–68.

Balfour, A., H.H. Scott, *Health Problems of the Empire*, London: W. Collins Sons & Co., 1924, 134.

Balfour, M., S.K. Talpade, 'Maternity Conditions of Women Mill-Workers in India,' *Indian Medical Gazette*, May 30, 1930, 241–249.

Bandyopadhyay, P., *Indian Famine and Agrarian Problems: A Study of the Administration of Lord George Hamilton, Secretary of State for India, 1895–1903*, Calcutta: Star Publishers, 1987.

Banerjee, H., *Agrarian Society of the Punjab, 1849–1901*, New Delhi: Manohar, 1982.

Barrier, N.G., 'The Punjab Disturbances of 1907: The Response of the British Government in India to Agrarian Unrest,' *Modern Asian Studies*, 1, 4, 1967, 353–383.

———, *Banned: Controversial Literature and Political Control in British India, 1907–1947*, New Delhi: Manohar, 1976.

Behal, R.P., P. Mohapatra, 'Tea and Money Versus Human Life: The Rise and Fall of the Indenture System in the Assam Tea Plantations 1840–1908,' *Journal of Peasant Studies*, 19, 3/4, 1992, 142–172.

Bengtsson, T., C. Campbell, J.Z. Lee, et al., *Life Under Pressure: Mortality and Living Standards in Europe and Asia, 1700–1900*, Cambridge, MA: MIT Press, 2004.

Bengtsson, T., M. Dribe, 'New Evidence on the Standard of Living in Sweden During the Eighteenth and Nineteenth Centuries: Long-Term Development of the Demographic Response to Short-Term Economic Stress,' in R.C. Allen, T. Bengtsson, M. Dribe, eds., *Living Standards in the Past: New Perspectives on Well-Being in Asia and Europe*, Oxford: Oxford University Press, 2005, 341–371.

Bentley, C.A., *Report of an Investigation into the Causes of Malaria in Bombay*, Bombay: Miscellaneous Official Publications, 1911.

———, 'A New Conception Regarding Malaria,' in *3rd Meeting of the General Malaria Committee Held at Madras, Nov 18–20, 1912*, Simla: Government Central Branch Press, 1913, 61–84.

———, 'Some Problems Presented by Malaria in Bengal,' in *Proceedings of the Third Meeting of the General Malaria Committee Held at Madras, Nov. 18–20, 1912*, Simla: Government Central Branch Press, 1913.

———, *Report on Malaria in Bengal: The Past and Present Distribution of Malaria in Bengal and its Influence Upon the Population*, Calcutta: Bengal Government Press, 1916.

———, 'Dr. Bentley on Amelioration of Malaria by Irrigation,' *Indian Medical Record*, Feb. 1922, 41–43.

———, 'Some economic aspects of Bengal malaria,' *Indian Medical Gazette*, Sept. 1922, 321–326.

————, *Malaria and Agriculture in Bengal: How to Reduce Malaria in Bengal by Irrigation*, Calcutta: Bengal Government Press, 1925.

Bhatia, B.M., *Famines in India*, Bombay: Asia Publishers House, 1963.

————, 'Famine and Agricultural Labour in India,' *Indian Journal of Industrial Relations*, 10, 1975, 575–594.

Bhattacharya, N., 'The Logic of Tenancy Cultivation: Central and South-east Punjab, 1870–1935,' *Indian Economic and Social History Review*, 20, 2, Apr.–June 1983, 121–170.

————, 'Agrarian Change in Punjab, 1880–1940,' unpublished PhD dissertation, Jawaharlal Nehru University, 1985.

————, 'Agricultural Labour and Production: Central and South-East Punjab, 1870–1940,' in K.N. Raj, et al., eds., *Essays on the Commercialization of Indian Agriculture*, New Delhi: Oxford University Press, 1985, 105–152.

————, 'Lenders and Debtors: Punjab Countryside, 1880–1940,' *Indian Economic and Social History Review*, 1, 2, n.s., 1985, 305–342.

————, 'Pastoralists in a Colonial World,' in D. Arnold, R. Guha, eds., *Nature, Culture, Imperialism: Essays on the Environmental History of South Asia*, New Delhi: Oxford University Press, 1998, 49–85.

Biswas, A., 'The Decay of Irrigation and Cropping in West Bengal, 1850–1925,' in B. Chattopadhyay, P. Spitz, eds., *Food Systems and Society in Eastern India*, Geneva: United Nations Research Institute for Social Development, 1987, 85–131.

Blaxter, K.L., ed., *Nutritional Adaptation in Man*, London: John Libbey, 1985, 13–30.

Blyn, G., *Agricultural Trends in India, 1891–1947*, Philadelphia: University of Pennsylvania Press, 1966.

Boserup, E., *The Conditions of Agricultural Growth*, Chicago: Aldine, 1965.

Bouma, M.J., H. van der Kaay, 'The El Niño Southern Oscillation and the Historical Malaria Epidemics on the Indian Subcontinent and Sri Lanka: An Early Warning System for Future Epidemics?' *Tropical Medicine and International Health*, 1, 1, Feb. 1996, 86–96.

Brennan, L., 'The Development of the Indian Famine Codes: Personalities, Politics and Policies,' in B. Currey, G. Hugo, eds., *Famine as a Geographic Phenomenon*, Dordrecht: D. Reidel Publishers, 1984, 91–111.

Brennan, L., L. Leathcote, A. Lucas, 'The Causation of Famine: A Comparative Analysis of Lombok and Bengal 1891–1974,' *South Asia*, 7, 1, 1984, 1–26.

Brennan, L., J. McDonald, R. Shlomowitz, 'Long-Term Change in Indian Health,' *South Asia: Journal of South Asian Studies*, n.s., 26, 1, 2003, 51–69.

Brown, P.J., 'Demographic and Socioeconomic Effects of Disease Control: The Case of Malaria Eradication in Sardinia,' *Medical Anthropology*, 7, 2, 1983, 63–87.

————, 'Malaria, *Miseria*, and Underpopulation in Sardinia: The "Malaria Blocks Development" Cultural Model,' *Medical Anthropology*, 17, 1997, 239–254.

Bynum, W.F., 'An Experiment that Failed: Malaria Control at Mian Mir,' *Parassitologia*, 36, 1–2, 1994, 107–120.

———, ' "Reasons for Contentment": Malaria in India,' *Parassitologia*, 42, 1998, 19–27.

———, 'Malaria in Inter-War British India,' *Parassitologia*, 42, 1–2, 2000, 25–31.

Calvert, H., *The Size and Distribution of Cultivators' Holdings in the Punjab*, Lahore: Bureau of Economic Inquiry, 1928.

Carmichael, A.G., 'Infection, Hidden Hunger, and History,' *Journal of Interdisciplinary History*, 14, 3, 1983, 249–264.

Carter, R., P.M. Graves, 'Gametocytes,' in W.H. Wernsdorfer, I.A. McGregor, eds., *Malaria: Principles and Practice of Malariology*, Edinburgh: Churchill Livingstone, 1988, 253–306.

Catanach, I., 'Plague and the Tensions of Empire: India, 1896–1918,' in D. Arnold, ed., *Imperial Medicine and Indigenous Societies*, Manchester: Manchester University Press, 1988, 149–171.

Celli, A., 'The Restriction of Malaria in Italy,' in *Transactions Fifteenth International Congress on Hygiene and Demography, Washington, September 23–28, 1912*, Washington, DC: Government Printing Office, 1913, 516–531.

Chambers, R., R. Longhurst, A. Pacey, eds., *Seasonal Dimensions to Rural Poverty*, London: Frances Pinter Publishers, 1981.

Chandavarkar, R., 'Plague Panic and Epidemic Politics in India, 1896–1914,' in T. Ranger, P. Slack, eds., *Epidemics and Ideas*, Cambridge: Cambridge University Press, 1992, 203–240.

Chaudhuri, B., 'Agricultural Production in Bengal, 1850–1900,' *Bengal Past and Present*, 88, 2, 1969, 152–206.

Chaudhuri, K.N., 'Foreign Trade and Balance of Payments,' in D. Kumar, ed., *Cambridge Economic History of India, vol. 2*, Cambridge: Cambridge University Press, 1983.

Chaytor White, J., 'Report on the Outbreak of Malarial Fever in the United Provinces During the Period September to December 1908,' *Records of the Malaria Survey of India*, 1, 2, Mar. 1930, 114–130.

Chen, M.A., *Coping with Seasonality and Drought*, New Delhi: Sage, 1991.

Chopra, R.N., *Evolution of Food Policy in India*, New Delhi: Palgrave Macmillan, 1981.

Christophers, S.R., 'Second Report of the Anti-Malarial Operations in Mian Mir, 1901–1903,' *Sci. Mem. Off. Med. San. Dep.*, 9, 1904.

———, 'A New Statistical Method of Mapping Epidemic Disease in India, with Special Reference to the Mapping of Epidemic Malaria,' *Proceedings of the Imperial Malaria Conference held in Simla, October 1909*, 16–21.

———, 'On Malaria in the Punjab,' *Proceedings of the Imperial Malaria Conference held in Simla, October 1909*, 29–47.

———, 'Suggestions on the Use of Available Statistics for Studying Malaria in India,' *Paludism*, 1, 1910, 16–32.

———, 'Malaria in the Punjab,' *Sci. Mem. Off. Med. San. Dep.*, 46, Calcutta: Superintendent Government Printing Office, 1911.

———, 'Epidemic Malaria of the Punjab, with a Note on a Method of Predicting Epidemic Years,' *Paludism*, 2, 1911, 17–26.

———, 'Malaria in the Andamans,' *Sci. Mem. Off. Med. San. Dep.*, 56, 1912.

————, 'The Spleen Rate and Other Splenic Indices: Their Nature and Significance,' *Indian Journal of Medical Research*, 2, 1914, 823–866.

————, 'A Revision of the Nomenclature of Indian Anophelini,' *Indian Journal of Medical Research*, 3, 2, 1916, 454–488.

————, 'Malaria: Endemiology and Epidemiology,' in W. Byam, R.G. Archibald, eds., *The Practice of Medicine in the Tropics*, London: Henry Frowde, Hodder, and Stoughton, 1922, 2, 1546–1554.

————, 'What Disease Costs India: A Statement of the Problem Before Medical Research in India,' *Indian Medical Gazette*, Apr. 1924, 196–200.

————, 'Note on Malaria Research and Prevention in India,' in *Report of the Malaria Commission on its Study Tour of India*, Geneva: LN, 1930, 11–26.

————, 'Measures for the Control of Malaria in India,' *Journal of the Royal Society of Arts*, Apr. 30, 1943, 285–295.

————, 'Sydney Price James,' *Obituary Notice of Fellows of the Royal Society*, 5, 1945–1948, 507–523.

————, 'Endemic and Epidemic Prevalence,' in M.F. Boyd, ed., *Malariology*, Philadelphia: W.B. Saunders Co. 1949, 698–721.

————, 'Policy in Relation to Malaria Control,' *Indian Journal of Malariology*, Dec. 1955, 297–303.

Christophers, S.R., C.A. Bentley, 'Black-Water Fever: Being the First Report to the Advisory Committee Appointed by the Government of India to Conduct an Enquiry Regarding Black-Water and Other Fevers Prevalent in the Duars,' *Sci. Mem. Med. Sanit. Dep.*, 35, 1908.

————, *Malaria in the Duars. Being the Second Report to the Advisory Committee Appointed by the Government of India to Conduct an Enquiry Regarding Blackwater and Other Fevers Prevalent in the Duars*, Simla: Government Monotype Press, 1909.

————, 'The Human Factor,' in W. E. Jennings, ed., *Transactions of the Bombay Medical Congress, 1909*, Bombay: Bennett, Coleman & Co., 1910, 78–83.

Christophers, J.A. Sinton, 'A Malaria Map of India,' *Indian Journal of Medical Research*, 14, 1, 1926, 173–178.

Christophers, S.R., J.A. Sinton, G. Covell, 'How to Take a Malaria Survey,' *Health Bulletin*, 14, Calcutta: GOI Press, 1928.

Clemesha, W.W., 'Note on the Influence of Railway Construction on Malaria,' in 'Collected Memoranda on the Subject of Malaria,' *Records of the Malaria Survey of India*, 1, 2, Mar. 1930, 163–170.

Connell, A.K., 'Indian Railways and Indian Wheat,' *Royal Statistical Society*, 48, June 1885, 236–276.

Corbellini, G., 'Acquired Immunity Against Malaria as a Tool for the Control of the Disease: The Strategy Proposed by the Malaria Commission of the League of Nations,' *Parassitologia*, 40, 1998, 109–115.

Cornish, W.R., *Report of the Sanitary Commissioner for Madras for 1877*, Madras: Government Central Branch Press, 1878.

Cotton, A., *The Madras Famine*, London: Simpkin, Marshall [1878]; reprinted in A. Cotton, *Famine in India*, New York: Arno Press, 1976.

Covell, G., 'The Malaria Survey of India, 1927–1937,' *Journal of the Malaria Institute of India*, 1, 1, Mar. 1938, 1–17.

——, 'A Brief Review of the History and Development of the More Important Antimalarial Drugs,' *Indian Journal of Malariology*, 1, 2, June 1947, 231–241.

——, 'Developments in Malaria Control Methods During the Past Forty Years,' *Indian Journal of Malariology*, Dec. 1955, 305–312.

Covell, G., J.D. Baily, 'The Study of a Regional Epidemic of Malaria in Northern Sind,' *Records of the Malaria Survey of India*, 3, 2, Dec. 1932, 279–321.

Cragg, F.W., 'The Zoophilism of *Anopheles* in Relation to the Epidemiology of Malaria in India: A Suggestion,' *Indian Journal of Medical Research*, 10, 3, 1923, 962–964.

Curley, D., 'Fair Grain Markets and Mughal Famine Policy in Late Eighteenth-Century Bengal,' *The Calcutta Historical Journal*, 7, 1, 1977, 1–27.

Currie, K., 'British Colonial Policy and Famines: Some Aspects and Implications of 'Free Trade' in the Bombay, Bengal and Madras Presidencies, 1860–1900,' *South Asia*, 14, 2, 1991, 23–56.

Curtis, L.P., 'MacDonnell, Antony Patrick (1844–1925),' *Dictionary of National Biography*, doi: 34714.

Dandekar, V.M., N. Rath, *Poverty in India*, Pune: Indian School of Political Economy, 1971.

Dandekar, V.M., V.P. Pethe, *A Survey of Famine Conditions in the Affected Regions of Maharashtra and Mysore, 1952–1953*, Bangalore: Gokhale Institute, 1972.

Darling, M.L., *At Freedom's Door*, London: Oxford University Press, 1949.

Das Gupta, M., 'Selective Discrimination Against Female Children in Rural Punjab,' *Population and Development Review*, 13, 1, 1987, 77–100.

Dasgupta, A.K., 'Agricultural Growth Rates in the Punjab, 1906–1942,' *Indian Economic and Social History Review*, 18, July–Dec. 1981, 341.

Davis, K., *The Population of India and Pakistan*, New York: Princeton University Press, 1951.

Davis, M., *Late Victorian Holocausts: El Niño Famines and the Making of the Third World*, London: Verso, 2001.

Dempster, T.E., 'Notes on the Disease of the Spleen as an Easy and Certain Method of Detecting Malarious Localities in Hot Climates, (1848),' *Records of the Malaria Survey of India*, 1, 2, Mar. 1930, 69–85.

den Tuinder, N., 'Population and Society in Kheda District (India), 1819–1921: A Study of the Economic Context of Demographic Developments,' Doctoral dissertation, University of Amsterdam, 1992.

Dial Das, *Vital Statistics of the Punjab, 1901–1940*, Board of Economic Inquiry, Punjab, 80, 1942, Appendix 1.

Digby, W., *The Famine Campaign in Southern India 1876–1878*, Vol. 2, London: Longmans Green, 1878.

——, *'Prosperous' British India: A Revelation from Official Records*, London: T. Fisher Unwin, 1901.

Dobson, M.J., M. Malowany, R.W. Snow, 'Malaria Control in East Africa: The Kampala Conference and Pare-Taveta Scheme: A Meeting of Common and High Ground,' *Parassitologia*, 42, 2000, 149–166.

Drèze, J., 'Famine Prevention in India,' in J. Dreze, A. Sen, eds., *The Political Economy of Hunger*, Vol. 2, Oxford: Clarendon Press, 1990, 13–122.

Drèze, J., A. Sen, *Hunger and Public Action*, Oxford: Clarendon Press, 1989.

Dutt, R., *Open Letter to Lord Curzon on Famines and Land Assessment in India*, London: Paul Kegan, 1900.

Dyson, T., 'The Historical Demography of Berar, 1881–1980,' in T. Dyson, ed., *India's Historical Demography: Studies in Famine, Disease and Society*, London: Curzon Press, 1989, 150–196.

———, 'On the Demography of South Asian Famines,' *Population Studies*, 45, 1991, Parts 1 & 2, 5–25, 279–297.

———, 'Infant and Child Mortality in the Indian Subcontinent, 1881–1947,' in A. Bideau, B. Desjardins, H. Brignoli, eds., *Infant and Child Mortality in the Past*, Oxford: Clarendon Press, 1997, 109–135.

Dyson, T., M. Das Gupta, 'Demographic Trends in Ludhiana District, Punjab, 1881–1981: An Exploration of Vital Registration Data in Colonial India,' in Ts'ui-jung Liu et.al., eds., *Asian Population History*, Oxford: Oxford University Press, 2001, 79–104.

Dyson, T., C. O'Grada, 'Introduction,' in *Famine Demography: Perspectives from the Past and Present*, Oxford: Oford University Press, 2002.

Dyson, T., M. Murphy, 'Macro-level study of socioeconomic development and mortality: adequacy of indicators and methods of statistical analysis,' in J. Cleland, A. Hill, eds., *The Health Transition: Methods and Measures*, Canberra: Australian National University, 1991, Health Transition Series No. 3, 147–164.

Evans, H., 'European Malaria Policy in the 1920s and 1930s: The Epidemiology of Minutiae,' *Isis*, 80, 1989, 40–59.

Farley, J., *To Cast Out Disease: A History of the International Health Division of the Rockefeller Foundation, 1913–1951*, New York: Oxford University Press, 2004.

———, *Brock Chisholm, the World Health Organization, and the Cold War*, Vancouver: University of British Columbia Press, 2008.

Fayrer, Sir Joseph, *On the Climate and Fevers of India*, Croonian Lectures, London: J. & A. Churchill, 1882, 96–97.

Fillol, F., et al., 'Impact of Child Malnutrition on the Specific Anti-*Plasmodium Falciparum* Antibody Response,' *Malaria Journal*, June 2, 2009.

Floate, H.F.G., 'The Mauritian Malaria Epidemic 1866–1868: Geographical Determinism One Hundred Years Ago,' *Journal of Tropical Geography*, 29, 1969, 10–20.

Floud, R., R. Fogel, B. Harris, Sok Chul Hong, eds., *The Changing Body: Health, Nutrition, and Human Development in the Western World since 1700*, Cambridge: Cambridge University Press, 2011.

Fogel, R., 'Second Thoughts on the European Escape from Hunger: Famines, Chronic Malnutrition, and Mortality Rates,' in S.R. Osmani, ed., *Nutrition and Poverty*, Oxford: Clarendon Press, 1992, 243–280.

———, *Explaining Long-Term Trends in Health and Longevity*, New York: Cambridge University Press, 2012.

Fontaine, R.E., A.E. Najjar, J.S. Prince, 'The 1958 Malaria Epidemic in Ethiopia,' *American Journal of Tropical Medicine and Hygiene*, 10, 795–803.

Frederiksen, H., 'Malaria Control and Population Pressure in Ceylon,' *Public Health Reports*, 75, 10, Oct. 1960, 865–868.

———, 'Determinants and Consequences of Mortality Trends in Ceylon,' *Public Health Reports*, 76, 8, Aug. 1961, 659–663.

Fry, A.B., 'The Role of Cattle in the Epidemiology of Malaria,' *Indian Medical Gazette*, Jan. 1922, 1–2.

Gangulee, N., *Health and Nutrition in India*, London: Faber and Faber, 1939.

Garenne, M. et al., 'The Demographic Impact of a Mild Famine in an African City: The Case of Antananarivo, 1985–1987,' in T. Dyson, C.Ó. Gráda, eds., *Famine Demography: Perspectives from the Past and Present*, Oxford: Oxford University Press, 2002.

Garnham, C., 'Christophers, Sir (Samuel) Rickard,' *Oxford Dictionary of National Biography*, doi: 30928.

Genton, B., 'Relation of Anthropometry to Malaria Morbidity and Immunity in Papua New Guinean Children,' *American Journal of Clinical Nutrition*, 68, 3, 1998, 734–741.

Ghosh, A.K. *Prices and Economic Fluctuations in India 1861–1947*, New Delhi: S. Chand, 1979.

Ghosh, K.K., *Agricultural Labourers in India: A Study in the History of their Growth and Economic Condition*, Calcutta: Indian Publications, 1969.

Giles, G. M., 'Cold Weather Notes on Mosquitoes from the United Provinces, India,' *Journal of Tropical Medicine*, May 16, 1904, 149–152.

Gill, C.A., 'The Personal Factor in Sanitation,' *Indian Medical Gazette*, Aug. 1911, 298–302.

———, 'Epidemic or Fulminant Malaria Together with a Preliminary Study of the Part Played by Immunity in Malaria,' *Indian Journal of Medical Research*, 2, 1, July 1914, 268–314.

———, 'The Role of Meteorology in Malaria,' *Indian Journal of Medical Research*, 8, 4, 1921, 633–693.

———, 'The Forecasting of Malaria Epidemics with Special Reference to the Malarial Forecast for the Year 1926,' *Indian Journal of Medical Research*, 15, 1, 1927, 265–276.

———, *The Genesis of Epidemics and Natural History of Disease*, London: Bailliere, Tindall & Cox, 1928.

Gillespie, J.A., 'Social Medicine, Social Security and International Health, 1940–1960,' in E. Rodríguez-Ocaña, ed., *The Politics of the Healthy Life: An International Perspective*, Sheffield: European Association for the History of Medicine and Health, 2002, 219–239.

Glover, H., *Erosion in the Punjab*, Lahore: Civil and Military Gazette, 1944.

Goodman, N., *International Health Organizations and their Works*, London: J. & A. Churchill, 1952.

Gopinath, R., 'Aspects of Demographic Change and the Malabar Economy, 1871–1921,' *Economic and Political Weekly*, Jan. 1987, PE-30–36.

Gourlay, J., *Florence Nightingale and the Health of the Raj*, Aldershot, Hants: Ashgate, 2003.

Gray, P., 'Famine and Land in Ireland and India, 1845–1880: James Caird and the Political Economy of Hunger,' *The Historical Journal*, 49, 1, 2006, 193–215.

Guha, S., 'Mortality Decline in Early Twentieth Century India: A Preliminary Inquiry,' Indian *Economic and Social History Review*, 28, 4, 1991, 371–392.

———, 'Introduction,' in S. Guha, ed., *Growth, Stagnation or Decline? Agricultural Productivity in British India*, New Delhi: Oxford University Press, 1992.

———, The Importance of Social Intervention in England's Mortality Decline: The Evidence Reviewed,' *Social History of Medicine*, 7, 1, 1994, 89–113.

———, 'Mortality Decline in Early Twentieth Century India: A Preliminary Enquiry,' in S. Guha, ed., *Health and Population in South Asia: From Earliest Times to the Present*, London: Hurst, 2001.

Guilmoto, G., 'Towards a New Demographic Equilibrium: The Inception of Demographic Transition South in India,' *Indian Economic and Social History Review*, 28, 3, 1992, 247–289.

Guntupalli, A.M., J. Baten, 'The Development and Inequality of Heights in North, West, and East India 1915–1944,' *Explorations in Economic History*, 43, 2006, 578–608.

Guz, D., 'Population Dynamics of Famine in Nineteenth Century Punjab, 1896–1897 and 1899–1900,' in T. Dyson, ed., *India's Historical Demography: Studies in Famine, Disease and Society*, London: Curzon Press, 1989.

Hamid, N., 'Dispossession and Differentiation of the Peasantry in the Punjab During Colonial Rule,' *Journal of Peasant Studies*, 10, 1, 1982.

Hamlin, C., 'Could You Starve to Death in England in 1839? The Chadwick-Farr controversy and the Loss of the "Social" in Public Health,' *American Journal of Public Health*, 85, 6, 1995, 856–866.

———, *Public Health and Social Justice in the Age of Chadwick*, Cambridge: Cambridge University Press, 1998.

———, *More Than Hot: A Short History of Fever*, Baltimore: Johns Hopkins University Press, 2014.

Hardiman, D., 'Usury, Dearth and Famine in Western India,' *Past and Present*, 152, Aug. 1996, 113–156.

Harrison, G., *Mosquitoes, Malaria and Man: A History of the Hostilities since 1880*, New York: E. P. Dutton, 1978.

Harrison, M., *Public Health in British India: Anglo-Indian Preventive Medicine 1859–1914*, Cambridge: Cambridge University Press, 1994.

———, ' "Hot Beds of Disease": Malaria and Civilization in Nineteenth-Century British India,' *Parassitologia*, 40, 1–2, 1998, 11–18.

———, *Climates and Constitutions: Health, Race Environment and British Imperialism in India*, New Delhi: Oxford University Press, 2002, 173–176.

Hehir, P., *Malaria in India*, London: Humphrey Milford, 1927.

Heston, A., 'National Income,' in D. Kumar, ed., *Cambridge Economic History of India, vol. 2*, Cambridge: Cambridge University Press, 1983, 376–462.

Hicks, E.P., S. Abdul Majid, 'A Study of the Epidemiology of Malaria in a Punjab District,' *Records of the Malaria Survey of India*, 7, 1, 1937, 1–43.

Hill, J.L., 'A.P. MacDonnell and the Changing Nature of British Rule in India 1885–1901,' in R.I. Crane, N.G. Barrier, eds., *British Imperial Policy in India and Sri Lanka, 1858–1912: A Reassessment*, New Delhi: Heritage Publishers, 1981.

Hirst, L.F., *The Conquest of Plague: A Study of the Evolution of Epidemiology*, Oxford: Clarendon Press, 1953.

Hume, J.C., 'Colonialism and Sanitary Medicine: The Development of Preventive Health Policy in the Punjab, 1860 to 1900,' *Modern Asian Studies*, 20, 4, 1986, 703–724.

Humphreys, M., *Malaria: Poverty, Race, and Public Health in the United States*, Baltimore: Johns Hopkins University Press, 2001.

Hurd, J.M., 'Railways and the Expansion of Markets in India, 1861–1921,' *Explorations in Economic History*, 12, 3, July 1975, 263–288.

Hurd, J.M., 'Railways,' in D. Kumar, ed., *Cambridge Economic History of India, vol. 2*, Cambridge: Cambridge University Press, 1983, 737–761.

Hutchinson, F.H.G., 'Note on the Supply of Quinine as an Anti-Malarial Measure,' [1920], reprinted in *Records of the Malaria Survey of India*, 1, 2, 1930, 193–195.

Iyengar, M.O.T, 'Studies on Malaria in the Deltaic Regions of Bengal,' *Journal of the Malaria Institute of India*, Dec. 1942, 435–446.

James, S.P., 'Malaria in India,' *Sci. Mem. Off. Med. Sanit. Dep.*, 2, 1902.

———, 'First Report on the Anti-Malaria Operations in Mian Mir, 1901–1903,' *Sci. Mem. Med. Sanit. Dep.*, 6, 1903.

———, 'Malaria in Mian Mir,' in W.E. Jennings, ed., *Transactions of the Bombay Medical Congress, 1909*, Bombay: Bennett, Coleman & Co., 1910, 84–93.

———, 'A Note on Some of the Measures that Have Been Taken to Make Quinine Available to the Poor in India,' *Paludism*, 3, 1911, 10–14.

———, Commentary, in R. Briercliffe; 'Discussion on the Malaria Epidemic in Ceylon 1934–1935,' *Proceedings of the Royal Society of Medicine*, 29, 1936, 537–562.

James, S.P., S.R. Christophers, 'The Success of Mosquito Destruction Operations,' *British Medical Journal*, Sept. 17, 1904, ii, 631–632.

James, S.P., S.R. Christophers, 'What Can the State Do to Prevent it?' *Lancet*, June 26, 1909, 1860–1862.

James, S.P., W.G. Liston, *The Anopheline Mosquitoes of India*, 2nd ed., Calcutta: Thacker, Spink & Co., 1911.

Jeffery, R., *The Politics of Health in India*, Berkeley: University of California Press, 1988.

Jennings, W.E., ed., *Transactions of the Bombay Medical Congress, 1909*, Bombay: Bennett, Coleman & Co., 1910, 84–93.

Jones, W.H.S., *Malaria, a Neglected Factor in the History of Greece and Rome*: Cambridge, Macmillan & Bowes, 1907.

Kamat, V., 'Resurgence of Malaria in Bombay (*Mumbai*) in the 1990s: A Historical Perspective,' *Parassitologia*, 42, 2000, 135–148, 2000.

Kaw, M.A., 'Famines in Kashmir, 1586–1819: The Policy of the Mughal and Afghan Rulers,' *Indian Economic and Social History Review*, 33, 1, 1966, 59–71.

Kazi, I., *Historical Study of Malaria in Bengal, 1860–1920*, Dhaka: Pip International Publishers, 2004.

Kessinger, T., *Vilyatpur 1848–1969, Social and Economic Change in a North Indian Village*, Berkeley: University of California Press, 1974.

Kielmann, A.A., C. McCord, 'Weight-for-Age as an Index of Risk of Death in Children,' *Lancet*, 311, 8076, June 10, 1978, 1247–1250.

King, W., 'The Prevention of Malaria,' *British Medical Journal*, June 3, 1911, 1348.

Klein, I., 'Malaria and Mortality in Bengal, 1840–1921,' *Indian Economic and Social History Review*, 9, 2, 1972, 132–160.

———, 'Death in India,' *Journal of Asian Studies*, Aug. 1973, 639–659.

———, 'When the Rains Failed: Famine, Relief, and Mortality in British India,' *Indian Economic and Social History Review*, 21, 2, 1984, 185–214.

———, 'Plague, Policy and Popular Unrest in British India,' *Modern Asian Studies*, 22, 4, 1988, 723–755.

———, 'Population Growth and Mortality in British India Part I: The Climacteric of Death,' *Indian Economic and Social History Review*, 26, 4, 1989, 387–403.

———, 'Population Growth and Mortality in British India Part II: The Demographic Revolution,' *Indian Economic and Social History Review*, 27, 1, 1990, 33–63.

———, 'Development and Death: Reinterpreting Malaria, Economics and Ecology in British India,' *Indian Economic and Social History Review*, 38, 2, 2001, 147–179.

Knight, H., *Food Administration in India 1939–1947*, Stanford: Stanford University Press, 1954.

Kolsky, E., ' "One Scale of Justice for the Planter and Another for the Coolie": Law and Violence on the Assam Tea Plantations,' in E. Kolsky, *Colonial Justice in British India*, New York: Cambridge University Press, 2010.

Korenromp, E.L. et al., 'Malaria Attributable to the HIV-I Epidemic, Sub-Saharan Africa,' *Emerging Infectious Diseases*, 11, 9, 2005, 1413.

Kumar, D., *Land and Caste in South India: Agricultural Labour in the Madras Presidency during the 19th Century*, Cambridge: Cambridge University Press, 1965.

———, 'The Fiscal System,' in D. Kumar, ed., *Cambridge Economic History of India, vol. 2*, Cambridge: Cambridge University Press, 1983, 905–944.

Kumar, A., 'The Indian Drug Industry under the Raj, 1860–1920,' in B. Pati, M. Harrison, eds., *Health, Medicine and Empire: Perspectives on Colonial India*, Hyderabad: Orient Longman, 2001.

Kunitz, S.J., 'Mortality Since Malthus,' in R. Scofield, D. Coleman, eds., *The State of Population Theory: Forward from Malthus*, Oxford: Basil Blackwell, 1986, 279–302.

Lal, D., *Cultural Stability and Economic Stagnation, India c. 1500 BC – AD 1980*, Oxford: Clarendon Press, 1988.

Lal, R.B., S.C. Seal, *General Rural Health Survey, Singur Health Centre, 1944*, Calcutta: All-India Institute of Hygiene and Public Health, GOI Press, 1949.

Langford, C., 'Reasons for the Decline in Mortality in Sri Lanka Immediately After the Second World War: A Re-Examination of the Evidence,' *Health Transition Review*, 6, 1996, 3–23, 15.

Lardinois, R., 'Deserted Villages and Depopulation in Rural Tamil Nadu c. 1780–1830,' in T. Dyson, ed., *India's Historical Demography: Studies in Famine, Disease and Society*, London: Curzon Press, 1989, 16–48.

———, 'Famine, Epidemics and Mortality in South India: A Reappraisal of the Demographic Crisis of 1876–1878,' *Economic and Political Weekly*, 20, Mar. 16, 1985, 454–465.

League of Nations, Malaria Commission, *Report of the Malaria Commission on its Study Tour of India*. Geneva: League of Nations, 1930.

Learmonth, A.T.A., 'Some Contrasts in the Regional Geography of Malaria in India and Pakistan,' *Transactions and Paper, Institute of British Geographers*, 23, 1957, 37–59.

Leslie, J.T.W., 'An Address on Malaria in India: Delivered at the Opening of the Malaria Conference, Simla, October 1909,' *Lancet*, Nov. 20, 1909, 1483–1486.

Lindauer, J., S. Singh, *Land Taxation and Indian Economic Development*, New Delhi: Kalyani Publishers, 1979.

Litsios, 'Malaria Control, the Cold War, and the Postwar Reorganization of International Assistance,' *Medical Anthropology*, 17, 1997, 255–278.

Livi-Bacci, M., *Population and Nutrition: An Essay on European Demographic History*, Cambridge: Cambridge University Press, 1991.

Lobo, L., *Malaria in the Social Context: A Study in Western India*, New Delhi: Routledge, 2010.

Lovat, F., *India Under Curzon and After*, Bombay: Times of India, 1911.

Loveday, A., *The History of Indian Famines*, London: G. Bell & Sons, 1914.

Lukis, C.P., 'Presidential Address at the Second Meeting of General Malaria Committee at Bombay, 16th and 17th November 1911,' *Paludism*, 4, 1912, 1–9.

Macdonald, G., 'Community Aspects of Immunity to Malaria,' in L.J. Bruce-Chwatt, V.J. Glanville, eds., *Dynamics of Tropical Disease: The Late George Macdonald*, London: Oxford University Press, 1973, 77–84.

———, 'The Analysis of Malaria Epidemics,' in L.J. Bruce-Chwatt, Glanville, eds., *Dynamics of Tropical Diseases: The Late George Macdonald*(London: Oxford University Press, 1973), 146–160.

Macdonald, G., J. Abdul Majid, 'Report on an Intensive Malaria Survey in the Karnal District, Punjab,' *Records of the Malaria Survey of India*, 2, 3, Sept. 1931, 423–477.

Macdonnell, A.P., *Report on the Food-Grain Supply and Famine Relief in Behar and Bengal, 1873–1874*, Calcutta: Bengal Secretariat Press, 1876.

Macleod, R., M. Lewis, eds., *Disease, Medicine and Empire*, London: Routledge, 1988.

McKeown, T., *The Modern Rise of Population*, London: Edward Arnold, 1976.

Maharatna, A., 'Regional Variation in Demographic Consequences of Famines in Late Nineteenth and Early twentieth Century India,' *Economic and Political Weekly*, June 4, 1994, 1399–1410.

——, *The Demography of Famines: An Indian Historical Perspective*, New Delhi: Oxford University Press, 1996.

——, 'Famines and Epidemics: An Historical Perspective,' in T. Dyson, C. Ó Gráda, eds., *Famine Demography: Perspective from the Past and Present*, Oxford: Oxford University Press, 2002, 113–141.

Mankodi, K., 'Political and Economic Roots of Disease: Malaria in Rajasthan,' *Economic and Political Weekly*, Jan. 27, 1996, PE-42–48.

Manson, P., *Tropical Diseases: A Manual of the Diseases of Warm Climates*, London: Cassell and Co., 1898.

Martorell, R., 'Child Growth Retardation: A Discussion of its Causes and Its Relationship to Health,' in J.C. Waterlow, K. Mathur, J.N, Gopal Jayal, eds., *Drought Policy and Politics in India*, New Delhi: Sage, 1993.

Mathur, K.K., et al., 'Epidemic of Malaria in Barmer Disrict (Thar Desert) of Rajasthan During 1990,' *Indian Journal of Malariology*, 29, Mar. 1992, 1–10.

Mayne, B., 'The Influence of Relative Humidity on the Presence of Parasites in the Insect Carrier and the Initial Seasonal Appearance of Malaria in a Selected Area in India,' *Indian Journal of Medical Research*, 15, 4, 1928, 1073–1084.

McAlpin, M., *Subject to Famine: Food Crises and Economic Change in Western India, 1860–1920*, Princeton: Princeton University Press, 1983.

McGregor, I.A., 'Malaria and Nutrition,' in W.H. Wernsdorfer, I.A. McGregor, eds., *Malaria: Principles and Practice of Malariology*, Edinburgh: Churchill Livingstone, 1988, 754–777.

——, R.J.M. Wilson, 'Specific Immunity: Acquired in Man,' in W.H. Wernsdorfer, McGregor, eds., *Malaria: Principles and Practice of Malariology*, Edinburgh: Churchill Livingstone, 1988, 559–619.

McKenzie Taylor, E., M.L. Mehta, 'Some Irrigation Problems in the Punjab,' *The Indian Journal of Agricultural Science*, 11, 2, 137–169.

Mehta, D.R., 'Malaria Control in the Punjab (India) with Special Reference to the National Malaria Control Programme,' *Indian Journal of Malariology*, 9, 4, Dec. 1955, 327–342.

Millman, S., R.W. Kates, 'Toward Understanding Hunger,' in L.F. Newman, ed., *Hunger in History: Food Shortage, Poverty, and Deprivation*, Cambridge, MA: Blackwell, 1990, 3–24.

Mills, I.D., 'The 1918–1919 Influenza Pandemic – the Indian Experience,' *Indian Economic and Social History Review*, 23, 1, 1986, 1–40.

Mody, A., 'Population Growth and Commercialisation of Agriculture: India, 1890–1940,' *Indian Economic and Social History Review*, 19, 3–4, 1982, 237–266.

Mohanty, B., 'Orissa Famine of 1866: Demographic and Economic Consequences,' *Economic and Political Weekly*, 28, Jan. 2–9, 1993, 55–66.

Mohapatra, P., 'Coolies and Colliers: A Study of the Agrarian Context of Labour Migration from Chotanagpur, 1881–1920,' *Studies in History*, 1, 2, n.s., 1985, 247–299.

Mooij, J., *Food Policy and the Indian State: The Public Distribution System in South India*, New Delhi: Oxford University Press, 1999.

Mukherjee, A., 'Scarcity and Crime: A Study of Nineteenth Century Bengal,' *Economic and Political Weekly*, 28, Feb. 6, 1993, 237–243.

Mukherjee, N., A. Mukherjee, 'Rural Women and Food Insecurity: What a Food Calendar Reveals,' *Economic and Political Weekly*, Mar. 12, 1994, 597–599.

Mukherjee, R., *Changing Face of Bengal: A Study in Riverine Economy*, Calcutta: University of Calcutta, 1938.

Muraleedharan, V.R., 'Malady in Madras: The Colonial Government's Response to Malaria in the Early Twentieth Century,' in D. Kumar, ed., *Science and Empire: Essays in Indian Context (1700–1947)*, New Delhi: Anamika Prakasshanin, 1991, 101–114.

———, 'Quinine (cinchona) and the Incurable Malaria,' *Parassitologia*, 42, 2000, 91–100.

———, 'Cinchona' Policy in British India: The Critical Early Years,' in A.K. Bagchi, K. Soman, eds., *Maladies, Preventives and Curatives: Debates in Public Health in India*, New Delhi: Tulika Books, 2005, 32–43.

Muraleedharan, V.R., D. Veeraraghavan, 'Anti-Malaria Policy in the Madras Presidency: An Overview of the Early Decades of the Twentieth Century,' *Medical History*, 36, 1992, 290–305.

Nájera, J.A., 'The Control of Tropical Diseases and Socioeconomic Development, with Special Reference to Malaria and its Control,' *Parassitologia*, 36, 1–2, Aug. 1994, 17–33.

———, 'Malaria Control: Achievements, Problems and Strategies,' *Parassitologia*, 43, 1–2, 1–89, 2001.

Nandi, J. et al., 'Anthropophily of Anophelines in Duars of West Bengal and other regions of India,' *Journal of Communicable Disease*, 32, 2, 2000, 95–99.

Nash, V., *The Great Famine*, London: Longmans Green, 1901.

Nathan, R., H.B. Thornhill, L. Rogers, *Report on the Measures Taken Against Malaria in the Lahore (Mian Mir) Cantonment*, Calcutta: Government Printing Office, 1910.

Newman, L.F., ed., *Hunger in History: Food Shortage, Poverty, and Deprivation*, Cambridge, MA: Blackwell, 1990.

Norman White, F., *Twenty Years of Plague in India with Special Reference to the Outbreak of 1917–1918*, Simla: Government Central Branch Press, 1929.

Obit., 'J.T.W. Leslie,' *British Medical Journal*, Apr. 8, 1911, 848–849.

O'Conor, J.E., *Prices and Wages in India*, Calcutta: GOI Press, 1886.

O'Meara, W.P. et al., 'Effect of a Fall in Malaria Transmission on Morbidity and Mortality in Kilifi, Kenya,' *Lancet*, 372, Nov. 1, 2008, 1555–1562.

Omvedt, G., *The Political Economy of Starvation: Imperialism and the World Food Crisis*, Bombay: Leela Bhosale, 1975.

Ortega Osona, J.A., 'The Attenuation of Mortality Fluctuations in British Punjab and Bengal, 1870–1947,' in Ts'ui-jung Liu, ed., *Asian Population History*, Oxford: Oxford University Press, 2001, 306–349.

Packard, R.M., 'Maize, Cattle and Mosquitoes: The Political Economy of Malaria Epidemics in Colonial Swaziland,' *Journal of African History*, 25, 1984, 189–212.

———, 'Malaria Dreams: Postwar Visions of Health and Development in the Third World,' *Medical Anthropology*, 17, 1997, 279–296.

———, ' "No Other Logical Choice": Global Malaria Eradication and the Politics of International Health in the Post-War era,' *Parassitologia*, 40, 1998, 217–229.

———, *The Making of a Tropical Disease: A Short History of Malaria*, Baltimore: Johns Hopkins University Press, 2007.

———, ' "Roll Back Malaria, Roll in Development"? Reassessing the Economic Burden of Malaria,' *Population and Development Review*, 35, 1, 2009, 53–87.

Pai, M. et al., 'Malaria and Migrant Labourers,' *Economic and Political Weekly*, Apr. 19, 1997, 838–842.

Parkes, E.A., *A Manual of Practical Hygiene, Prepared Especially for Use in the Medical Service of the Army*, London: John Churchill, 1866.

Parthasarathi, P., 'Rethinking Wages and Competitiveness in the Eighteenth Century: Britain and South Asia,' *Past and Present*, 158, Feb. 1998, 79–109.

Parthasarathy, B., N.A. Sontakke, A.A. Monot, D.R. Kothawale, 'Droughts/Floods in the Summer Monsoon Season Over Different Meteorological Subdivisions of India for the Period 1871–1984,' *Journal of Climatology*, 7, 1987, 57–70.

Patel, S.J., *Agricultural Labourers in Modern India and Pakistan*, Bombay: Current Book House, 1952.

Pati, B., M. Harrison. *Health, Medicine and Empire: Perspectives on Colonial India*, London: Sangam Books, 2001.

Paustian, P.W., *Canal Irrigation in the Punjab*, New York: Columbia University Press, 1930.

Peile, J.B., 'Notes of the Economic Condition of the Agricultural Population of India,' in *Famine Commission Report*, London: HMSO, 1880, Appendix I, Miscell. Papers, 162–166.

Phillips, J.A.S., 'On the Results of Anti-Malaria Measures in Five Towns in the United Provinces,' *Indian Medical Gazette*, May 1924, 221–228.

Polu, S., *Infectious Disease in India, 1892–1940: Policy-Making and the Perceptions of Risk*, London: Palgrave Macmillan, 2012.

Post, J.D., 'Nutritional Status and Mortality in Eighteenth-Century Europe,' in L.F. Newman, ed., *Hunger in History: Food Shortage, Poverty, and Deprivation*, Cambridge, MA: Blackwell, 1990, 241–280.

Rajasekhar, D., 'Famines and Peasant Mobility: Changing Agrarian Structure in Kurnool District of Andhra 1871–1900,' *Indian Economic and Social History Review*, 28, 2, 1991, 121–150.

Ramachandra Rao, T., *Anophelines of India*, 1st ed., New Delhi: Malaria Research Centre, *Indian Council of Medical research*, 1984.

Ramanna, M., 'A Mixed Record: Malaria Control in Bombay Presidency, 1900–1935,' in D. Kumar, R. Sekhar Basu, eds., *Medical Encounters in British India*, New Delhi: Oxford University Press, 2013, 208–231.

Ramasubban, R., 'Imperial health in British India, 1857–1900,' in R. Macleod, M. Lewis, eds., *Disease, Medicine and Empire*, London: Routledge, 1988, 38–60.

———, *Public Health and Medical Research in India: Their Origins under the Impact of British Colonial Policy, SAREC report R4*, Stockholm: SIDA, 1982.

Ramaswamy, C., *Review of Floods in India during the Past 75 Years*, New Delhi: Indian National Science Academy, 1985.

———, *Meteorological Aspects of Severe Floods in India, 1923–1979*, New Delhi: India Meteorological Department, Hydrology Monograph No. 10, 1987.

Rangasami, A., 'Systems of Limited Intervention: An Evaluation of the Principles and Practice of Relief Administration in India,' in J. Floud, A. Rangasami, eds., *Famine and Society*, New Delhi: Indian Law Institute, 1993, 185–198.

Robb, P., 'New Directions in South Asian History,' *South Asia Research*, 7, 2, Nov. 1987, 133.

Ross, R., 'The Anti-Malaria Experiment at Mian Mir,' *British Medical Journal*, Sept. 17, 1904, ii, 632–635.

———, 'Mosquitoes and Malaria: A Campaign that Failed,' *Lancet*, Apr. 10, 1909, 1074–1075.

———, 'Malaria Prevention at Mian Mir, *Lancet*, July 3, 1909, 43–45.

———, 'The Practice of Malaria Prevention,' in W.E. Jennings, ed., *Transactions of the Bombay Medical Congress*, Bombay: Bennett, Coleman & Co., 1910, 67–74.

———, *The Prevention of Malaria*, London: John Murray, 1910.

———, *Memoirs: The Great Malaria Problem and its Solution*, London: John Murray, 1923.

———, 'Malaria and Feeding,' *Journal of Tropical Medicine and Hygiene*, May 1, 1929, 132.

Rotberg, R.I., 'Nutrition and History,' *Journal Interdisciplinary History*, 14, 3, 1983, 199–204.

Rowlands, M.G.M. et al., 'Seasonality and the Growth of Infants in a Gambian Village,' in R. Chambers, R. Longhurst, A. Pacey, eds., *Seasonal Dimensions to Rural Poverty*, London: Frances Pinter, 1981.

Rushbrook Williams, L.F., *India in the Year 1919*, Calcutta: Superintendent Government Printing Office, 1920.

Russell, A.J.H., 'Quinine Supplies in India,' *Records of the Malaria Survey of India*, 7, 4, Dec. 1937, 233–244.

Russell, P.F., 'Malaria in India: Impressions from a Tour,' *Americal Journal of Tropical Medicine*, 16, 6, 1936, 653–664.

———, 'Malaria Due to Defective and Untidy Irrigation,' *Journal of the Malaria Institute of India*, 1, 4, 1938, 339–349.

Russell, P., L.S. West, R.D. Manwell, *Practical Malariology*, Philadelphia: W.B. Saunders, 1946.

Samanta, A., *Malaria Fever in Colonial Bengal, 1820–1939: Social History of an Epidemic*, Kolkata: Firma KLM, 2002.

Sami, L., 'Starvation, Disease and Death: Explaining Famine Mortality in Madras, 1876–1878,' *Social History of Medicine*, 24, 3, 2011, 700–719.

Sandeep, K., 'Control, Eradication and Resurgence of Malaria in Kerala during the post 50 years,' *Kerala Medical Journal*, 1, 2, Dec. 2008.

Scrimshaw, N.S., 'The Phenomenon of Famine,' *American Review of Nutrition*, 7, 1987, 1–21.

Scrimshaw, N.S., C.E. Taylor, J.E. Gordon, *Interactions of Nutrition and Infection*, Geneva: World Health Organization, 1968.

Sen, A., *Poverty and Famines: An Essay on Entitlement and Deprivation*, Oxford: Oxford University Press, 1981.

Sen, S., *Women and Labour in Late Colonial India: The Bengal Jute Industry*, Cambridge: Cambridge University Press, 1999.

Sen, S.R., *Growth and Instability in Indian Agriculture*, New Delhi: Ministry of Food and Agriculture, 1967.

Senior White, R., *Studies in Malaria as It Affect Indian Railways*, Indian Research Fund Association, Technical Paper, 258, Calcutta: Central Publications Branch, 1928.

Sewell, E.P., 'The Results of the Campaign Against Malaria in Mian Mir,' *British Medical Journal*, Sept. 1904, 635–636.

Sharma, S., *Famine, Philanthropy and the Colonial State*, New Delhi: Oxford University Press, 2001.

Sharma, V.P., 'Determinants of Malaria in South Asia,' in E.A. Casman, H. Dowlatabadi, eds., *The Contextual Determinants of Malaria*, Washington, DC: Resources for the Future, 2002, 110–132.

Sharma, V.P., 'Malaria and Poverty,' *Current Science*, 84, 2003, 513–515.

Sharma, V.P., K.N. Mehotra, 'Malaria Resurgence in India: A Critical Study,' *Social Science Medicine*, 22, 1986, 835–845, 836.

Shiva, M., 'Mewat Calling: A Brief Report pf the Malaria Outbreak in Mewat,' *Health for the Millions*, Mar.–Apr. 1997, 11–12.

Siddiqui, J., *World Health and World Politics: The World Health Organization and the UN System*, London: Hurst, 1995.

Singh, K.S., 'The Famine Code: The Context and Continuity,' in J. Floud, A. Rangasami, eds., *Famine and Society*, New Delhi: Indian Law Institute, 1993, 139–162.

Singh, N., Starvation and Colonialism: A Study of Famines in the Nineteenth Century British Punjab 1858–1901, New Delhi: National Book Organisation, 1996.

Sinha, R.P., *Food in India: An Analysis of the Prospects for Self-Sufficiency by 1975–1976*, Bombay: Oxford University Press, 1961.

Sinton, J.A., 'A Bibliography of Malaria in India,' *Records of the Malaria Survey of India*, Oct. 1929, 1–200.

———, 'What Malaria Costs India, Nationally, Socially and Economically,' *Records of the Malaria Survey of India*, 5, 3, Sept. 1935, 223–264; 4, 4, Dec. 1935, 413–489; 6, 1, Mar. 1936, 91–169.

Slater, L.B., *War and Disease, Biomedical Research on Malaria in the Twentieth Century*, New Brunswick: Rutgers University Press, 2009.

Sotiroff-Junker, J., *Behavioural, Social and Economic Aspects of Malaria and its Control*, Geneva: World Health Organization, 1978.

Srivastava, H.S., *The History of Indian Famines, 1858–1918*, Agra: Sri Ram Mehra, 1968.

Stephens J.W.W., S.R. Christophers, 'An Investigation into the Factors Which Determine Malarial Endemicity,' *Reports to the Malaria Committee of the Royal Society*, 7th series, Aug. 15, 1902, 23–45.

———, 'The Occurrence of Blackwater Fever in India,' *Reports to the Malaria Committee of the Royal Society*, 8, 1902, 3–13.

Strickland, G.T. et al., 'Endemic Malaria in Four Villages of the Pakistani Province of Punjab,' *Transactions of the Royal Society of Tropical Medicine and Hygiene*, 81, 1, 1987, 36–41.

Sur, S.N., *Malaria Problem in Bengal*, Calcutta: Bengal Public Health Department, 1929, 188.

Swellengrebel, N.H., 'Some Aspects of the Malaria Problem in Italy,' in League of Nations Health Organisation. Malaria Commission, *Report on its Tour of Investigation in Certain European Countries in 1924*, C.H. 273, Geneva, Mar. 26, 1925, Annex 11, 168–171.

Thorburn, S.S., *The Punjab in Peace and War*, Edinburgh: Blackwood, 1904.

Thorner, D., 'Long Term Trends in Output in India,' in S. Kuznets et al., eds., *Economic Growth: Brazil, India, Japan*, Durham: Duke University Press, 1955.

Timbres, H.G., 'Studies on Malaria in Villages in Western Bengal,' *Records of the Malaria Survey of India*, 5, 4, Dec. 1935, 366.

Torry, W.I., 'Drought and the Government-Village Emergency Food Distribution System in India,' *Human Organization*, 45, 1, 1986, 11–23.

———, 'Mortality and Harm: Hindu Peasant Adjustments to Famines,' *Social Science Information*, 25, 1, 1986, 125–160.

Trevaskis, H.K., *Land of the Five Rivers*, Oxford: Oxford University Press, 1928.

———, *The Punjab of Today*, Vol. 2, Lahore: Civil and Military Gazette Press, 1931–1932.

Twomey, M., 'Employment in Nineteenth Century Indian Textiles,' *Explorations in Economic History*, 20, 1983, 35–57.

Vasavi, A.R., 'The Millet Drought': Oral narratives and the Cultural Grounding of Famine-Relief in Bijapur,' *South Indian Studies*, 2, July–Dec. 1996, 205–233.

Venkat Rao, V., 'Review of Malaria Control in India,' *Indian Journal of Malariology*, 3, 4, Dec. 1949, 313–326.

Viswanathan, D.K., 'A Study of the Effects of Malaria and of Malaria Control Measures on Population and Vital Statistics in Kanara and Dharwar Districts as Compared with the Rest of the Province of Bombay,' *Indian Journal of Malariology*, 3, 1, Mar. 1949, 69–99.

Wakimura, K., 'Epidemic Malaria and "Colonial Development": Reconsidering the Cases of Northern and Western India,' Economic History Congress XIII, Buenos Aires, Argentina, July 2002, mimeo.

Walter, J., R. Schofield, eds., *Famine, Disease and the Social Order in Early Modern England*, Cambridge: Cambridge University Press, 1989.

Watson, M., 'The Lesson of Mian Mir,' *Journal of Tropical Medicine and Hygiene*, July 1, 1931, 183–189.

Watts, S., 'British Development Policies and Malaria in India 1897-c.1929,' *Past and Present*, 165, 1999, 141–181.

Webb, J.L.A., *Humanity's Burden: A Global History of Malaria*, New York: Cambridge University Press, 2009, 27–41.

———, *The Long Struggle Against Malaria in Tropical Africa*, New York: Cambridge University Press, 2014.

Whitcombe, E., *Agrarian Conditions in Northern India*, Berkeley: University of California Press, 1972.

———, 'Irrigation,' in *Cambridge Economic History of India, vol. 2*, Cambridge: Cambridge University Press, 1983.

———, 'Famine Mortality,' *Economic and Political Weekly*, 28, June 5, 1993, 1169–1179.

———, 'The Environmental Costs of Irrigation in British India: Waterlogging, Salinity, Malaria,' in D. Arnold, R. Guha, eds., *Nature, Culture, Imperialism: Essays on the Environmental History of south Asia*, New Delhi: Oxford University Press, 1995, 237–259.

World Health Organization, *World Malaria Report*, Geneva, 2009.

Will, P.E., B. Wong, *Nourish the People: The State Civilian Granary System in China, 1650–1850*, Ann Arbor: University of Michigan, 1991.

Worboys, M., 'The Discovery of Colonial Malnutrition Between the Wars,' in D. Arnold, ed., *Imperial Medicine and Indigenous Societies*, Manchester: Manchester University Press, 1988, 208–225.

———, 'Manson, Ross and Colonial Medical Policy: Tropical Medicine in London and Liverpool, 1899–1914,' in R. Macleod, M. Lewis, eds., *Disease, Medicine and Empire: Perspectives on Western Medicine and the Experience of European Expansion*, London: Routledge, 1988, 21–37.

———, 'Germs, Malaria and the Invention of Mansonian Tropical Medicine: From "Diseases in the Tropics" to "Tropical Diseases",' in D. Arnold, ed., *Warm Climates in Western Medicine: The Emergence of Tropical Medicine, 1500–1900*, Amsterdam: Redopi, 1996, 181–207.

———, 'Colonial Medicine,' 67–80, in R. Cooter, J. Pickstone, eds., *Medicine in the Twentieth Century*, Amsterdam: Harwood Academic Publishers, 2000.

Yacob, M., S. Swaroop, 'The Forecasting of Epidemic Malaria in the Punjab,' *Journal of the Malaria Institute of India*, 5, 3, 1944, 319–335.

———, 'Investigation of Long-Term Periodicity in the Incidence of Epidemic Malaria in the Punjab, *Journal of the Malaria Institute of India*, 6, 1, 1945, 39–51.

———, 'Malaria and Rainfall in the Punjab,' *Journal of the Malaria Institute of India*, 6, 3, 1946, 273–284.

———, 'Malaria and Spleen Rate in the Punjab,' *Indian Journal of Malariology*, 1, 4, 1947, 469–489.

——, 'Preliminary Forecasts of the Incidence of Malaria in the Punjab,' *Indian Journal of Malariology*, 1, 4, 1947, 491–501.

Zurbrigg, S., '*Rakku's Story: Structures of Ill-health in Rural India*,' Bangalore: Centre for Social Action, 1984.

——, 'Hunger and Epidemic Malaria in Punjab, 1868–1940,' *Economic and Political Weekly*, Jan. 12, 1992, PE 2–26.

——, 'Re-Thinking the "Human Factor" in Malaria Mortality: The Case of Punjab, 1868–1940,' *Parassitologia*, 36, 1–2, 1994, 121–136.

——, 'Did Starvation Protect from Malaria? Distinguishing Between Severity and Lethality of Infectious Disease in Colonial India,' *Social Science History*, 21, 1, 1997, 27–58.

Index

Acton, H.W. 193
Africa, holoendemic malaria in
45n82, 281, 412–413
agrarian unrest 224
Agricultural credit (takavi) 345,
348–349, 353–354
Agricultural Labour Enquiry
(1952) 354
Amrith, Sunil 413
Amritsar 42, 80–81, 177–181, 198
Andaman Islands 191
Andersen, O. 408
Anderson, M. 230
An. gambiae 230
An. minimus 93n97, 227
Anopheles culicifacies 12, 21,
51, 64–65, 197, 205n74, 218,
221–222, 227
An. rossii (An. subpictus) 221
An. stephensi 89n1, 254
Arnold, David xviii, 19, 366n122
Ayurveda, view of malaria 15

Baker-Dempster report 101,
215, 283
Bengal 22, 31, 41n54, 153, 275,
293, 313; Permanent Settlement
(1793) 275–276; see also
Burdwan fever; famines
Bentley, C.A. 9, 31, 80, 191, 195,
211, 226–231, 241–243, 254,
266, 274–276, 280, 411
Bhatia, B.M. 30, 118n49, 308, 350
Bhattacharya, Neeladri xvi, 97–98,
111–113, 118n44, 118n56,

119n59, 197, 351, 361n33,
368n154
blackwater fever 211, 216,
226–227, 231, 241–242; in West
Africa 216–217
Bombay (municipality): anti-malaria
efforts in 22, 241–242, 254, 280;
see also Malaria in Bombay
Bombay Medical Congress (1909)
210, 212, 214, 239, 241–243, 247
bonification 241, 251, 283, 297
British Medical Association
conference (1904) 219–220,
266n1
Burdwan fever 43n69, 229,
274–276, 408
Bynum, William 21, 43n65, 43n67,
233n29, 235n45, 245, 272n98,
272n105

calorie consumption per capita 109,
120n71, 317, 325n37, 347, 354,
365n95, 392
canal irrigation 12, 21–22, 143,
149, 209, 221, 245; abolition as
malaria control measure 221, 223,
280–281; adverse effects on soil
19, 87, 99, 283–284, 300n72;
irrigated area, trend 155n21, 283,
338; and malaria mortality 12, 22,
64, 82, 87, 164, 255; see also well
irrigation; West Jumna Canal
case fatality rate xxii, 8, 28, 46n97,
81, 406
Celli, Angelo 9, 213, 228, 241, 244